Progress in
Cancer Research and Therapy
Volume 27

PATHOGENESIS OF LEUKEMIAS AND LYMPHOMAS: ENVIRONMENTAL INFLUENCES

Progress in Cancer Research and Therapy

Progress in
Cancer Research and Therapy
Volume 27

Pathogenesis of Leukemias and Lymphomas: Environmental Influences

Editors

Ian Magrath
Pediatric Branch
National Cancer Institute
National Institutes of Health
Bethesda, Maryland 20205

Gregory T. O'Conor
Office of International Affairs
National Cancer Institute
National Institutes of Health
Bethesda, Maryland 20205

Bracha Ramot, M.D.
Chaim Medical Center
Tel-Hashomer and Sackler School of Medicine
Tel-Aviv University, Israel

Raven Press ■ New York

Raven Press, 1140 Avenue of the Americas, New York, New York 10036

Library of Congress Cataloging in Publication Data
Main entry under title:

Pathogenesis of leukemias and lymphomas.

   (Progress in cancer research and therapy ; v. 27)
   Includes index.
   1. Leukemia—Addresses, essays, lectures.   2. Lymphoma
—Addresses, essays, lectures.   3. Environmentally
induced diseases—Addresses, essays, lectures.
4. Epidemiology—Addresses, essays, lectures.   I. Magrath,
Ian.   II. O'Conor, Gregory T.   III. Ramot, Bracha,
1927–   .   IV. Series.   [DNLM: 1. Leukemia—Etiology—
Congresses.   2. Leukemia—Occurrence—Congresses.
3. Lymphoma—Etiology—Congresses.   4. Lymphoma—
Occurrence—Congresses.   W1 PR667M v.27 / QZ 350 P297 1982]
RC643.P36   1984   616.99′419071   82-42584
ISBN 0-89004-901-7

Preface

In the last few years progress in the biological sciences has accelerated dramatically as a consequence of the development of two new technologies, namely the production of large quantities of monoclonal antibodies and recombinant DNA technology. These have led to major advances in the understanding of a number of diseases, paramount among them the hematologic malignancies. In the major centers, leukemias and lymphomas are now characterized on the basis of their expression of a number of surface proteins, such that their cell lineage is known with a degree of precision unimagined by pioneer histopathologists. The characterization of transforming genes in retroviruses, and the recognition that very similar genes exist in all normal cells have led to new insights and approaches in the unraveling of the complex sequence of events which leads ultimately to the altered cellular behavior which characterizes malignant neoplasia.

This book represents a first step in an attempt to develop a more organized approach to the study of the pathogenesis of human hematologic malignancies. We hope that this volume will promote cross-fertilization between fields as diverse as epidemiology and molecular biology, and foster collaboration among scientists and clinicians with, at first sight, completely different interests. We believe that progress in understanding the cause or causes of human cancer will be accelerated dramatically by this kind of interdisciplinary communication.

This book is divided into four main sections. The first consists of a number of papers summarizing the spectrum of lymphoid neoplasia encountered in various parts of the world. Since in many of the developing countries sophisticated immunological analysis of tumor cell lineage has not so far been carried out, many of these descriptions still rely heavily upon histopathology. It seems highly probable that many new observations will be made when these tumors are characterized immunologically. The second section focuses on the immunological classification of lymphoid neoplasia. Considerable emphasis has been given to acute lymphoblastic leukemia in children and to its immunological subdivisions. This disease provides an excellent example of how an immunological perspective may sharpen the focus of the epidemiologist, and permit observations to be made which would otherwise be overlooked. In the third section, overviews of the epidemiology of lymphoid neoplasia are provided and some particularly interesting and pertinent topics are discussed, including the development of lymphoproliferative syndromes and lymphoid neoplasia in immunodeficient individuals and the association of Epstein-Barr virus with some of these syndromes and with Burkitt's lymphoma. In the final section, pertinent animal models are described and the subject of viral oncogenesis, and in particular the role of viral and cellular oncogenes in the genesis of neoplasia, is discussed. This field is moving forward at a dramatic rate, and a considerable amount of new information has been published since the National Institutes of Health (NIH) workshop. In particular, the finding that the c-myc oncogene is present on chromosome 8 and is translocated into chromosomal regions bearing immunoglobulin genes in Burkitt's lymphoma is likely to be a seminal observation. In summary, the data presented demonstrate that differences in hematologic malignancies do exist in different parts of the world. A number of possible factors which may influence the development of leukemias and lymphomas are considered, and particular emphasis is given to the role of viruses and the molecular changes which may accompany the malignant state.

Because of its multidisciplinary approach, this volume should have appeal to both physicians and scientists who are interested in the pathogenesis of human lymphoid neoplasia, including clinicians, pathologists, epidemiologists, immunologists, virologists, cell biologists and molecular biologists. The probable multifactorial nature of the cause(s) of human cancer and the need for a concerted, but multi-targeted approach, preordain that the traditional boundaries between the various medical sciences must be breached if continued progress is to be made. Just as the management of patients with cancer requires a team approach, so too is team work required in the exploration of the very nature of cancer, which, apart from the intellectual challenge, possesses the potential bonus of permitting more rational approaches to intervention.

Ian Magrath, M.B., M.R.C.P.

Acknowledgments

The meeting that produced the chapters in this volume was sponsored by the Fogarty International Center; The National Cancer Institute, Bethesda, Maryland; and Ortho Diagnostic Systems, Inc., Raritan, New Jersey. We gratefully acknowledge the assistance of Dr. Earle Chamberlayne, Dr. Peter Condliffe, and Ms. Nancy Shapiro of the Fogarty International Center in organizing the international meeting. The program committee consisted of Dr. R. W. Miller, Dr. A. S. Levine, Dr. D. Poplack, Dr. G. Reaman, Dr. W. A. Blattner, and the editors of this volume. Special thanks are owed to Ms. Laurene Kuhar and Ms. Mary Belle Jordan for tireless secretarial assistance.

Contents

Variations in Acute Lymphoblastic Leukemia and Non-Hodgkin's Lymphoma Phenotypes in Subpopulations

Epidemiology and Pathogenesis of Leukemias and Lymphomas

Recent Advances and New Approaches in the Search for a Viral Etiology of Human Lymphoid Neoplasia

Contributors

Dharam Ablashi
*Laboratory of Cellular and Molecular
  Biology
National Cancer Institute
National Institutes of Health
Bethesda, Maryland 20205*

M. I. Aboul-Enein
*National Cancer Institute
Cairo University
Cairo, Egypt*

K. Al Rubei
*Department of Haematology
The Children's Hospital
Ladywood Middleway
Ladywood, Birmingham B16 8ET,
  United Kingdom*

Gary Armstrong
*Laboratory of Cellular and Molecular
  Biology
National Cancer Institute
National Institutes of Health
Bethesda, Maryland 20205*

Susan M. Astrin
*The Institute for Cancer Research
Fox Chase Cancer Center
Philadelphia, Pennsylvania 19111*

E. A. Bamgboye
*Medical Statistics Unit
Department of Preventive and Social
  Medicine
University College Hospital
Ibadan, Nigeria*

I. Ben-Bassat
*Institute of Hematology
Chaim Medical Center
Tel-Aviv University
Tel-Hashomer 52621 Israel*

Thomas Bechtold
*Department of Pathology and Laboratory
  Medicine
University of Nebraska Medical Center
Omaha, Nebraska 68105*

William A. Blattner
*Family Studies Section
Environmental Epidemiology Branch
National Cancer Institute
National Institutes of Health
Bethesda, Maryland 20205*

Douglas W. Blayney
*Family Studies Section
Environmental Epidemiology Branch
National Cancer Institute
National Institutes of Health
Bethesda, Maryland 20205*

J. Bosco
*Department of Medicine
University Hospital
University of Malaya
Kuala Lumpur, Malaysia*

W. Paul Bowman
*Division of Hematology-Oncology
St. Jude Children's Research Hospital
Memphis, Tennessee 38101*

James Boyett
*Pediatric Oncology Group
Veterans Administration Medical Center
Gainesville, Florida 32602*

Marie Campbell
*Department of Pathology
University of the West Indies
Kingston 7, Jamaica*

Daniel Catovsky
Medical Research Council Leukaemia Unit
Royal Postgraduate Medical School
London W12OHS, United Kingdom

L. Chan
University Department of Medicine
National University of Singapore and
 Singapore General Hospital
Singapore 0316

S. H. Chan
University Department of Medicine
National University of Singapore and
 Singapore General Hospital
Singapore 0316

R. Cherian
Department of Pathology
University Hospital
University of Malaya
Kuala Lumpur, Malaysia

Max D. Cooper
Cellular Immunobiology Unit
University of Alabama
Birmingham, Alabama 35294

Jeffrey Cossman
Hematopathology Section
Laboratory of Pathology
National Cancer Institute
National Institutes of Health
Bethesda, Maryland 20205

William Crist
Division of Hematology-Oncology
Department of Pediatrics
University of Alabama
University Station
Birmingham, Alabama 35294

A. Crockard
Medical Research Council Leukaemia Unit
Royal Postgraduate Medical School
London W12OHS, United Kingdom

U. Datta
Department of Immunopathology
Postgraduate Institute of Medical
 Education and Research
Chandigarh-160012, India

Barry Dowell
Division of Immunology
Duke University Medical Center
Durham, North Carolina 27710

M. N. El-Bolkainy
National Cancer Institute
Cairo University
Cairo, Egypt

M. Essex
Department of Microbiology
Harvard University School of Public
 Health
Boston, Massachusetts 02115

E. M. Essien
Department of Haematology
University College Hospital
Ibadan, Nigeria

Jan van Eys
Division of Oncology
Department of Pediatrics
M.D. Anderson Hospital
University of Texas Cancer Center
Houston, Texas 77030

Alberto Faggioni
Laboratory of Cellular and Molecular
 Biology
National Cancer Institute
National Institutes of Health
Bethesda, Maryland 20205

John M. Falletta
Division of Hematology-Oncology
Department of Pediatrics
Duke University Medical Center
Durham, North Carolina 27710

A. H. Filipovich
Immunodeficiency Cancer Registry
University of Minnesota Hospitals
Minneapolis, Minnesota

Stuart C. Finch
Cooper Medical Center
Rutgers Medical School
Camden, New Jersey 08103

G. E. Francis
Department of Haematology
Royal Free Hospital
London W12OHS, United Kingdom

N. Gad-El-Mawla
National Cancer Institute
Cairo University
Cairo, Egypt

Robert C. Gallo
Laboratory of Tumor Cell Biology
National Cancer Institute
National Institutes of Health
Bethesda, Maryland 20205

D. A. G. Galton
Medical Research Council Leukaemia Unit
Royal Postgraduate Medical School
London W12OHS, United Kingdom

Stephen L. George
Division of Biostatistics
St. Jude Children's Research Hospital
Memphis, Tennessee 38101

W. N. Gibbs
Department of Pathology
University of the West Indies
Kingston 7, Jamaica

Melvyn F. Greaves
Membrane Immunology Laboratory
Imperial Cancer Research Fund
London WC2A 3PX, England

A. Grover
Department of Radiotherapy
Postgraduate Institute of Medical
_ Education and Research_
Chandigarh-160012, India

D. R. Gulati
Department of Neurosurgery
Postgraduate Institute of Medical
_ Education and Research_
Chandigarh-160012, India

B. D. Gupta
Department of Radiotherapy
Postgraduate Institute of Medical
_ Education and Research_
Chandigarh-160012, India

Denman Hammond
Childrens Cancer Study Group
Operations Office
University of Southern California
_ Comprehensive Cancer Center_
Los Angeles, California 90031

B. Hanchard
Department of Pathology
University of the West Indies
Kingston 7, Jamaica

Shinji Harada
Department of Pathology and Laboratory
_ Medicine_
University of Nebraska Medical Center
Omaha, Nebraska 68105

F. G. H. Hill
Department of Haematology
The Children's Hospital
Ladywood Middleway
Ladywood, Birmingham, B16 8ET,
_ United Kingdom_

Richard Honour
Childrens Cancer Study Group
Operations Office
University of Southern California
_ Comprehensive Cancer Center_
Los Angeles, California 90031

G. Bennett Humphrey
University of Oklahoma Health Sciences
_ Center_
Oklahoma Children's Memorial Hospital
Oklahoma City, Oklahoma 73126

Elaine S. Jaffe
Hematopathology Section
Laboratory of Pathology
National Cancer Institute
National Institutes of Health
Bethesda, Maryland 20205

S. E. Johnson
Medical Research Council Leukaemia Unit
Royal Postgraduate Medical School
London W12OHS, United Kingdom

V. S. Kalyanaraman
Department of Cell Biology
Litton Bionetics, Inc.
Kensington, Maryland 20895

Henry S. Kaplan
Department of Radiology
Cancer Biology Research Laboratory
Stanford University School of Medicine
Stanford, California 94305

J. H. Kersey
Immunodeficiency Cancer Registry
University of Minnesota Hospitals
Minneapolis, Minnesota 55455

S. Krishnamurthi
Cancer Institute
Adyar, Madras-600020, India

Y. K. Kueh
University Department of Medicine
National University of Singapore and
  Singapore General Hospital
Singapore 0316

Faith Kung
Department of Pediatrics
University of California San Diego
Medical Center
San Diego, California 92103

Rick Lamb
Department of Pediatrics
University of California San Diego
Medical Center
San Diego, California 92103

I. Lampert
Department of Histopathology
Royal Postgraduate Medical School
London W12OHS, United Kingdom

Sanford L. Leikin
Department of Hematology/Oncology
Children's Hospital National Medical
  Center, and
Department of Child Health and
  Development
George Washington University School of
  Medicine
Washington, D.C. 20010

Gilbert M. Lenoir
International Agency for Research on
  Cancer
69372 Lyons cedex 08, France

Carolyn Level
Childrens Cancer Study Group
Operations Office
University of Southern California
  Comprehensive Cancer Center
Los Angeles, California 90031

Arthur S. Levine
National Institute of Child Health and
  Human Development
Intramural Research Program
National Institutes of Health
Bethesda, Maryland 20205

H. P. Lin
Department of Paediatrics
University Hospital
University of Malaya
Kuala Lumpur, Malaysia

W. S. Lofters
Department of Pathology
University of the West Indies
Kingston 7, Jamaica

Dan Longo
Medicine Branch
National Cancer Institute
National Institutes of Health
Bethesda, Maryland 20205

K. F. Lui
University Department of Medicine
National University of Singapore and
  Singapore General Hospital
Singapore 0316

Ian T. Magrath
Pediatric Branch
National Cancer Institute
National Institutes of Health
Bethesda, Maryland 20205

Susan L. Melvin
Division of Pathology
St. Jude Children's Research Hospital
Memphis, Tennessee 38101

Richard Metzgar
Division of Immunology
Duke University Medical Center
Durham, North Carolina 27710

Robert W. Miller
Clinical Epidemiology Branch
National Cancer Institute
National Institutes of Health
Bethesda, Maryland 20205

Oscar Misad
Department of Pathology
Instituto Nacional de Enfermedades
Neoplasicas
Lima, Peru

M. Modan
Institute of Epidemiology
Chaim Sheba Medical Center
Tel-Hashomer 52621, and
Sackler School of Medicine
Tel-Aviv University
Israel

O. S. Morgan
Department of Medicine
University of the West Indies
Kingston 7, Jamaica

C. O'Brien
Department of Histopathology
Royal Postgraduate Medical School
London W12OHS, United Kingdom

M. O'Brien
Medical Research Council Leukaemia Unit
Royal Postgraduate Medical School
London W12OHS, United Kingdom

Gregory T. O'Conor
Office of International Affairs
National Cancer Institute
National Institutes of Health
Bethesda, Maryland 20205

Laura Olivares
Departments of Statistics and Epidemiology
Instituto Nacional de Enfermedades
Neoplasicas
Lima, Peru

Y. W. Ong
University Department of Medicine
National University of Singapore and
Singapore General Hospital
Singapore 0316

C. J. Oon
University Department of Medicine
National University of Singapore and
Singapore General Hospital
Singapore 0316

R. Owor
Department of Pathology
Makerere University Medical School
Kampala, Uganda

T. Pang
Department of Medical Microbiology
University Hospital
University of Malaya
Kuala Lumpur, Malaysia

Gary Pearson
Mayo Clinic
Rochester, Minnesota 55901

Thierry Philip
Centre Léon Bérard
Pediatric Oncology Department
69374 Lyons cedex 08, France

M. Popovic
Laboratory of Tumor Cell Biology
National Cancer Institute
National Institutes of Health
Bethesda, Maryland 20205

Gerald Presbury
Division of Hematology-Oncology
St. Jude Children's Research Hospital
Memphis, Tennessee 38101

D. Jeanette Pullen
Division of Hematology-Oncology
Department of Pediatrics
University of Mississippi Medical Center
Jackson, Mississippi 39216

David Purtilo
Department of Pathology and Laboratory
   Medicine
Pediatrics and Eppley Institute for
   Research in Cancer and Allied Diseases
University of Nebraska Medical Center
Omaha, Nebraska 68105

Luis Quiroz
Clinical Laboratories Service
Instituto Nacional de Enfermedades
   Neoplasicas
Lima, Peru

K. R. Rajalakshmi
Cancer Institute
Adyar, Madras-60020, India

Bracha Ramot
Holding the Yechiel and Helen Lieber
   Chair for Cancer Research at the Tel
   Aviv University
Chaim Sheba Medical Center
Tel-Hashomer 52621, and Sackler School
   of Medicine
Tel-Aviv University, Israel

Gregory H. Reaman
Department of Hematology/Oncology
Children's Hospital National Medical
   Center, and
Department of Child Health and
   Development
George Washington University School of
   Medicine
Washington, D.C. 20010

Marvin S. Reitz, Jr.
Laboratory of Tumor Cell Biology
National Cancer Institute
National Institutes of Health
Bethesda, Maryland 20205

Marjorie Robert-Guroff
Department of Cell Biology
Litton Bionetics, Inc.
Kensington, Maryland 20895

Geraldine Rogers
Department of Pathology and Laboratory
   Medicine
University of Nebraska Medical Center
Omaha, Nebraska 68105

Maryann Roper
Division of Hematology-Oncology
Department of Pediatrics
University of Alabama
University Station
Birmingham, Alabama 35294

Ugo G. Rovigatti
Fox Chase Cancer Center
The Institute for Cancer Research
Philadelphia, Pennsylvania 19111

Ivor Royston
Department of Medicine
University of California San Diego
School of Medicine and Veterans
   Administration Medical Center
La Jolla, California 92161

T. G. Sagar
Cancer Institute
Adyar, Madras-600020, India

Avery A. Sandberg
Roswell Park Memorial Institute
Buffalo, New York 14263

Prem Sarin
Laboratory of Tumor Cell Biology
National Cancer Institute
National Institutes of Health
Bethesda, Maryland 20205

M. G. Sarngadharan
Laboratory of Tumor Cell Biology
National Cancer Institute
National Institutes of Health
Bethesda, Maryland 20205

K. Sasikala
Cancer Institute
Adyar, Madras-600020, India

Harland Sather
Childrens Cancer Study Group
Operations Office
University of Southern California
    Comprehensive Cancer Center
Los Angeles, California 90031

S. Sehgal
Department of Immunopathology
Postgraduate Institute of Medical
    Education and Research
Chandigarh-160012, India

Beerelli Seshi
Department of Pathology and Laboratory
    Medicine
University of Nebraska Medical Center
Omaha, Nebraska 68105

V. Shanta
Cancer Institute
Adyar, Madras-600020, India

J. Sharp
Department of Haematology
Kings College Hospital Medical School
London, United Kingdom

Joseph V. Simone
Division of Hematology-Oncology
St. Jude Children's Research Hospital
Memphis, Tennessee 38101

Susan Slovin
Department of Pathology
Tufts University School of Medicine
Boston, Massachusetts 02111

I. Sng
University Department of Medicine
National University of Singapore and
    Singapore General Hospital
Singapore 0316

Roger Sohier
International Agency for Research on
    Cancer
69372 Lyons cedex, France

Andres Solidoro
Department of Medicine
Instituto Nacional de Enfermedades
    Neoplasicas
Lima, Peru

Geetha Soman
Cancer Institute
Adyar, Madras-600020, India

B. D. Spector
Immunodeficiency Cancer Registry
University of Minnesota Hospitals
Minneapolis, Minnesota 55455

Richard Sposto
Childrens Cancer Study Group
Operations Office
University of Southern California
    Comprehensive Cancer Center
Los Angeles, California 90031

Taizan Suchi
Department of Pathology and Clinical
    Laboratories
Aichi Cancer Center Hospital
Tashiro-cho, Chikusa-ku
Nagoya 464, Japan

M. S. Sukumaran
Cancer Institute
Adyar, Madras-600020, India

R. Suri
University Department of Medicine
National University of Singapore and
    Singapore General Hospital
Singapore 0316

Kazuo Tajima
Division of Epidemiology
Aichi Cancer Center Research Institute
Tashiro-cho, Chikusa-ku
Nagoya 464, Japan

C. L. Tan
Department of Medicine
National University of Singapore and
    Singapore General Hospital
Singapore 0316

Y. O. Tan
University of Medicine
National University of Singapore and
 Singapore General Hospital
Singapore 0316

H. N. Tawfik
National Cancer Institute
Cairo University
Cairo, Egypt

P. A. Trumper
Department of Haematology
The Children's Hospital
Ladywood Middleway
Ladywood, Birmingham B16 8ET,
 United Kingdom

Philip Tsichlis
Laboratory of Tumor Virus Genetics
National Cancer Institute
National Institutes of Health
Bethesda, Maryland 20205

Eric H. Westin
Laboratory of Tumor Cell Biology
National Cancer Institute
National Institutes of Health
Bethesda, Maryland 20205

C. K. Oladipupo Williams
Department of Haematology
University College Hospital
Ibadan, Nigeria

F. Wong-Staal
Laboratory of Tumor Cell Biology
National Cancer Institute
National Institutes of Health
Bethesda, Maryland 20205

Joanne Yetz
Department of Pathology and Laboratory
 Medicine
University of Nebraska Medical Center
Omaha, Nebraska 68105

Alice Yu
Department of Pediatrics
University of California San Diego
Medical Center
San Diego, California 92103

Nancy Zeller
Laboratory of Tumor Virus Genetics
National Cancer Institute
National Institutes of Health
Bethesda, Maryland 20205

Katharine A. Zener
Family Studies Section
Environmental Epidemiology Branch
National Cancer Institute
National Institutes of Health
Bethesda, Maryland 20205

D. Zerbe
Immunodeficiency Cancer Registry
University of Minnesota Hospitals
Minneapolis, Minnesota 55455

Introduction

In 1981, while serving as a Fogarty International Scholar at the National Institutes of Health, Dr. Bracha Ramot gave a lecture in which she described some interesting changes she had observed in the pattern of leukemia and lymphoma in young Gaza Strip Arabs. Over a period of approximately 12 years, during which time there was a dramatic improvement in socioeconomic conditions, Burkitt's lymphoma, which had originally been the commonest malignancy in children, was gradually superseded in frequency by acute lymphoblastic leukemia (ALL). Moreover, a much higher proportion of the now predominant ALL was shown to be of T-cell type than is the case in Europe and North America. Although the numbers of patients involved were small, this observation stimulated a series of discussions involving the editors of this volume and contributor Dr. R. Miller. We were impressed by the similarity of the earlier Gaza Strip pattern—a high frequency of Burkitt's lymphoma and low frequency of acute leukemia—with the pattern in Equatorial African children. Moreover, the change in relative frequency of different lymphoid malignancies which accompanied socioeconomic development in the Gaza Strip suggested that the environment may be more important than racial factors in determining the pattern of lymphoid neoplasia. Finally, we were intrigued by the high fraction of T-cell ALL in the later Gaza Strip pattern and, thinking that this pattern might be representative of "intermediate" socioeconomic level populations or subpopulations, began to look for additional evidence to support this.

Blacks in the USA have been recognized for some years as a subpopulation in which there is a lower incidence of ALL, but a worse prognosis than Whites. A preliminary poll of nearby institutions suggested that there was, as in the Arabs, a greater proportion of T-cell ALL in Blacks than Whites. Further, there is evidence, some of which is presented in this book, that the incidence of sub-types of ALL in Blacks is changing, presumably as a result of socioeconomic development. If this is so, the characteristics of ALL in Blacks today may be similar to those which pertained in Whites in the past. Indeed, one might envisage the current pattern of ALL phenotypes in the less developed parts of the world as similar to that in Europe and America perhaps as recently as 60–100 years ago. This notion is supported by the observations made by Court-Brown and Doll in 1961. They showed that the incidence of acute leukemia in children living in England and Wales increased markedly between 1911 and 1951. This increase occurred predominantly in children below 4 years of age and resulted in the development of the early age peak so characteristic of childhood ALL, and recently recognized, as shown by Greaves in this volume, to consist almost entirely of common ALL. The evidence suggests quite strongly that the latter disease is a concomitant of advancing prosperity and/or industrialization. Interestingly, an early age peak appears now to have developed

xxv

in some Asian and South American countries and is also present in at least some Black populations in the United States, although this was not the case until very recently.

These interesting observations suggest that it will be uniquely rewarding to study prospectively the incidence and phenotypic characteristics of ALL in selected populations or subpopulations undergoing rapid social, economic and industrial development. ALL, however, is but one example, and geographical studies of lymphoid neoplasia in general (and probably of many other diseases), represent a valuable approach to the collection of information pertinent to etiology, or at least to an improved understanding of environmental factors which may influence the development of specific diseases. Further, more detailed studies in developing countries might well bring to light previously unrecognized diseases and possibly also lead to the identification of new, potentially pathogenic agents, as exemplified by the exciting studies carried out at clinical, epidemiological and virological levels on "Adult T-cell leukemia/lymphoma" (ATLL) in Southern Japan and parts of the Caribbean. In this regard, the enormous contribution that has already been made to virology, immunology and cell biology by the description and study of African Burkitt's lymphoma should also be cited. Indeed, the karyotypic changes first detected in this tumor coupled with molecular studies of gene rearrangements show promise of revealing at a molecular level the nature of the genetic changes which lead to the altered cellular behavior characteristic of this neoplasm. In spite of its rarity throughout most of the world, Burkitt's tumor has proved to be a model tumor with regard to our comprehension of cancer.

At the present time considerably more is known about the pathogenesis of animal tumors than is the case with their human counterparts. The major reason for this, of course, is the possibility of exposing animals experimentally to viruses or carcinogenic chemicals. In humans a quite different approach must be adopted, and epidemiological studies become of critical importance for the provision of clues which may lead ultimately to the recognition of factors involved in tumor pathogenesis. In the context of hematologic malignancies there are a number of indications that the spectrum of disease differs markedly in different parts of the world, and that these differences relate predominantly to the environment. In effect, a series of *natural experiments* have been performed which will surely provide fertile soil for progress in understanding the pathogenesis of leukemias and lymphomas. Yet at the present time this huge scientific resource is left virtually untapped, and will remain only partially utilized until diagnostic precision and demographic descriptions are improved in Africa, Asia and South America.

If prospective studies of the epidemiology and pathogenesis of human malignancy in various parts of the world are to be carried out successfully, there seems little doubt that a team approach is essential. Not only must all possible diagnostic means be brought to bear on the recognition of disease entities, but demographic studies on the one hand, and sophisticated molecular studies of the tumor cells on the other, need to be included in current and future investigations. Particularly important in this regard are immunological studies, for it is inconceivable that neoplasms of the immune system can be understood without recourse to immunological characterization. The newer insights into ALL phenotypes, including the recent demonstration of immunoglobulin gene rearrangements in common ALL, provide an excellent example of the enormous contribution to understanding (and hence to diagnosis, including sub-categorization, and potentially to improvement in treatment) which can be made by immunological studies. The necessity for precise diagnosis, that is, recognition of individual pathological entities, cannot be overemphasized, for epidemiological studies will always be of questionable value if individual diseases are not studied separately. In light of the above comments, it appears to be inappropriate to group ALL subtypes together for epidemiological purposes, let alone ALL and chronic lymphocytic leukemia; yet many studies have been published in which "lymphoid" or "lymphocytic" leukemias are lumped together. Immunological characterization may be of particular value in classifying the many tumors around the world currently classified as "diffuse, histiocytic" or "diffuse, poorly differentiated lymphocytic" lymphomas. The immunological phenotypes of these histological categories may well vary markedly with geographic location. Illustrative of this probability is the recent observation that the lymphomas of mature T-cell malignancies, including peripheral T-cell lymphoma and ATLL are not readily distinguished from B-cell diffuse lymphomas on the basis of histology alone (see Chapters by Gibbs, et al., Catovsky et al., and Cossman and Jaffe), but can easily be distinguished from mixed cell and large cell lymphomas of B-cell origin by immunological testing. It remains possible that the so-called "Japanese" ATLL is also common in many other parts of the world.

These considerations convinced us that there is much to be gained from geographical studies of lymphoid malignancy, and we decided, as a prelude to the possible institution of a multi-centered, international project with this objective, to hold a workshop at the National Institutes of Health on the influence of the environment in the pathogenesis of leukemias and lymphomas. We felt it important to bring together not only pathologists and clinicians from different parts of the world, but also epidemiologists, virologists, immunologists, and molecular biologists, in order both to create a data base from which to work, and also to estimate the degree of interest and the potential difficulties in developing such a prospective multidisciplinary epidemiological study.

This meeting took place in May, 1982. In addition to the formal papers, much valuable discussion took place informally between the sessions. Participants from the developing countries were able to point out some of the major difficulties facing them in carrying out detailed studies of the kind envisioned. Such difficulties range from the limited demographic information available in many of the countries, to the relative lack of laboratory expertise and facilities. These participants also conveyed, however, a contagious enthusiasm, and demonstrated by their presentations that a considerable amount can be accomplished even with severely limited resources, given sufficient motivation and application. Presentations from several centers within the United States and Europe demonstrated that there is also much to be learned from horizontal studies of discrete populations within individual countries. In this regard the emphasis was upon ALL in Blacks compared with Whites, for reasons already discussed. All of the conference participants hopefully benefited from presentations of the latest developments in such diverse fields as immunological phenotyping, potential physical and chemical oncogens, the importance of immunosuppression to the development of lymphoid malignancy, the potential relevance of karyotypic changes to the pathogenesis of neoplasia, animal models of virus induced leukemia and lymphoma, and molecular mechanisms of oncogenesis, with the emphasis on the role of oncogenes in neoplasia.

This volume provides a record of the May workshop. It consists of the presented papers and rapporteur's comments for the four main sessions. The final session of the meeting consisted of general discussion directed towards the possibility of developing the multidisciplinary epidemiological study alluded to above. That discussion has not been reproduced here. Suffice to say that there was considerable enthusiasm, particularly on the part of the participants from developing countries, for a much expanded level of collaboration in the future. Needs were expressed for the provision of reagents and the training of personnel in order that immunological phenotyping could be carried out in the major centers in the developing countries themselves. Many of the clinicians also expressed a desire for a greater degree of collaboration in the establishment of standardized therapeutic protocols, and in some cases, assistance in obtaining drugs for therapeutic studies such that the results of treatment of these diseases could be incorporated into the total framework of the proposed study. All agreed upon the need for accurate documentation of epidemiological and clinical information accompanied by careful histological and immunological studies. In addition, the establishment of banks for serum and tissue storage would doubtless provide an invaluable resource to virologists and molecular biologists in furthering their studies of the potential role of viruses and oncogenes in the pathogenesis of human neoplasia. Since the meeting, considerable further progress has been made towards initiating such a project and a feasibility study, sponsored by the International Agency for Research in Cancer, will be commenced in the near future.

In order to enhance the value of this book to readers who may be less familiar with the known patterns of lymphoid neoplasia in the developed countries, an appendix has been provided that gives selected epidemiological information for leukemias and lymphomas in the USA (derived predominantly from the SEER program of the National Cancer Institute, Bethesda, MD). This will hopefully enable the reader to better interpret the significance of some of the observations reported in this volume.

Ian Magrath, M.B., M.R.C.P.

PATHOGENESIS OF LEUKEMIAS AND LYMPHOMAS: ENVIRONMENTAL INFLUENCES

Pathogenesis of Leukemias and Lymphomas:
Environmental Influences, edited by
I. T. Magrath, G. T. O'Conor, and B. Ramot.
Raven Press, New York © 1984.

Geography of Lymphoid Neoplasia: An Overview

Gregory T. O'Conor

Office of International Affairs, National Cancer Institute, National Institutes of Health, Bethesda, Maryland 20205

International and interregional differences in tumor incidence have traditionally suggested important etiological leads. Such comparisons have provided a basis for the formulation of testable hypotheses and the design of rational field and laboratory investigations. The value of comparative data derived from cancer registries, vital statistics records, or other health records largely depends on the accuracy of demographic definition, reliability of diagnosis, and a reasonable degree of uniformity in nomenclature and classification. This introductory chapter discusses these requirements.

CLASSIFICATION OF LYMPHOMAS

The first objective of disease classification must be the definition of biological entities, and classification systems should have clinical and/or etiological relevance. The classification of neoplastic diseases has historically been based on cellular morphology and on histogenesis. In general, this approach has been effective, because there is, in most instances, a relationship among the morphological characteristics of tumor cells, the tissue of origin, and recognized clinical entities. From experience, we have learned to relate histology and cytology to prognosis and response to treatment. Furthermore, our lack of insight into the cause of most tumors precludes a meaningful classification on an etiological basis.

The classification of lymphoid neoplasms has long been controversial and confusing. Although a variety of terms have been used, the older systems generally recognized four major groups: lymphosarcoma, reticulosarcoma, Hodgkin's disease, and lymphatic leukemia. Lymphosarcoma was often divided into nodular and diffuse types, based on the architectural pattern in tissue sections. The data in the last edition of *Cancer Incidence in Five Continents* (17) have been compiled under the rubrics of the International Classification of Disease, ICD-8, which combines lymphosarcoma and reticulosarcoma and, therefore, refers to only three major categories: lymphosarcoma and reticulosarcoma—200, Hodgkin's disease—201, and lymphatic leukemia—204. This very limited classification does allow for the identification of some variations in the geographic distribution of these broad categories, but in the light of current knowledge, such information is inadequate and cannot

1

significantly contribute to the design of the type of analytical investigations, clinical or epidemiological, that are now indicated.

In recent years, the application of increasingly sophisticated biochemical and immunological techniques has permitted the recognition of functional components of the lymphoreticular system and a more precise definition of the origin, maturation, and function of the specific cellular elements in these components (6,10). These have, in turn, led to a spate of new classification systems for the lymphoid neoplasms and particularly for solid tumors of the non-Hodgkin's type (13). These new systems introduced many unfamiliar terms and sometimes attempted to combine morphological and functional parameters. Although each of these classifications had merit for specialists in a rapidly evolving field, they proved to be a further source of frustration to clinical oncologists concerned primarily with the evaluation of therapeutic trials, where uniformity and a constancy of nomenclature, as well as clinical relevance, are essential to a useful classification system.

In response to this clinical need, the National Cancer Institute sponsored an international effort involving extensive review and analysis of both histological material and clinical records, which resulted in what is called a "Working Formulation" for non-Hodgkin's lymphoma (11) (Table 1). The intent was not to develop and promulgate a new classification but rather to establish a common language base with terminology that can be widely accepted. The Working Formulation permits ready translation to or from existing classifications. It is necessarily based on morphology, because the use of marker studies is still somewhat limited and the methodology for such studies is insufficiently standardized for routine use. The Working Formulation does not, therefore, distinguish between B- and T-cell tumors, except where morphological correlations with function are well established, as in follicular tumors and Burkitt's tumor, which are always of B-cell origin.

Although the Working Formulation evolved from a clinical demand and is structured for clinical relevance, it serves equally well for etiological studies, because it includes, or at least permits the identification of, the presently recognized disease entities that may have epidemiological as well as clinical significance. Preferred ICD-O code numbers (19) are being assigned to each of the terms in the Working Formulation to facilitate further the comparison of data from diverse sources. It is hoped and expected that the Working Formulation will indeed prove to be a key reference point and a means for achieving uniformity in terminology and for making valid comparisons of data.

CANCER REGISTRY DATA

As a further preface to the reports on lymphoid tumor distribution in the following chapters, some historical data are provided here that are representative of the existing information in cancer registries relating to the geographic distribution of the non-Hodgkin's lymphomas. Table 2 lists the relative frequency, incidence, and relative importance of non-Hodgkin's lymphoma in the spectrum of neoplasms for males in eight countries. In general, these tumors are more common in males, except in

TABLE 1. *Working formulation for non-Hodgkin's lymphomas*

LOW GRADE
  Malignant lymphoma, small lymphocytic (SLC)
      Consistent with chronic lymphocytic leukemia (CLL)
      Plasmacytoid
  Malignant lymphoma, follicular, small cleaved cell (FSC)
  Malignant lymphoma, follicular, mixed small cleaved and large cell (FMC)

INTERMEDIATE GRADE
  Malignant lymphoma, follicular, large cell (FLC)
  Malignant lymphoma, diffuse, small cleaved cell (DSC)
  Malignant lymphoma, diffuse, mixed small and large cell (DMC)
      Epithelioid component (Lennert's)
  Malignant lymphoma, diffuse large cell (DLC)
      Cleaved cell
      Noncleaved cell

HIGH GRADE
  Malignant lymphoma, large cell, immunoblastic (IBL)
      Plasmacytoid
      Clear cell
      Polymorphous
      Epithelioid component (Lennert's)
  Malignant lymphoma, lymphoblastic (LBL)
      Convoluted cell
      Nonconvoluted cell
  Malignant lymphoma, small noncleaved cell (undifferentiated)
      Burkitt's
      Non-Burkitt's
  Miscellaneous
      Composite
      Mycosis fungoides
      Histiocytic
      Extramedullary plasmacytoma
      Unclassifiable
      Other

Cali, Colombia, and in Singapore, where a slight female predominance is recorded. I must emphasize that these data are for non-Hodgkin's lymphoma as a group and make no provision for the many known and separate disease entities included within this generic term. Also, the rates and ratios given are for males of all ages and do not reflect the large variations in age distribution that occur and that have great epidemiological significance. In Table 3, the ratio of non-Hodgkin's lymphoma to total cancer incidence is calculated using the data from these representative cancer registries.

Both tables indicate that, except in Nigeria, non-Hodgkin's lymphomas are everywhere uncommon and represent only a small fraction of all tumors. One might further suspect that the overall incidence of these tumors as a group is fairly constant throughout the world and that small recorded variations are the result of the occurrence of a particular type of tumor in very high frequency within very localized geographic perimeters. This is certainly true in Nigeria, where non-Hodgkin's lymphomas have a total incidence of 5.9/100,000, constitute 18% of all tumors, and are the most common form of neoplasia. This high rate and relative frequency

TABLE 2. *Non-Hodgkin's lymphoma (NHL[a])*: geographic comparisons of relative frequency and incidence in males

Location	NHL frequency rank	NHL incidence (per 100,000)	Incidence of most common tumor (per 100,000)	
Nigeria	1	5.9	Liver (#2)	4.9
Israel	9	8.7	Lung	30
Colombia	10	1.9	Stomach	20
Singapore	10	1.4	Liver	7.4
Connecticut	12	5.8	Lung	61
Japan	13	1.8	Stomach	80
Denmark	18	3.6	Lung	54
Jamaica	18	1.6	Stomach	14

[a]NHL in this context refers to ICD code 200, lymphosarcoma and reticulosarcoma.
Based on data from ref. 17.

TABLE 3. *Non-Hodgkin's lymphoma as a percentage of total cancer in males*

Location	Percentage
Nigeria	18
Israel	4
Colombia	2.3
Singapore	3.1
Connecticut	1.8
Japan	1.1
Denmark	1.2
Jamaica	1.6

Based on data from ref. 17.

for the total population are, however, only a reflection of the unusual incidence of Burkitt's tumor in Nigerian children.

It is said that in the Middle East, notably in Saudi Arabia, lymphomas are also among the commonest tumors, but published registry data are not available. Unpublished data from the registry in Kuwait indicate that non-Hodgkin's lymphomas are, indeed, among the commonest tumors in both males and females (J. Omar, *personal communication*). In Japan and India (not included in these tables), both Hodgkin's and non-Hodgkin's lymphomas are of notably low incidence (2). In Singapore, Colombia, and Jamaica, non-Hodgkin's lymphomas also appear to be relatively uncommon compared with the incidence data from Israel, the United States, and Europe. The Israeli rate, which is for all Jews, may reflect the suspected high incidence in the Mediterranean region and the Middle East, as well as a high incidence in U.S. and European immigrants.

It is clearly not possible to draw many conclusions from crude data presented in this fashion. They serve to illustrate that for any fruitful investigation of tumors that as a group are so uncommon, the precise definition of specific disease entities within the group and accurate demographic descriptions are absolutely critical. The collection of information of this kind in a prospective manner using, so far as possible, the newer techniques for characterizing tumor types is desperately needed.

GEOGRAPHIC DIFFERENCES

Despite the obvious limitations to descriptive epidemiology, the documentation of geographic differences in the incidence of specific types of lymphoid tumors has led to important observations and, in some cases, to a better understanding of etiological mechanisms. A few brief, and general comments that highlight some of these differences and their possible significance are appropriate to this overview. For the non-Hodgkin's lymphomas, tumor categories and/or specific entities are identified within the reference frame of the Working Formulation (Table 1).

Acute lymphocytic leukemia (ALL) is primarily a disease of children and young adults. In the white populations of Western industrialized societies, a very pronounced and sharp peak occurs in the age-specific rates during the first quinquennium and usually between two and four years of age (16). This peculiar age distribution, absent in most other populations, is very distinctive and is largely unexplained. The great majority, if not all, of the cases in the United States, which account for this characteristic distortion of the age distribution curve, are classified as "common ALL" because they lack the usual immunological markers for B or T cells. Recent techniques that permit definition of genetic rearrangements during early cell maturation indicate that these cells are, in fact, committed to the B-cell line of differentiation and may, thus, be considered "pre-B cells" (9). In populations without this early age peak, many of the cases of ALL may be of the T-cell type.

Chronic lymphocytic leukemia and malignant lymphomas of the small lymphocytic type are very rare in children and are uncommonly diagnosed in developing countries or in non-Western populations. These related neoplasms are predominantly tumors of B cells.

Follicular lymphomas, whether of small cleaved cells, mixed cells, or large cells, are by definition B-cell tumors, since they arise from the cells of the germinal center. They also are primarily tumors of adults, and in the United States and most European countries, they represent a large proportion of all malignant lymphomas. In contrast, they are far less common in Japan and Latin America and are rarely identified in African countries.

The diffuse malignant lymphomas are a much more heterogenous group and, with the exception of Burkitt's tumor, can be of either B-cell or T-cell type. In general, one may say that the diffuse mixed, and particularly the diffuse large-cell lymphomas, as well as the immunoblastic lymphomas, are more common in developing countries in both children and adults.

The cases of adult T-cell lymphoma/leukemia reported with such high relative frequency in Japan (15) appear to correspond, at least in part, to a spectrum of lymphomas seen in the United States and referred to as peripheral T-cell lymphomas. In the Working Formulation, they fall into the diffuse mixed-cell, diffuse large-cell, or immunoblastic categories. Preliminary observations suggest a possible etiological association of the recently identified human type C retrovirus (HTLV) with many of these cases (7).

Immunoproliferative small intestinal disease (IPSID) is a very specific entity with endemicity in Iraq, Iran, and some of the adjacent countries of the Mediterranean region (18). It is often a precursor of a malignant lymphoma classifiable within the immunoblastic category and may be further characterized by a monoclonal gammopathy of the alpha heavy chain type. Severe malnutrition in infancy, associated with diarrhea and perhaps with specific infectious agents, has been postulated to be critical to the development of IPSID (3).

Little epidemiological information is available relating to lymphoblastic lymphoma, other than that it occurs primarily in children and young adults, and when bone marrow and peripheral blood manifestations are prominent, it may be indistinguishable from ALL. There is often a thymic tumor, and the neoplastic cells may be typed as of B- or T-cell origin.

The familiar distribution of Burkitt's tumor is perhaps the classic example of how geographic pathology may contribute to the identification of risk factors and to the further study of pathogenetic mechanisms in tumorigenesis. There can be little doubt that in the endemic areas as well as in some cases from nonendemic areas, the Epstein-Barr virus plays an important role in the oncogenic process. Genetic factors, in addition to other environmental factors such as hyperendemic malaria, may, by their effect on host susceptibility, be critical to tumorigenesis (8,12).

ETIOLOGICAL IMPLICATIONS

Lymphoid cells of whatever type are the principal functioning elements of the immune system, and malignant lymphomas and lymphoid leukemias are the neoplasms of this system. It is, therefore, logical, if not a truism, that host or environmental factors that directly or indirectly result in aberrations of the immune response must be considered in the pathogenesis of lymphoid tumors and that disturbances of immune regulation may represent precancerous conditions. Genetic or acquired defects in the immunoregulatory apparatus are thus determinant risk factors (4).

Environmental factors that are known to alter immune response, and therefore to influence the development of lymphoreticular neoplasms experimentally and in humans, include nutrition, infectious agents, and chemical compounds. There is evidence to suggest a dose-response relationship in the pathogenesis of at least some lymphoid neoplasms. That is, the risk of disease is proportional to the intensity and length of exposure and the degree to which the risk factors provoke an aberrant response of the immune system. This seems to be true for most cancers into which we have some etiological insight. Tobacco and smoking have not yet been seriously considered as risk factors for the lymphomas and leukemias. The evidence to date suggests that radiation may be of etiological importance in some cases of ALL, but only at an early age and a high exposure level.

Socioeconomic status is often implicated in the pathogenesis of many types of lymphoma. Poor nutrition and increased exposure to infectious agents are two of the major consequences of underprivilege, and both are known to profoundly influence the development and effective response of the immune system (5,14). Burkitt's tumor, adult T-cell lymphoma, and the immunoblastic lymphoma associated with IPSID are examples of tumors in which specific and nonspecific infectious agents are suspect. Nutrition is thought to be an important factor in IPSID and may also play a role in the other lymphomas.

Although Hodgkin's disease is not a major subject in this volume, there is good epidemiological evidence that nutritional factors and immune competence may affect incidence, age distribution, and the morphological expression of this type of malignant lymphoma (1).

The authors of the following chapters represent countries in which specific environmental factors, as well as racial factors, vary widely. In many instances, the data they present, relating to incidence, age and sex distribution, and other epidemiological parameters of lymphoreticular neoplasms, are largely based on a morphological interpretation of histological material without the benefit of immunological or biochemical markers. Nevertheless new etiological information has surfaced, and on this we can build an extended international collaboration directed to better our understanding of the neoplastic process in general and the ultimate prevention of this group of tumors in particular.

SUMMARY

Geographic variations in incidence and in the age and sex distribution of lymphoid neoplasms provide an important basis for generating etiological hypotheses and for designing analytical studies. Although these tumors of the immune system do not represent a large component of the total tumor burden in most countries, they are by their very nature particularly suited for studying the interactions of genetics, other host factors, and environmental factors in carcinogenesis. Uniformity of diagnostic criteria and a classification system that defines the biological entities are prerequisites for the collection of comparable data that will have value in this context. The availability of cytogenetic, immunological, and biochemical markers and probes provides an unprecedented opportunity to gain new insights into the natural history of these tumors through interdisciplinary and international collaboration.

REFERENCES

1. Correa, P., and O'Conor, G. T. (1971): Epidemiological patterns of Hodgkin's disease. *Int. J. Cancer*, 8:192–201.
2. Correa, P., and O'Conor, G. T. (1973): Geographic pathology of lymphorecticular tumors. Summary of survey from the Geographic Pathology Committee of the International Union Against Cancer. *JNCI*, 50:1609–1617.

3. Dutz, W., Borochovitz, D., Kohout, E., and Vessal, K. (1980): The two basic forms of primary intestinal lymphoma. In: *Proceedings of the 3rd International Symposium on Detection and Prevention of Cancer*, Part II, Vol. 2. Marcel Dekker, New York.

4. Greene, M. H. (1982): Non-Hodgkin's lymphoma and mycosis fungoides. In: *Cancer Epidemiology and Prevention*, edited by D. Schottenfeld and J. F. Fraumeni, pp. 754–778. W. B. Saunders Co., Philadelphia.

5. Gross, R. L., and Newberne, P. M. (1980): Role of nutrition in immunologic function. *Physiol. Rev.*, 60(I):188–302.

6. Jaffe, E. S., and Green, I. (1977): Neoplasms of the immune system. In: *Mechanisms of Tumor Immunity*, edited by I. Green, S. Cohen, and R. T. McCluskey. John Wiley & Sons, New York.

7. Kalyaweroman, V. S., Sorngadharan, M. G., Bunn, P. A., Minna, J. D., and Gallo, R. C. (1981): Antibodies in human sera reactive against an internal structural protein of human T-cell lymphoma virus. *Nature*, 294:271–273.

8. Klein, G. (1976): Lymphoma development in mice and humans: Diversity of initiation is followed by convergent cytogenetic evolution. *Proc. Natl. Acad. Sci. USA*, 76:2442–2446.

9. Korsmeyer, S. J., Heiter, P. A., Ravetch, J. V., Poplack, D. G., Waldman, T. H., and Leder, P. (1981): Developmental hierarchy of immunoglobulin gene rearrangements in human leukemic pre-B cells. *Proc. Natl. Acad. Sci. USA*, 78:7096–7100.

10. Mann, R. B., Jaffe, E. S., and Berard, C. W. (1979): Malignant lymphomas: a conceptual understanding of morphological diversity. *Am. J. Pathol.*, 94:105–192.

11. The Non-Hodgkin's Lymphoma Pathologic Classification Project (1982): National Cancer Institute sponsored study of classifications of non-Hodgkin's lymphomas: Summary and description of a working formulation for clinical usage. *Cancer*, 49:2112–2135.

12. O'Conor, G. T. (1970): Persistent immunologic stimulation as a factor in oncogenesis with special reference to Burkitt's tumor. *Am. J. Med.*, 48:278–285.

13. O'Conor, G. T., and Sobin, L. H. (1977): Meeting reports: EORTC-CNRS. International colloquium on lymphoid neoplasms. *Biomedicine*, 26:385–386.

14. Richie, E., and Copeland, E. M. (1978): Relationship between nutrition and immunity: an overview. *Cancer Bull.*, 30(3):78–84.

15. The T- and B-cell Malignancy Study Group (1981): Statistical analysis of immunologic, clinical and histopathologic data on lymphoid malignancies in Japan. *Jpn. J. Clin. Oncol.*, 11(I):15–38.

16. Vianna, N. J. (1975): *Lymphoreticular Malignancies, Epidemiological and Related Aspects*. University Park Press, Baltimore.

17. Waterhouse, J., Muir, C. S., Correa, P., and Powell, J., editors (1976): *Cancer Incidence in Five Continents*, Vol. 3. *International Agency for Research on Cancer Scientific Publication*. 15, Lyons, France.

18. World Health Organization (1976): Alpha-heavy chain disease and related small intestinal lymphoma: A memorandum. *Bull. WHO*, 54:615–624.

19. World Health Organization (1976): *ICD-O, International Classification of Diseases for Oncology*. WHO, Geneva.

Pathogenesis of Leukemias and Lymphomas:
Environmental Influences, edited by
I. T. Magrath, G. T. O'Conor, and B. Ramot.
Raven Press, New York © 1984.

Epidemiology of Lymphoma and Leukemia in Egypt

M. N. EL-Bolkainy, N. Gad-El-Mawla, H. N. Tawfik, and M. I. Aboul-Enein

National Cancer Institute, Cairo University, Cairo, Egypt

Malignant lymphoma is relatively common in Egypt (5) as well as in other countries of the Middle East (25). In this region, the disease presents some special features, including young age incidence, predominance of unfavorable histologic types, presentation at late stages, and high frequency of intestinal lymphomas (25). An etiologic link has been postulated between low socioeconomic status, malnutrition, the prevalence of parasitic as well as viral infections, and the development of lymphoma (6,9,25). In this chapter we review the experience of a large institute in Cairo so that this experience may be compared with findings in other countries.

The National Cancer Institute (NCI) in Cairo is a comprehensive cancer center to which patients are referred from both urban and rural areas of Egypt. At the NCI, malignant lymphoma was diagnosed in 7.8% and leukemia in 2.7% of 11,626 cancer patients registered during 1970–1974. In a recent series of 8,010 patients registered during 1977–1980, the relative frequencies were 8.8% for lymphoma and 3.8% for leukemia. Thus, lymphoma continues to be more common than leukemia, but the relative frequency varies with age. The lymphoma to leukemia ratio is 3.1:1 in adults and only 1.3:1 in children under 16. Lymphoma and leukemia together rank as the third most frequent malignant disease in Egypt after carcinoma of the urinary bladder (29%) and breast (14%).

Even higher relative frequencies for lymphoreticular neoplasms have been reported from other centers in Egypt. At Kasr El-Aini Center of Radiation Oncology and Nuclear Medicine, lymphoma constituted 11% of all cancers registered (17). The figures reported from the Cancer Registry for the metropolitan Cairo area were 11.1% for lymphoma and 5% for leukemia (4); these figures represent pooled data from five university hospitals.

MALIGNANT LYMPHOMA

In a large pathology series of 2,010 patients reported from the NCI by Tawfik and Aboul-Ella (22), non-Hodgkin's lymphomas predominated and constituted 68.3% of all cases of lymphoma. However, in pediatric patients below the age of 18, Hodgkin's disease was more frequent, representing 73.1% of all lymphomas.

Age and Sex Distribution

The mean age of Egyptian patients with non-Hodgkin's lymphoma was reported to be 41.7 years, the median age 45.4 years, and the male-female ratio 2.3:1 (22). Patients with Hodgkin's disease, however, had a mean age of 29.8 years, a median age of 25.8 years, and a male-female ratio of 3.4:1. The median ages of Egyptian patients with Hodgkin's disease and non-Hodgkin's lymphoma are approximately 10 years lower than those reported in Western literature (24). This difference is attributed mainly to the population structure in Egypt—53% of the population is below the age of 20 years and only 14% is in the age group 40 to 59 years.

The age distribution curve for non-Hodgkin's lymphoma in Egyptian patients (Fig. 1) shows a progressive increase in frequency with age, with a peak at the age of 45 years. The curve for Hodgkin's disease (Fig. 1) is bimodal, with peaks at ages 15 and 35 years.

Pathologic Subtypes

The unfavorable histologic types of lymphoma are more common among Egyptians (22) than among patients from Western countries. Thus, in Hodgkin's disease, the mixed cellularity type predominates (Table 1). Non-Hodgkin's lymphomas are more commonly diffuse than nodular, and diffuse lymphomas were most frequently classified as poorly differentiated lymphocytic (Table 2). This subtype is a heterogeneous group; the majority are small cleaved cells, but the lymphoblastic and the monomorphic peripheral T subtypes are included. Chronic lymphocytic leukemia was excluded from the well-differentiated lymphocytic group. The histiocytic group

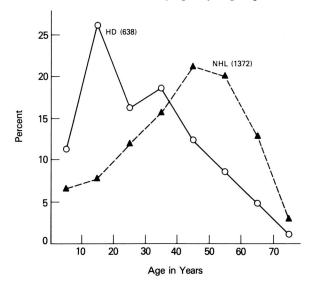

FIG. 1. Age distribution of Egyptian patients with malignant lymphoma, National Cancer Institute, Cairo. 1972–1981. HD = Hodgkin's disease; NHL = non-Hodgkin's lymphoma. Numbers in parentheses are number of patients.

TABLE 1. *Histopathologic types of Hodgkin's disease, National Cancer Institute, Cairo, 1972–1981*

Type	No. of cases	Percentage
Lymphocyte predominance	107	16.8
Nodular sclerosis	114	17.9
Mixed cellularity	382	59.9
Lymphocyte depletion	35	5.5
Total	638	100.0

TABLE 2. *Histopathologic types of non-Hodgkin's lymphoma, National Cancer Institute, Cairo, 418 patients, 1976–1980*

Type	Nodular	Diffuse
WDL[a]	1 (0.2%)	29 (6.9%)
PDL[b]	35 (8.4%)	178 (42.6)
Histiocytic	14 (3.3%)	62 (14.8%)
Mixed	22 (5.3%)	48 (11.5%)
Others	— (0.0%)	29 (6.9%)
Total	72 (17.2%)	346 (82.8%)

[a]Well-differentiated lymphocytic, excluding chronic lymphocytic leukemia.
[b]Poorly differentiated lymphocytic.

included large cleaved, large noncleaved, and immunoblastic subtypes. The lymphomas are commonly of B-cell type on the basis of examination of surface immunoglobulin; in 64 patients with non-Hodgkin's lymphoma in which marker studies were performed by Aboul-Ella (3), 90.6% were of the B-cell type. Burkitt's lymphoma is believed to be rare in Egypt.

Clinical Stage

Egyptian patients with lymphoma usually present at an advanced stage of the disease (Table 3). In a pediatric series of 114 patients staged according to the Ann Arbor system, 73% of cases were stages III and IV (12). Moreover, large tumor masses are common at initial clinical presentation. This is attributed to the delay of patients in seeking treatment, as well as to the predominance of aggressive types of lymphomas.

The association of malignant lymphoma and bilharzial hepatosplenomegaly is not uncommon in Egyptian patients, which sometimes creates difficulties in the clinical staging (21). It was possible to evaluate this problem by comparing the clinical stage with the pathologic stage determined after celiotomy. Thus, in two studies, schistosomiasis caused a false positive error in the clinical evaluation of

TABLE 3. *Clinical stage of lymphomas,*
National Cancer Institute, Cairo

Stage[a]	Hodgkin's (462 patients) (%)	Non-Hodgkin's (418 patients) (%)
I	17.3	14.4
II	15.8	10.5
III	34.9	27.0
IV	32.0	48.1

[a]Ann Arbor classification.

splenic involvement by lymphomas in 24% (23) and 53% (21) of patients, respectively. In the clinical assessment of liver involvement, schistosomal disease resulted in 23% false positives (21). Difficulties may also arise in the interpretation of liver biopsies in view of the presence of bilharzial granulomas that may simulate Hodgkin's disease. Finally, abnormal enzymatic liver function tests [serum glutamic oxaloacetic transaminase (SGOT), serum glutamic pyruvic transaminase (SGPT), and alkaline phosphatase] may also occur in patients with bilharzial hepatic fibrosis; hence, an elevated level does not necessarily denote lymphomatous involvement in these patients (14).

INTESTINAL LYMPHOMA

Primary gastrointestinal lymphomas are relatively common in Egypt (7), representing 5.6% of all lymphomas and 28.5% of extranodal lymphomas (1). In a series of 53 patients reported by Abdel-Latif (1), the most common gastrointestinal site of origin was the small intestine (38%), followed by stomach (34%) and colon (28%). In lymphomas of the small intestine, the mean age of patients was 29 years, males predominated with a sex ratio of 1.9:1, and the ileum was affected more frequently than the jejunum. This site distribution of gastrointestinal lymphomas observed in Egypt differs from that reported in Western literature, where gastric lymphoma markedly predominates (8,16,19,20). In a series of 538 North American patients reported by Freeman et al. (8), the most common site was the stomach (64%), followed by small intestine (21%) and colon (15%).

The histopathologic types of the 53 patients with intestinal lymphomas reported by Abdel-Latif (1) included 32 cases of poorly differentiated lymphocytic lymphoma, 11 cases of histiocytic lymphoma, nine cases of mixed lymphohistiocytic lymphoma, and only one case of Hodgkin's disease, which involved the anal canal. The lymphomas were diffuse in 50 patients and nodular in three patients. In nine patients, plasmacytoid change was a prominent feature in the tumor.

The so-called Mediterranean lymphoma reported in other countries of the Middle East (18) was not encountered in the NCI material and appears to be rare in Egypt. However, in 8 of 29 Egyptian patients with disseminated nodal non-Hodgkin's lymphoma (stage III and IV), alpha-heavy chain protein was elevated in the sera (11,13), but IgA and IgG were not elevated. These patients showed evidence of intestinal malabsorption by the D-xylose test and radiography. Peroral intestinal biopsy showed plasma cell infiltrate in the mucosa, but it was of mild degree. Malabsorption in these patients was probably caused by the widespread intestinal and/or mesenteric lymph node involvement by lymphoma.

LEUKEMIA

The age and sex distribution patterns of 220 patients with different types of leukemia treated at NCI, Cairo (15) are presented in Table 4. Gad-El-Mawla et al. (10) also reviewed a series of 141 cases of acute leukemia in children below the age of 16 years treated at NCI, Cairo. This series included 123 patients with acute lymphatic leukemia (ALL) (87.2%) and 18 patients with acute nonlymphatic leukemia (ANLL). The age distribution of these children with ALL is presented in Fig. 2. The peak incidence is at the age of six years, with two other lesser peaks at three and 10 years. This differs from the earlier age peak for ALL of children

TABLE 4. *Age and sex distributions of leukemias, National Cancer Institute, Cairo, 220 patients, 1977–1978*

Type	Frequency		Median age (years)	Male:female
	Number	Percentage		
ALL[a]	98	44.5	11.0	2.4:1
ANLL[b]	41	18.6	24.8	2.1:1
CML[c]	48	21.8	37.9	1.8:1
CLL[d]	33	15.0	53.9	3.1:1

[a]Acute lymphatic leukemia.
[b]Acute nonlymphatic leukemia.
[c]Chronic myeloid leukemia.
[d]Chronic lymphocytic leukemia.

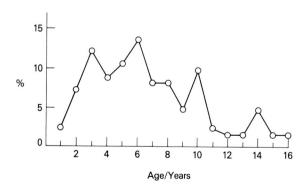

FIG. 2. Age distribution of 123 Egyptian children with acute lymphoblastic leukemia treated at National Cancer Institute, Cairo, 1977–1981 (10).

reported in the United States and England. Moreover, the most frequent type of ALL in Egyptian patients is L2, according to the French-American-British (FAB) classification, in contrast to the predominance of L1 type in the United States. Immunologic typing was reported on a series of 18 pediatric Egyptian patients with ALL, using surface immunoglobulin and E-rosette test (2). Fourteen cases were null-cell type (i.e., they neither expressed surface immunoglobulin nor formed E rosettes), three were B-cell type, and one was T-cell type.

The 41 patients with ANLL (Table 4) included 26 myeloid, eight monocytic, five myelomonocytic, and two stem cell. The median age of ANLL is 24.8 years, much younger than that reported in the West (24). The relative paucity of acute leukemia in the older age groups in Egypt (Fig. 3) appears to be unrelated to the population structure and represents a real difference from that reported in North Americans. The median age of chronic lymphocytic and chronic myeloid leukemias (CLL and CML) is also two decades younger than that reported in Western literature (24). This is believed to reflect the relatively younger Egyptian population structure rather than a real rate increase of either CLL or CML. In Egypt, both types of chronic leukemia occur more often in males than in females.

Clustering of leukemia cases in time and place has been reported in Egypt (15), with peaks during January and July and a high prevalence in Cairo and Port Said governorates. This study included all types of leukemia and used statistical tests in the evaluation of data, which indicated that this phenomenon was real rather than apparent.

DISCUSSION

The epidemiologic and pathologic features of malignant lymphoma and leukemia in Egypt are different from those observed in some tropical countries and in affluent

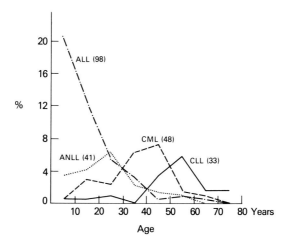

FIG. 3. Age distribution of Egyptian patients with various types of leukemia, National Cancer Institute, Cairo, 220 patients, 1977–1979 (15). ALL = acute lymphocytic leukemia, ANLL = acute nonlymphatic leukemia; CML = chronic myeloid leukemia; CLL = chronic lymphocytic leukemia. Numbers in parentheses are number of patients.

societies such as the United States and Western European countries. In Egypt, lymphoma is more common than leukemia, but this lymphoma predominance is more marked in adults (3.1:1) than in children (1.3:1). Non-Hodgkin's lymphoma is more common than Hodgkin's disease in adults, but the reverse is true in children. The median age incidence of both Hodgkin's disease and non-Hodgkin's lymphoma is one decade earlier than that observed in the United States, which may be in part the result of the age structure of the population in Egypt.

The predominance of unfavorable histologic types is another distinctive feature of our material. Thus, in Hodgkin's disease, the mixed cellularity subtype predominates (60%), whereas nodular sclerosis (18%) and lymphocyte depletion (6%) subtypes are less frequent. This pattern is in sharp contrast to the predominance of nodular sclerosis in the United States and of lymphocyte depletion in some tropical African countries. Non-Hodgkin's lymphoma is commonly diffuse (83%) and frequently classified as poorly differentiated lymphocytic subtype, which is a rather heterogeneous group. Burkitt's lymphoma and lymphoblastic lymphoma are rare in Egypt. Immunologic cell-typing studies done so far on Egyptian material are preliminary but reveal that the majority of cases of non-Hodgkin's lymphoma are of the B-cell type. More detailed studies are currently underway and may generate valuable information for international comparison.

Mediterranean lymphoma (immunoproliferative small intestinal disease) is extremely rare in Egypt, and the intestinal lymphomas observed appear to arise *de novo*. Malabsorption, when it occurs, is usually seen in patients with advanced-stage lymphoma and widespread nodal involvement.

Acute leukemia is common in Egyptian children. The majority of cases are ALL (87%), commonly of the L2 subtype in the FAB classification. This contrasts with the predominance of the L1 subtype in patients from the United States and Europe. The age peak for ALL in Egyptian children occurs at six years, which is slightly later than that reported from the United States and Western Europe.

REFERENCES

1. Abdel-Latif, N. M. (1977): *Extranodal Lymphoma, a Pathological Study*. M.D. Thesis, Cairo University.
2. Abdelhadi, S. (1982): *Lymphocyte Subpopulations and Viral Hepatitis B in Childhood Acute Lymphoblastic Leukemia Types According to FAB Classification*. M.D. Thesis, Cairo University.
3. Aboul-Ella, F. (1978): *Immunological, Histochemical, Cytological and Histological Features of Malignant Lymphomas, Application of New Methods of Classification*. Ph.D. Thesis, El-Azhar University, Cairo.
4. Aboul-Nasr, A. L. (1979): *The Cancer Registry for the Metropolitan Cairo Area, Progress Report 5*. Cairo University Press, Cairo.
5. Aboul-Nasr, A. L., Tawfik, H. N., and Abou El-Einen, M. (1973): Lymphoreticular tumors and leukemias in Egypt. *JNCI*, 50:1619–1621.
6. El-Mishad, A. M., and Ezzat, I. (1979): Antibodies to Epstein-Barr virus in head and neck neoplasms and control groups. *Med. J. Cairo Univ.*, 47:369–375.
7. El-Said, A. A., El-Bolkainy, N., and Zaki, M. S. (1974): Primary lymphomas of the gastrointestinal tract. *Med. J. Cairo Univ.*, 42:269–279.
8. Freeman, C., Berg, J., and Cutler, S. (1972): Occurrence and prognosis of extranodal lymphomas. *Cancer*, 29:252–260.
9. Gaafar, R. M. (1980): *Australia and Anti-Australia Antigen in Lymphomas and Leukemias*. M.D. Thesis, Cairo University.

10. Gad-El-Mawla, N., Aboul-Enein, M., Abdel-Hadi, S., El-Deeb, B., Abu-Gabal, A., Kamel, A., El-Serafy, M., and Hamza, R. (1983): Acute leukemia in Egyptian children. *(in press)*.
11. Gad-El-Mawla, N., Attia, M. A. M., Salen, E., El-Rouby, O., Osman, A., El-Bolkainy, M. N., and El-Serafi, M. (1978): Alpha-chain disease in patients with malignant lymphoma. *Egypt J. Hematol.* 3:59–67.
12. Gad-El-Mawla, N., El-Morsey, B. A., Sherif, M., Osman, A., Ezzat, I., and Awaad, H. K. (1974): Malignant lymphoma in children: clinicopathologic study of 114 cases. *Gaz. Egypt. Paediatr. Assoc.*, 22:197–208.
13. Gad-El-Mawla, N., Osman, A., El-Rouby, O., El-Rouby, A., Sabet, S., Sherif, M., and Awaad, H. (1974): Study of the malignant lymphoma in the bilharzial patient: the absorptive function of the small intestine. *Med. J. Cairo Univ*, 42:111–118.
14. Gad-El-Mawla, N., Salem, E., Ashmawy, S., and El-Rouby, A. (1973): Studies on the lymphomas in the bilharzial patient: enzymatic study and liver function tests. *J. Egypt. Med. Assoc.*, 56:423–432.
15. Hamza, M. R., Ibrahim, A. S., Mansour, M. A., Iskander, I. R., Gad-El-Mawla, N., and Khalil, I. F. (1982): Clinicopathologic study of leukemia: anlaysis of 220 cases managed at the National Cancer Institute. *J. Egypt. Natl. Cancer Inst.*, 1:29–37.
16. Loehr, W. J., Mujahed, Z., Zahn, F. D., Gray, G. F., and Thorbjarnarson, B. (1969): Primary lymphoma of the gastrointestinal tract: a review of 100 cases. *Ann. Surg.*, 170:232–238.
17. Mahfouz, M., El-Ghamrawy, K., Zaki, O., Risk, S., and Aboul-Enein, M. (1983): Clinicoepidemiologic features of malignant lymphomas in Egypt. *Med. J. Cairo Univ. (in press)*.
18. Rappaport, H., Ramot, B., Hulu, N., and Park, J. K. (1972): The pathology of so-called Mediterranean abdominal lymphoma with malabsorption. *Cancer*, 29:1502–1511.
19. Rosenfelt, F., and Rosenberg, S. A. (1980): Diffuse histiocytic lymphoma presenting with gastrointestinal tract lesions, the Stanford experience. *Cancer*, 45:2188–2193.
20. Rundles, R. W. (1974): Malignant lymphomas of the gastrointestinal tract. *Cancer*, 34:948–950.
21. Sherif, M., Gad-El-Mawla, N., El-Bolkainy, N., Badawi, S., and Awwad, H. (1975): Clinical staging of malignant lymphoma in patients suspected to have hepatosplenic schistosomiasis. *J. Trop. Med. Hyg.*, 78:67–70.
22. Tawfik, H. N., and Aboul-Ella, F. (1982): Malignant lymphoma, pathological features of 2010 Egyptian cases. *J. Egypt. Natl. Cancer Inst.*, 1:1–11.
23. Tawfik, H. N., Maebed, H., Ibrahim, A. S., and El-Sayed, L. (1979): Pathological staging of malignant lymphomas. *Med. J. Cairo Univ.*, 47:39–48.
24. Waterhouse, J. A. H. (1974): *Cancer Handbook of Epidemiology and Prognosis*, pp. 178–190. Churchill Livingstone, Edinburgh.
25. World Health Organization (1975): *Report on the Symposium on Lymphomas, Hammamet, Tunisia, 1974*, EMRO 8501/R. WHO Regional Office for the Eastern Mediterranean, Alexandria.

*Pathogenesis of Leukemias and Lymphomas:
Environmental Influences*, edited by
I. T. Magrath, G. T. O'Conor, and B. Ramot.
Raven Press, New York © 1984.

Trends in Leukemia Incidence in Ibadan, Nigeria

*C. K. Oladipupo Williams, *E. M. Essien, and **E. A. Bamgboye

*Department of Haematology and **Medical Statistics Unit, Department of Preventive
and Social Medicine, University College Hospital, Ibadan, Nigeria*

Reports from various areas of Black Africa on the clinical manifestations of human leukemia subtypes in indigenous African populations indicate features that are unique and common to the various ethnic groups thus far studied. These features include (a) rarity of acute lymphoblastic leukemia (ALL) in the zero- to four-year age group, and peak frequency of diagnosis between five and 14 years of age (1,2,5,6,11–13,17); (b) frequent occurrence of acute myelogenous leukemia (AML) in children and common association with chloromas (4,6,9,18); and (c) high frequency of chronic lymphocytic leukemia (CLL) in African women below the age of 45 (7,9,10), whereas among people older than 50, the disease occurs predominantly in men. It therefore seems reasonable to attribute these unifying features in different ethnic groups to etiological factors that are shared by virtue of similar environmental influences.

Within the past two decades, significant socioeconomic changes have taken place at different rates in various areas of the continent. Consequent upon these changes, one would expect to observe a change in the pattern of environmentally conditioned diseases. In this chapter, we seek to identify such a change in the pattern of leukemia variants by analyzing and comparing trends in the frequency of diagnosis and age-specific incidence of leukemia subtypes at the University College Hospital (UCH), Ibadan, Nigeria, for the periods 1958–1968 and 1978–1982. We also attempt to relate possible socioeconomic influences to the observed changes.

MATERIALS AND METHODS

During 1958–1968 and 1978–1982, there was considerable interest in the study of leukemia in Ibadan. Part of the intervening period coincided with a time of civil turmoil and less reliable documentation of these diseases. Cases of acute and chronic leukemia diagnosed in patients seen at UCH from 1958 to 1968 inclusive (11 years) were identified retrospectively through their medical records. The characteristics of these patients and their diseases have been reported by Essien (6,7). Cases of leukemia seen at the same institution from July 1, 1978 to March 31, 1982 (45 months) and referred to the Department of Haematology were studied prospectively. Other cases that escaped the referral services were identified through a detailed search of hematological laboratory records at UCH.

The diagnosis of the leukemia subtypes was established primarily by routine hematological indexes in both studies. Occasionally, special cytochemical stains were used to confirm the subtype. Cytogenetic examinations were not available during the two study periods. During the later but not the earlier period of study, it was possible to support the diagnosis of CLL in cases of doubtful lymphocytosis by the estimation of IgM and lymphocyte transformability with phytohemagglutinin (19), thereby excluding cases of tropical splenomegaly syndrome, which, because of associated lymphocytosis, can mimic CLL (8).

The incidence of acute leukemia in the various age groups of inhabitants of Ibadan and its environs was derived for the 1958–1968 period from population figures obtained from the national census of 1963 and the number of acute leukemia cases identified during that period. Because no reliable census figures are available for Nigeria after 1963, in calculating the incidence of leukemia subtypes in 1978–1982 it was necessary to project the population of Ibadan from the 1963 census data, assuming a steady growth rate of 2.5 to 5% (16). These figures have been recommended for the economic planning of the Nigerian states and urban areas by the Federal Office of Statistics. Although a growth rate of 2.5% is generally considered too conservative for Ibadan, 5% has been considered rather high, and the true growth rate probably lies between these limits.

Patients in the prospective observation group (1978–1982) were characterized socioeconomically by level of education and profession. They were subdivided into five groups on a socioeconomic status scale (SES) ranging from 1 (the highest) to 5 (the lowest). Grouped in SES 1 were highly educated individuals, senior public officers, and business executives. SES 2 included persons with postsecondary school education and middle-level public officers. SES 3 consisted of individuals with postprimary school education, lower level public officers or institutional staff, and skilled handworkers. SES 4 included those persons with a primary school education and unskilled handworkers. The SES 5 group were illiterate peasant farmers and petty traders.

The study population was entirely African but included a number of different ethnic groups. The majority of patients in both study groups belonged to the Yoruba ethnic group, which is the dominant resident group in Ibadan. Ibadan is believed to be the largest city in West Africa and has at present an estimated population of between 1 and 2 million, depending on whether a growth rate of 2.5% or 5% since 1963 is assumed.

Odebiyi (15) and investigators at the Nigerian Institute of Social and Economic Research (16) have studied the social structure of Ibadan and its environs. From the results of such studies, it is estimated that approximately 10 to 15% of the population of Ibadan can be categorized as SES 1 or 2 approximately 10 to 15% as SES 3, and the remaining 70 to 80% as SES 4 or 5. It also has been established that the lower the socioeconomic status, the less the willingness to use modern health facilities (15). Thus, underdiagnosis of disease and presentation at a late stage of disease are more likely in patients of lower socioeconomic status.

A recent World Bank report gave the age structure of the Nigerian population as 47.2% for 0 to 14 years, 50.3% for 15 to 64 years, and 2.5% for 65 years and above (21); according to the 1963 census, the percentage distribution was 29, 69.8, and 12% for the three age groups, respectively. A projection of the current sizes of five-year age groups within the population based on an assumption of a uniform growth rate for all ages would, therefore, tend to underestimate the size of the groups below 14 years and above 65 years and overestimate the size of the age groups between 15 and 64 years. In estimating the leukemia incidence for 1978–1982, therefore, we have projected population sizes assuming a steady growth rate of 2.5% and 5% for the entire population but have assumed that the population of Ibadan is distributed as suggested by the World Bank study. We have taken the two extremes of the four incidence values thus obtained to represent a probable range of leukemia incidence.

RESULTS

Acute Leukemia

During 1958–1968, 26 and 57 cases of ALL and AML, respectively, were seen at UCH, compared to 30 and 31 cases, respectively, in 1978–1982. Thus, the annual accrual rate of ALL increased by approximately 250% in the later study period, whereas AML increased by 60%. Table 1 lists the annual accrual rates of the different leukemia subtypes by age group during the two study periods. There was a trend toward an increased frequency of diagnosis of ALL in young children, especially below the age of five years. ALL was not observed after the age of 49 years, nor AML after the age of 64 years, during either study period.

Table 2 shows the socioeconomic status of patients with the various leukemia subtypes in relation to the age groups. Childhood AML was observed most frequently in children of low socioeconomic background (SES 4 and 5). ALL was diagnosed significantly more frequently than AML in children of SES 2 and 3 ($p \leqslant 0.05$). No remarkable difference appeared, however, in the frequency of diagnosis of ALL and AML among adult (i.e., 15 to 64 years) patients of SES 1–5. Childhood ALL and AML showed a marked male predominance (male-female ratios were approximately 5:2 and 5:1, respectively). Adult ALL was also more common in males (male-female ratio of 7:2), whereas adult AML was diagnosed in nine males and eight females.

Ranges of leukemia incidence, derived as explained above, are shown in Table 3. A comparison of the incidence of acute leukemia (AL) in 1958–1968 with the incidence in 1978–1982 suggests an increased incidence, especially for the zero-to 14-year age group, where an increase of three- to 10-fold appeared likely (Table 3). Because the 1958–1968 incidence data for AL were not broken down for subtypes, the incidence of ALL and AML could not be directly compared for the

TABLE 1. Average annual accrual rates of leukemia subtypes[a] diagnosed at the University College Hospital, Ibadan, Nigeria, 1958–1968 and 1978–1982

Five year age group	ALL		AML		Ten- to 15-year age group	CLL		CML	
	1958–68	1978–82	1958–68	1978–82		1958–68	1978–82	1958–68	1978–82
0–4	0.27	2.1	0.09	0	0–15	0.27	0	0.36	0.53
5–9	0.45	1.6	0.90	2.93					
10–14	0.64	1.87	0.82	0.53	16–25	0.36	0	1.45	2.93
15–19	0.27	0.53	0.90	0.80					
20–24	0.18	1.07	0.36	0.27					
25–29	0.27	0.53	0.82	0.80	26–35	0.82	1.6	2.55	4.0
30–34	0.09	0	0.09	0.27					
35–39	0	0	0.09	0.80	36–45	2.0	2.13	1.45	1.6
40–44	0	0	0.18	0.53					
45–49	0.18	0.27	0.18	0.27	46–55	2.09	1.33	0.91	1.33
50–54	0	0	0.09	0.53					
55–59	0	0	0.55	0.27	56–65	1.55	2.13	0.36	0.8
60–64	0	0	0.09	0					
65–79	0	0	0	0	66–75	0.36	1.07	0.09	0.8
Total	2.35	7.79	5.16	8.0	Total	7.45	8.26	7.17	12.0

[a]Acute lymphocytic leukemia (ALL), acute myelogenous leukemia (AML), chronic lymphocytic leukemia (CLL), and chronic myelogenous leukemia (CML).

TABLE 2. Socioeconomic status[a] of leukemia patients seen at the University College Hospital, Ibadan, Nigeria, 1978–1982

Age group (years)	ALL	AML	CLL	CML
0–4	3.8 (3–5)	—	—	—
5–9	4.25 (3–5)	4.6 (4–5)[b]	—	—
10–14	4.43 (2–5)	5 (5,5)[c]	—	5
15–19	4.5 (4,5)	4 (4,4)	—	4 (4,4)
20–24	3.75 (2–5)	5[d]	—	2.7 (2–4)
25–29	4.5 (4,5)	3.3 (2–4)	5	4.5 (4–5)
30–34	—	5	5	3.6 (1–5)
35–39	—	3.6 (2–5)	4 (2–5)	5
40–44	5	1	5 (5,5)	4.7 (4–5)
45–49	—	—	5	4
50–54	—	4.5 (4,5)	5 (5,5)	5
55–59	—	4	5	5
60–64	—	—	5	5
65–69	—	—	—	—
70–74	—	—	5	—
75–79	—	—	3	2.5 (1–5)
Total	4.19 (2–5)	4.19 (1–5)	4.82 (2–5)	4.18 (1–5)

[a]Mean and range (in parentheses) of the socioeconomic status scale (SES). ALL = acute lymphocytic leukemia, AML = acute myelogenous leukemia, CLL = chronic lymphocytic leukemia, CML = chronic myelogenous leukemia.
[b]Five cases of chloroma-associated AML (CA-AML), with a mean SES of 4.6 and a SES range of 4–5.
[c]Two cases of CA-AML, both with SES of 5.
[d]One case of CA-AML (SES 5).

two study periods. However, differences in the annual accrual rates for the two subtypes show clearly that most of the increased incidence of AL in 1978–1982 is due to ALL.

The most common symptoms among the AL patients on admission were weakness, fever, and abnormal bleeding. Four of the AML patients presented apparently primarily because of the chloromatous swelling associated with their disease, whereas in three other AML patients, chloromas were found only on examination. High white-cell count (above 10^{10}/liter) was present in 80 to 90% of both ALL and AML patients. But although the level of white blood cells (WBC) was correlated with the presence of tissue invasion in ALL, there was no such correlation between WBC and chloroma in AML. These and other clinical and laboratory findings in Ibadan children have recently been published (20).

Chronic Leukemia

Table 1 shows changes in annual accrual rates of cases of CLL and chronic myelogenous leukemia (CML) seen in 1958–1968 and 1978–1982. As in AML,

TABLE 3. *Estimated range of incidence[a] of acute leukemia[b] in Ibadan, Nigeria, 1958–1968 and 1978–1982*

Age group	ALL		AML		AL	
	1958–1968	1978–1982	1958–1968	1978–1982	1958–1968	1978–1982
0–4	NA	<0.35–0.69	NA	<0.11–0.23	NA	<0.45–0.90
5–9	NA	<0.41–0.82	NA	<1.0–2.19	NA	<1.5–3.0
10–14	NA	<0.80–1.6	NA	<0.16–0.32	NA	<0.96–1.92
0–14	NA	0.29–0.99	NA	0.27–0.90	0.19	0.55–1.90
0–64	NA	0.18–0.37	NA	0.27–0.55	0.35	0.45–0.92
0–74	NA	~0.37–0.76[c]	NA	~0.5–1.0[d]	NA	~0.89–1.80[e]

[a]Number of cases per 100,000.
[b]ALL = acute lymphocytic leukemia, AML = acute myelogenous leukemia, AL = acute leukemia. NA = not available.
[c]All lymphoid leukemias.
[d]All myeloid leukemias.
[e]All subtypes.

the changes are much less marked than those observed over the same periods in ALL. During both study periods, CLL was most frequently encountered in women between 26 and 49 years old. However, the retrospective (1958–1968) observation of cases of CLL in the age group of 0 to 25 years could not be confirmed prospectively between 1978 and 1982. CML was observed in all 15-year age groups (Table 1) up to age 75 years in both study periods. There was a small trend toward increased annual accrual rate of CML in the later study period, especially in the age group 56 to 75 years.

CML predominated in male patients by a ratio of 13:8. CLL below 50 years predominated in females (male-female ratio of 1:6), whereas at 50 years and above, the male-female ratio was approximately 2:1. The clinical and laboratory features of CLL in Ibadan patients under the age of 50 years are shown in Table 4. The variant of the disease occurring in patients above 50 years showed similar laboratory features but was more frequently associated with marked lymphadenopathy, skin manifestations, a poorer response to chemotherapy, and a shorter survival. Thus, this variant of CLL appears to be a more aggressive disease than that found in middle-aged women.

Only two of 29 CLL, compared to 18 of 45 CML patients, were of SES 1–3, indicating a significant association of CLL with low socioeconomic status (SES 4–5) ($p<0.05$).

The incidences of CLL and CML in the zero to 64 age groups for 1978–1982 were similar: 2.2 to 4.4/1,000,000 and 2.3 to 4.9/1,000,000, respectively. The incidences of all subtypes of leukemia in the 35 to 64 and zero to 64 age groups were estimated at 2.8 to 5.7/100,000 and 0.9 to 1.8/100,000, respectively.

DISCUSSION

Improved health care delivery and other changes in the social milieu of traditional African communities can be expected to lead to increased diagnosis of various subtypes of leukemia and other rare diseases. However, the marked differences in the rates of increase observed in Ibadan between 1958–1968 and 1978–1982 with respect to various leukemia subtypes, as well as the differences in age-specific rates, suggest that factors besides improved disease recognition were responsible for the observed phenomenon. For example, improved disease recognition alone is unlikely to explain the difference between the increase recorded in the later study period in annual accrual rates in ALL (250%) compared to AML (60%). We suggest therefore that the changes are related at least in part to real changes in the incidence of the leukemia subtypes in the population.

Differences between Ibadan and the developed countries in the clinical manifestations of childhood acute leukemia led to the suggestion that the environment influences leukemogenesis (20). The association established in this study between low socioeconomic status and CLL (especially the variant occurring in women under 50) and chloroma-associated AML (CA-AML) lends some support to this view. Low socioeconomic status as used in the context of this report is generally

TABLE 4. Clinical and laboratory features of chronic lymphocytic leukemia in patients under 50 years of age seen at the University College Hospital, Ibadan, Nigeria, 1978–1982

Patient number	Age	Sex	Lymphadenopathy	Liver[a]	Spleen[b]	PCV[c]	Lymphocytes ($\times 10^9$/liter)	Platelet count ($\times 10^9$/liter)	BML[d,e]	Response to chemotherapy[f]	Survival (months)[g]
1	35	F	Present	9	23	27	396.0	Normal	NE	Good	? (Def.)
5	33	F	Present	?	?	22	315.0	ND[j]	NE	Good	? (Def.)
6	33	F	Absent	0	22	31	54.0	?	+ve	?	? (Def.)
7	40	F	Absent	9	20	49	100.0	108.0	NE	?	? (Def.)
9	45	F	Present	5	25	28	120.0	70.0	NE	Good	>36
11	36	F	Absent	0	20	28	640.0	?	NE	Good	40 (Died)
20	42	F	Absent	4	0	35	25.0	?	+ve	NT	>30
29	30	M	?	5	24	26	97.0	145.0	NE	NT	? (Def.)
37	42	F	Absent	8	20	33	25.0	Normal	NE	NT	? (Def.)
38	31	F	Absent	5	25	23	157.0	Reduced	NE	Good	>12
39	45	F	Absent	7	5	26	50.0	81.0	NE	Good	? (Def.)
45	37	M	Present	0	0	42	14.5	51.0	+ve	NT	>28
51	47	F	Absent	4	25	27	53.0	Reduced	+ve	NT	<1[h]
57	45	F	Present	6	10	29	11.0	Normal	NE	Splenect.[i]	? (Def.)
65	26	F	Marked	10	10	18	36.0	190.0	+ve	Poor	4 (Died)

[a]Centimeters below the right costal margin.
[b]Centimeters below the left costal margin.
[c]Packed cell volume.
[d]Bone marrow lymphocytosis.
[e]NE = not evaluated; +ve = positive.
[f]NT = not treated.
[g]? (Def) = not evaluated because patient defaulted on follow-up.
[h]Patient died accidentally because of default on follow-up.
[i]Splenectomy.
[j]ND = not determined.

associated with a low literacy level as well as poor living conditions. People in this socioeconomic group usually live in overcrowded, poorly ventilated houses with unsanitary surroundings, and malnutrition is common among them. Because individuals of low socioeconomic status are most likely to use modern medical facilities only as a last resort, it is probable that the strong association noted in this report between low SES and CLL as well as CA-AML is a real one and that there is indeed a high prevalence of both diseases in this group. The frequent occurrence of chloroma may be a manifestation of late presentation but is conceivably a unique manifestation of AML. The more frequent observation of CML in individuals of higher socioeconomic strata may be interpreted to imply that this condition affects all social strata uniformly but that because of their social habits, the affected individuals in higher social strata are more likely to seek medical advice and come to hospitals.

Our observation that the incidence of ALL in the zero- to four-year age group has increased markedly between the 1958–1968 and 1978–1982 periods suggests a shift in the direction of the age-related incidence pattern of developed countries (20). There is a trend (although not statistically significant) toward higher socioeconomic status with decreasing age among our ALL children. Furthermore, the SES of the ALL children is significantly higher that that of AML children ($p<0.05$), which signifies an association between higher socioeconomic status and increased incidence of ALL in this study. The association may be spurious, reflecting lower infant mortality through better care of the children in these socioeconomic strata. It could, however, be a real association in that families of higher socioeconomic level, on account of their status, are exposed selectively to factors that predispose them to develop ALL.

It previously has been noted that cases of ALL in Ibadan children are associated with poor risk factors. In fact, "standard-risk ALL" is rarely seen in Ibadan (20), which suggests that ALL in Ibadan children is different from the type seen in developed countries. Furthermore, the data presented suggest that there are at least two types of AML in Ibadan: the chloroma-associated variant afflicting mainly male children and young adults, usually of low socioeconomic status (Table 2), and the "adult type," occurring roughly equally in men and women of mixed socioeconomic backgrounds. Thus, although the former type appears to be related to environmental conditions, we found no indication of linkage of the latter type to a particular lifestyle. Note that CA-AML occurs most commonly in the same age group as Burkitt's lymphoma and that Epstein-Barr virus has been implicated by Cavdar et al. (3) in CA-AML in Turkish children.

Our observations also suggest that there may be two CLL variants in Ibadan: a variant afflicting predominantly middle-aged women, and another, apparently more aggressive in nature, afflicting predominantly older men. Low socioeconomic status appears to be common to the two groups of patients. The reason for the marked sex difference in CLL occurring below the age of 50 years is not clear. However, Fleming (10) has speculated on the possible role of oncogenic agents, including malaria, as predisposing factors acting in conjunction with pregnancy-induced depression of cell-mediated immunity.

Leukemia incidence in Nigeria has been difficult to determine because of the lack of a reliable statistical data base. The estimates presented in this report are based on projection of population sizes, using criteria recommended by national and international organizations. Note that the results of this exercise bear some similarity to incidence data reported by Surveillance, Epidemiology, and End Results (SEER) (22). The estimated cumulative annual leukemia incidence of approximately 0.9 to 1.8/100,000 for zero to 74 years for Ibadan is not remarkably different from 0.8/100,000 reported for U.S. Whites and 0.7/100,000 for U.S. Blacks, which suggests that the overall leukemia incidences in Ibadan and the United States are similar. However, important differences are recognizable. For instance, the virtual absence of leukemia in Ibadan people over 60 stands in sharp contrast to the high leukemia incidence in Americans in the same age group. The obvious reason for this is the small size of the population at risk in Ibadan.

The most striking difference between the leukemia incidence pattern in Ibadan and U.S. populations is seen in childhood. ALL in the zero- to four-year age group is more than six times and two times as common in U.S. White and Black children, respectively, as in Ibadan children. This is despite the use, in the comparison, of an incidence figure for Ibadan children that is believed to be grossly inflated, thus making it unlikely that the difference is the result of underdiagnosis alone. We have recently observed a low ALL-Wilms' tumor ratio in both Ibadan and U.S. Black children compared to their Caucasian counterparts, further supporting the probability that the low incidence of ALL in Ibadan children is not owing to underdiagnosis alone (20). The incidence of ALL is, however, similar in U.S. Black, U.S. White, and Ibadan children of 10 to 14 years old. Despite the recent trends in the ALL incidence pattern in Ibadan, with more cases being seen below the age of five years, the peak incidence of the disease remained in the 10- to 14-year age group. It will be interesting to see whether the ALL pattern in Ibadan evolves in the coming decades into one with a peak incidence in the zero- to four-year age group, as seen in developed countries, or whether the present pattern persists. Continued observations will therefore help to determine whether the present pattern is caused by differences in lifestyles dictated by differences in the socio-economic status of the people, or whether genetic susceptibility plays a role in the phenomenon.

The relatively high incidence of AML in Ibadan boys five to nine years old (1.0 to 2.19/100,000) appears to be another unique feature of leukemia in Ibadan. This disease and CLL in Ibadan middle-aged women are strongly associated with low socioeconomic status and therefore appear to be related to some environmental factors prevalent in Ibadan people in general and in its poorer citizens in particular. If these are, indeed, examples of environmental influence on leukemogenesis, they would be expected to disappear with the further socioeconomic development of Ibadan.

ACKNOWLEDGMENTS

We are grateful to Dr. Donald Okpala and Mrs. Karola Williams of the Nigerian Institute of Social and Economic Research, University of Ibadan, for useful discussions on the social structure of Ibadan. We also thank Mrs. O. A. Ajani for secretarial assistance in the preparation of the manuscript.

REFERENCES

1. Allan, N. C., and Watson-Williams, B. J. (1963): A study of leukaemias among Nigerians in Ibadan. In: *Proceedings of the 9th Congress of the European Society of Haematology*, pp. 906–915. S. Karger, Basel.
2. Amsel, G., and Nambembezi, J. S. (1964): Two-year survey of haematologic malignancies in Uganda. *JNCI*, 52:1397–1401.
3. Cavdar, A. O., Arcassoy, A., Gozdasoglu, S., Babacan, E., and Fraumeni, J. F. (1975): AMML in Turkish children with chloroma-like ocular manifestations. In: *Proceedings of International Meeting of Therapy of Acute Leukaemia, Rome, Dec. 6–8, 1973*. Editizioni Minerva Medica, Torino, Italy.
4. Davies, J. N. P., and Owor, R. (1965): Chloromatous tumors in African children. *Br. Med. J.*, 2:405.
5. Edington, G. M. (1970): *Cancer Incidence in Five Continents*, edited by R. Doll, C. S. Muir, and J. A. H. Waterhouse, pp. 90–95. International Union Against Cancer, Geneva.
6. Essien, E. M. (1972): Leukaemia in Nigerians. Part I. The acute leukaemias. *Afr. J. Med. Med. Sci.*, 3:117–130.
7. Essien, E. M. (1976): Leukaemia in Nigerians: The chronic leukaemias. *East Afr. Med. J.*, 53:96–103.
8. Fakunle, Y. M. (1981): Tropical splenomegaly. *Clin. Haematol.*, 10:963–973.
9. Fleming, A. F. (1978): Leukaemia in the Guinea savanna of northern Nigeria. In: *Advances in Comparative Leukaemia Research*, edited by P. Bentvelzen, J. Hilgers, and D. S. Yohn, pp. 53–54. Elsevier/North-Holland Biomedical Press, Amsterdam.
10. Fleming, A. F. (1979): Epidemiology of the leukaemias in Africa. *Leuk. Res.*, 3:51–59.
11. Jeoffrey, C., and Gelfand, M. (1972): Leukaemia in Rhodesian Africa. *J. Trop. Med. Hyg.*, 75:176–179.
12. Kasili, E. G., and Taylor, J. R. (1970): Leukaemia in Kenya. *East Afr. Med. J.*, 47:461–468.
13. Lothe, F. (1967): Leukaemia in Uganda. *Trop. Geogr. Med.*, 19:163–171.
14. O'Conor, G. T., and Davies, J. N. P. (1960): Malignant tumors in African children with special reference to malignant lymphoma. *J. Pediatr.*, 56:526–535.
15. Odebiyi, A. I. (1980): Socio-economic status, illness, behaviour and attitudes toward disease etiology in Ibadan. *Niger. Behav. Sci. J.*, 3:172–186.
16. Onibokun, P., Adesokan, R. B., and Bello, I. (1981): *Oyo State: A Survey of Resources for Development*. Nigerian Institute of Social and Economic Research, University of Ibadan, Ibadan, Nigeria.
17. Sonnet, J., Michaux, J. L., and Hekster, C. (1966): Incidence and forms of leukaemia among Congolese Bantus. *Trop. Geogr. Med.*, 18:272–286.
18. Templeton, A. C. (1973): Leukaemia. *Recent Results Cancer Res.*, 41:298–301.
19. Ukaejiofo, E. O., and David-West, A. S. (1979): The use of lymphocyte transformation and IgM estimation as diagnostic aids in leukaemoid reactions. *J. Trop. Med. Hyg.*, 82:197–200.
20. Williams, C. K. O., Folami, A. O., Laditan, A. A. O., and Ukaejiofo, E. O. (1982): Childhood acute leukaemia in a tropical population. *Br. J. Cancer*, 46:89–94.
21. World Bank (1981): *Nigeria—Country Economic Memorandum*. Report 3279. World Bank, Washington, D.C.
22. Young, J. L., Jr., Percy, C. L., and Asire, A. J., editors (1981): *Surveillance, Epidemiology and End Results: Incidence and Mortality Data, 1973–1977*. National Cancer Inst. Monogr. 57. National Cancer Institute, Bethesda, MD.

Pathogenesis of Leukemias and Lymphomas:
Environmental Influences, edited by
I. T. Magrath, G. T. O'Conor, and B. Ramot.
Raven Press, New York © 1984.

Geographic Distribution of Malignant Lymphomas and Leukemias in Uganda

R. Owor

Department of Pathology, Makerere University Medical School, Kampala, Uganda

The high frequency of lymphomas, particularly Burkitt's lymphoma, and the low frequency of leukemias in Ugandan children and tropical Africa as a whole has been repeatedly reported (1,6). The low frequency of leukemias is difficult to explain but may, at least in part, simply be the result of underdiagnosis. The geographical distribution of Burkitt's lymphoma in Uganda is well documented; most cases come from the West Nile and the northern region of the country. This distribution has been related to endemicity of malaria (3,4). On the other hand, other types of lymphoma do not show any particular geographical distribution. Previous studies in Uganda have shown that not only are leukemias uncommon, but among the acute leukemias the myeloid type is more frequent than the lymphoblastic type (7).

The present communication presents an assessment of the frequency and geographical distribution of lymphomas and leukemias in Uganda during 1977–1980. All cases of lymphomas and leukemias registered by the Kampala Cancer Registry (KCR) during the period were analyzed. The Registry records all cancer cases seen in the country; this is possible because the Makerere University Department of Pathology provides histopathology service for the whole country. Specimens are received from all government and private hospitals as well as private practitioners. Outside the capital city of Kampala, the health services are sparse but evenly distributed. Kampala and the surrounding districts have relatively better medical facilities.

RESULTS

When KCR data for lymphomas and leukemias from 1964 to 1968 and from 1977 to 1980 are compared (see Table 1), it is apparent that the total number of cases registered was significantly less during 1977–1980. Because the number of cancers and the population at risk are not well known, incidence rates cannot be provided. The proportional rates, however, have not changed much between the two review periods. The reduction in the number of registered cases reflects the reduction of medical services in the country because of social unrest and war.

The geographical distribution of the different types of non-Burkitt's lymphomas remains generally uniform throughout the country. Although the number of Burkitt's

TABLE 1. *Frequency of lymphomas and leukemias,*
Kampala Cancer Registry

Type	1964–1968		1977–1980	
	Number	Percentage	Number	Percentage
Total cancers	7,347	100	4,477	100
Burkitt's lymphoma	272	3.7	118	2.6
Hodgkin's disease	131	1.8	68	1.5
Other lymphomas	301	4.1	225	5.0
Leukemias	200	2.7	116	2.6

TABLE 2. *Age distribution of Burkitt's lymphoma,*
Kampala Cancer Registry, 1977–1980

Age group (years)	Number of cases	Age group (years)	Number of cases
0–5	23	31–35	0
6–10	53	36–40	2
11–15	22	41–45	0
16–20	6	46–50	0
21–25	0	51–55	0
29–30	0	56–60	1

lymphomas fell during 1977–1980, most of those seen came from the northern region of the country. The greatest fall was in West Nile, where medical services were much more affected. The age distribution of Burkitt's lymphoma patients in 1977–1980 (Table 2) is similar to that for the 1964–1968 period (9). Recent disturbances in the country have precluded any assessment of whether the geographical distribution pattern of Burkitt's lymphoma has changed significantly.

In recent years, since the establishment of the Uganda Cancer Institute in Kampala, interest in leukemias has been increasing. The number of leukemias registered annually by KCR has remained constant during the period. Table 3 shows the age distribution of 114 leukemia cases (in two cases, the age was not recorded). There is no significant difference in the sex ratio for any of the leukemias. The average age for the acute leukemias indicates that all types occur predominantly in young individuals. The majority of patients with acute lymphoblastic leukemia are below 10 years of age, whereas those with acute myeloid leukemia tend to be older (only four of 22 cases were below the age of 10).

DISCUSSION

Previous surveys in Uganda showed that acute myeloid leukemia was more common than the lymphoblastic type. The present survey shows that lymphoblastic leukemia is more commonly seen, and if this trend continues the pattern will be similar to that in Western Europe and North America. We are not able to explain

TABLE 3. *Age distribution of 114 leukemia cases, Kampala Cancer Registry*

Subtype	Age (years)															Average
	0–5	6–10	11–15	16–20	21–25	26–30	31–35	36–40	41–45	46–50	51–55	56–60	61–65	66–70	71–75	
Acute lymphatic	7	8	6	3	1	0	0	2	0	0	1	0	0	0	0	12.7
Acute myeloid	1	3	7	4	1	2	0	0	2	1	0	0	1	0	0	22.4
Chronic lymphatic	0	0	0	0	1	3	1	4	8	7	2	7	1	0	2	47.7
Chronic myeloid	0	3	1	1	2	6	2	5	1	1	1	2	0	1	0	33.0
Monocytic	0	0	0	1	0	0	0	0	0	0	0	0	0	0	0	—
Unclassified	1	0	0	0	0	0	0	0	0	0	0	0	0	0	0	—

this apparent change in pattern. This survey shows that about 25% of the acute myeloid leukemias were associated with chloromas, a similar percentage to that reported earlier from Uganda by Davies and Owor (2). For many years there has been speculation about why lymphoreticular tumors in the tropics tend to be solid—for instance, Burkitt's lymphoma and chloroma—whereas leukemias predominate in the Western world. We still have no explanation for this peculiarity, but subtyping of these tumors may give us a clue.

The geographical distribution of leukemias in Uganda is difficult to assess. Whenever and wherever there are interested clinicians or pathologists, the numbers tend to increase (5,8). Lacor Hospital in Gulu and Mulago Hospital in Kampala report the most leukemias, because clinicians send blood films and bone marrows to pathologists for diagnosis.

Because Kampala and surrounding districts have better medical facilities than other areas in the country, it is to be expected that most cases of leukemia are likely to be diagnosed in this region. Previous workers (5,7) showed that in the Kampala area, leukemia was most frequent in Busiro County; as may be seen in Table 4, Kyadondo County now has more cases. In fact, during 1977–1980, Busiro had only 22% of the cases reported from Kyadondo. These two counties are adjacent. The previous high frequency in Busiro County has not been explained, nor do we now have an explanation for either the high frequency in Kyadondo or the lower frequency in Busiro.

The geographical distribution of lymphomas and leukemias in Uganda raises some questions: Why is Burkitt's lymphoma, which continues to be the most common lymphoid malignancy, much more frequent in West Nile and the northern regions of Uganda? Other factors besides the endemicity of malaria may be playing a part. Although the numbers are small, acute lymphoblastic leukemia appears to be becoming more common than acute myeloid leukemia. This will be an important trend to follow and to characterize in more detail, particularly in regard to which age groups and immunological subtypes are predominantly affected. Why is Kyadondo County reporting more cases of leukemias than Busiro County, whereas the reverse was true about 10 years ago? These apparent changes in frequency and

TABLE 4. *Distribution of leukemias in Kyadondo (Kampala) and adjacent counties, 1977–1980*

County	No. cases
Kyadondo	27
Kyaggwe	9
Busiro	6
Bulemezi	3
Bugerere	1
Mawokota	1

geographical distribution should stimulate us to analyze these parameters according to the subtypes of lymphomas and leukemias.

REFERENCES

1. Davies, J. N. P. (1965): Leukemia in children in tropical Africa. *Lancet*, 2:65–67.
2. Davies, J. N. P., and Owor, R. (1965): Chloromatous tumours in African children in Uganda. *Br. Med. J.*, 2:405–407.
3. Kafuko, G. W., Baingana, N., Knight, E. M., and Tibemenya, J. (1969): Association of Burkitt's tumour and holoendemic malaria in West Nile District, Uganda: malaria as a possible aetiologic factor. *East Afr. Med. J.*, 46:414–436.
4. Kafuko, G. W., and Burkitt, D. P. (1970): Burkitt's lymphoma and malaria. *Int. J. Cancer*, 6:1–9.
5. Lothe, F. (1967): Leukaemia in Uganda. *Trop. Geogr. Med.*, 19:163–171.
6. O'Conor, G. T., and Davies, J. N. P. (1960): Malignant tumors in African children with special reference to malignant lymphoma. *J. Pediatr.*, 56:526–535.
7. Templeton, A. C. (1973): Leukaemia. In: *Tumours in a Tropical Country*, edited by A. C. Templeton, pp. 298–301. Springer-Verlag, Berlin.
8. Vanier, T. M., and Pike, M. C. (1967): Leukaemia incidence in tropical Africa (letter). *Lancet*, 1:512–513.
9. Wright, D. H. (1973): Lymphoreticular neoplasms. In: *Tumours in a Tropical Country*, edited by A. C. Templeton, pp. 270–291. Springer-Verlag, Berlin.

Pathogenesis of Leukemias and Lymphomas: Environmental Influences, edited by
I. T. Magrath, G. T. O'Conor, and B. Ramot.
Raven Press, New York © 1984.

Lymphoid Neoplasias at the Cancer Institute, Madras

V. Shanta, M. S. Sukumaran, T. G. Sagar, K. Sasikala,
Geetha Soman, K. R. Rajalakshmi, and S. Krishnamurthi

Cancer Institute, Adyar, Madras-600020, India

The Cancer Institute, Madras, is a comprehensive cancer center devoted to the study and treatment of malignant disease. It draws patients not only from Tamil Nadu where it is located but also from the neighboring states of Andhra Pradesh, Kerala, and Karnataka and a few from other states. The population of this area is nearly 100 million. This does not, however, imply that all cases in this area attend the Institute. The socioeconomic conditions in the area are poor, and an appreciable number of patients are probably not seen in a hospital but are treated locally by various indigenous systems of medicine, which are prevalent. Data from the Institute are therefore representative of a sample population of southern India.

This chapter reports a retrospective analysis of malignant lymphomas and leukemias seen at the Institute during a 10-year period (1970–1980), with reference to age, sex, histologic pattern, anatomical distribution in relation to histology, and results of treatment. Epidemiologic data in regard to ethnic derivation, religion, urban-rural distribution, socioeconomic status, diet, and heredity are briefly reviewed.

Malignant lymphomas and leukemias constitute 2.7% of all malignancies treated at the Institute (Table 1). In adults, they are among the rarer malignancies, occupying the 10th position. In the pediatric age group (less than 15 years), however, they are the second most common tumor types after retinoblastoma.

TABLE 1. *Frequency of lymphomas and leukemias, Cancer Institute, Madras, (1960–1979)*

Type	Overall	Male	Female
All malignancies	36,416	15,853	20,563
Malignant lymphomas, including Hodgkin's disease	748 (2.05%)	597 (3.8%)	151 (0.7%)
Leukemias	289 (0.8%)	190 (1.2%)	99 (0.5%)

MALIGNANT LYMPHOMAS

Hodgkin's disease (HD) constituted 46.8% and non-Hodgkin's lymphoma (NHL) 53.2% of 487 malignant lymphomas treated during period 1970–1980 (Table 2).

Age and Sex Distribution

The pediatric-adult ratio in HD of 1:2.3 (Table 2) is higher than is usually reported in the Caucasian races (2). The incidence reaches a peak in the five- to 14-year age group and falls off steadily through adolescence and young adult life to a low plateau in middle age and a sharp decline after the age of 55. In NHL, the pediatric-adult ratio is 1:5.4. The peak incidence in NHL is above the age of 40, with a steady rise in incidence with increasing age. The age distribution curves for both HD and NHL differ from those reported from Europe and America (Fig. 1).

In HD, the overall male-female ratio is 4.3:1, but in the pediatric group, the male preponderance rises sharply to 8.7:1. In NHL, the overall sex ratio is similar to that in HD (4.4:1) but does not change in the pediatric group, remaining at 4:1. The male preponderance and the overall low incidence in females in both HD and NHL is obvious (Fig. 1), but the explanation for this unequal distribution is obscure.

Epidemiologic Data

The distribution of lymphomas in the different ethnic groups (Tamil, Andhra, Kerala, Karnataka, and others) within the patient population did not reveal any specific ethnic susceptibility. Similarly, no clear trend was discerned with regard to socioeconomic status (using monthly family income as the base line), urban versus rural lifestyles, religion, or dietary habits. The frequency distribution pattern for both HD and NHL generally followed the population trend; a slightly higher proportion of urban dwellers (41.9% and 46.9% for HD and NHL, respectively, compared with the census figure of 20%) could probably be accounted for by the easier access urban dwellers have to the hospital facilities.

Clinical Stage and Histology

For HD, we used the Ann Arbor staging system (1) and the Rye classification for histopathologic typing (4) (Tables 3 and 4).

TABLE 2. *Age distribution of major types of malignant lymphomas, Cancer Institute, Madras, 1970–1980*

Type	Total (percentage)	Pediatric	Adult	Pediatric-adult ratio
Hodgkin's disease	228 (46.8%)	68	160	1:2.4
Non-Hodgkin's lymphomas	259 (53.2%)	40	219	1:5.5
Total	487	108	379	

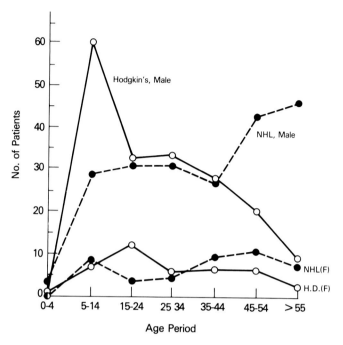

FIG. 1. Age and sex distribution for malignant lymphomas, Cancer Institute, Madras. HD = Hodgkin's disease; NHL = non-Hodgkin's lymphoma; F = female.

TABLE 3. *Stage distribution in Hodgkin's disease,*
Cancer Institute, Madras, 1970–1980

Age group	Total	Stage I	Stage II	Stage III	Stage IV
Pediatric	68	2	23	34	9
Adult	160	11	53	60	36
Total	228	13 (5.7%)	76 (33.3%)	94 (41.2%)	45 (19.7%)

The stage, histologic subtypes, and clinical presentation for the 259 cases of NHL in our series are displayed in Tables 5 to 7. Histologic classification is more complex and difficult for NHL than for HD. Numerous classifications using different nomenclatures are available. We have used the following criteria in our series: Basically, the tumors are either diffuse or nodular. Tumors with small, round, lymphoid cells with round, regular, densely staining nuclei, inconspicuous nucleoli, and minimal cytoplasm are designated as well-differentiated lymphomas. The presence of both a diffuse and a nodular pattern in the same section is not uncommon, and such lymphomas are classified as nodular.

TABLE 4. *Histologic subtypes[a] in Hodgkin's disease, Cancer Institute,*
1970–1980

Age group	Total	LP	NS	MC	LD	Type not available
Pediatric	68	1 (1.5%)	—	40 (58.9%)	23 (33.8%)	4 (5.9%)
Adult	160	8 (5.0%)	4 (2.5%)	71 (44.4%)	66 (41.25)	11 (6.9%)
Total	228	9 (3.9%)	4 (1.8%)	111 (48.7%)	89 (39.0%)	15 (6.6%)

[a]LP = lymphocyte predominance; NS = nodular sclerosis; MC = mixed cellularity; LD = lymphocyte depletion.

Many of the cases designated as diffuse, poorly differentiated lymphomas could be lymphoblastic lymphomas. Because we have not done immunologic typing, it is not possible to say what fraction of these tumors are T-cell malignancies.

Tumors with round or ovoid nuclei, dispersed chromatin with one or two nucleoli, and variable amounts of cytoplasm are designated reticulum cell sarcoma. These are large-cell lymphomas and most probably correspond to what is called diffuse histiocytic lymphoma.

Therapeutic Policy and Results of Treatment

All patients receive a meticulous pretreatment evaluation of stage of disease, including routine hematologic and biochemical evaluation, marrow aspiration and biopsy, careful histologic subtyping, radiologic studies, and pedal lymphography. Staging laparotomy and splenectomy were done routinely in all Hodgkin's cases, unless the patient declined surgery or was unfit on medical grounds. In NHL, staging laparotomy was done only under special circumstances and was not a routine procedure.

Our treatment policy in HD is extended field radiation, cytotoxic therapy, or a combination of the two, depending on stage of disease. Radiation is administered using 4 to 5 MeV X-rays—mantle radiation, mantle and upper abdomen, and inverted Y or inverted hockey stick or whole abdomen (3). Multidrug cytotoxic therapy using cyclophosphamide (Cytoxan®), vincristine sulfate (Oncovin®), procarbazine, and prednisolone is the standard schedule employed. In case of nonresponse, change of schedule to include an anthracycline derivative or vinblastine is attempted (5).

In NHL, initial cytotoxic therapy using cyclophosphamide, vincristine sulfate, and prednisone; cyclophosphamide, cytarabine (Cytosar®), vincristine sulfate, and prednisone; or cyclophosphamide, doxorubicin (adriamycin), vincristine sulfate, prednisone, and bleomycin is used. In most cases, a combination of cytotoxic therapy and radiotherapy is used.

TABLE 5. *Stage distribution of non-Hodgkin's lymphoma, Cancer Institute, Madras*

Age group	Total	Stage I	Stage II	Stage III	Stage IV	Visceral	Intraabdominal	Extranodal
Pediatric	40	2	2	7	17	3	4	5
Adult	219	2	22	85	79	9	14	8
Total	259	4 (1.5%)	24 (9.3%)	92 (35.5%)	96 (37.1%)	12 (4.6%)	18 (6.9%)	13 (5.0%)

TABLE 6. *Histologic subtypes[a] of non-Hodgkin's lymphoma, Cancer Institute, Madras*

Age group	Total	Diffuse			Nodular			RCS	NC
		WD	MD	PD	WD	MD	PD		
Pediatric	40	11	5	13	3	1	—	4	3
Adult	219	54	21	78	7	4	4	33	18
Total	259	65 (25.1%)	26 (10.1%)	91 (35.2%)	10 (3.9%)	5 (1.9%)	4 (1.5%)	37 (14.3%)	21 (8.0%)

[a]WD = well differentiated; MD = moderately differentiated; PD = poorly differentiated; RCS = reticulum cell sarcoma; NC = not classified.

TABLE 7. *Clinical presentation, non-Hodgkin's lymphoma, 259 cases*

Clinical presentation	Total	Adult	Pediatric
Lymphadenopathy but without mediastinal involvement	165 (63.7%)	145 (66.2%)	20 (50.0%)
Lymphadenopathy including mediastinal adenopathy	45 (17.4%)	38 (17.4%)	7 (17.5%)
Mediastinal adenopathy only	6 (2.3%)	5 (2.3%)	1 (2.5%)
Intraabdominal disease	18 (6.9%)	14 (6.4%)	4 (10.0%)
Visceral	12 (4.6%)	9 (4.1%)	3 (7.5%)
Extranodal	13 (5.0%)	8 (3.7%)	5 (12.5%)
Total	259	219	40

TABLE 8. *Three-year survival with no evidence of disease, Hodgkin's disease, Cancer Institute, Madras, 1970–1979*

Age group	Stage I	Stage II	Stage III	Stage IV	Overall
Pediatric	1/1 (100%)	15/16 (93.8%)	16/21 (76.2%)	1/7 (14.3%)	33/45 (73.3%)
Adult	5/5 (100%)	29/35 (82.9%)	23/39 (59.0%)	3/29 (10.3%)	60/108 (55.6%)
Overall	6/6 (100%)	44/51 (86.3%)	39/60 (65.0%)	4/36 (11.1%)	93/153 (60.78%)

TABLE 9. *Five-year survival with no evidence of disease, Hodgkin's disease, Cancer Institute, Madras, 1970–1977*

Age group	Stage I	Stage II	Stage III	Stage IV	Overall
Pediatric	1/1 (100%)	12/13 (92.3%)	11/14 (78.6%)	0/3 (0%)	24/31 (77.4%)
Adult	3/3 (100%)	21/25 (84.0%)	18/26 (69.2%)	2/20 (10.0%)	44/74 (59.5%)
Overall	4/4 (100%)	33/38 (86.8%)	29/40 (72.5%)	2/23 (8.7%)	68/105 (64.76%)

Three- and five-year survival data for HD are tabulated in Tables 8 and 9. Three-year survival data for NHL are shown in Table 10.

DISCUSSION

The clinicopathologic presentation in our HD cases was similar to the Type I disease described by the geographic pathology committee of the International Union

TABLE 10. *Three-year survival with no evidence of disease, non-Hodgkin's lymphoma,*
Cancer Institute, Madras, 1970–1979

Age group	Total	Stage I	Stage II	Stage III	Stage IV	Visceral	Intraabdominal	Extranodal	Overall
Pediatric	32	1/1	—	3/7	0/15	0/3	1/3	0/3	5/32 (15.6%)
Adult	165	1/1	9/15	16/58	3/70	3/7	0/7	4/7	36/165 (21.8%)
Total	197	2/2	9/15	19/65	3/85	3/10	1/10	4/10	41/197 (20.8%)

Against Cancer (2) and which occurs in the poorer economies in South America and Africa. Sixty percent of our cases were Stage III or IV (Table 3), one-third of the patients were children (predominantly male), and 87.7% had an unfavorable histologic subtype (mixed cellularity or lymphocyte depletion) (Table 4). The low frequency of the nodular sclerosis subtype in HD is significant (6).

Biologically, however, our cases differ from Type I HD in that the results of treatment were certainly satisfactory. The overall three- and five-year survival rates with no evidence of disease are 60.78% (93/153) and 64.76% (68/105), respectively (Tables 8 and 9), despite the fact that more than 60% of cases were Stages III or IV. The response to treatment in the pediatric age group was significantly better than that in the adult age group in all stages of disease. Children appear to have a better tolerance to intensive treatment than adults. The critical factors in survival seem to be the stage of disease and the type of treatment administered. The histologic subtype, in our experience, did not really seem to have an impact on survival.

The clinical presentation of NHL (Table 7), in over 50% of cases, was generalized lymphadenopathy. Mediastinal involvement was present in only 17% of cases. Mediastinal adenopathy as the main presentation was low (2.3%). Intraabdominal presentation and visceral lymphomas constituted only 6.9% and 4.6% of all cases, respectively. This is quite different from the experiences in Africa and America. The paucity of abdominal lymphomas, especially in the pediatric group, is striking.

The unfavorable histologic subtypes of NHL in our series far outweigh the favorable types (Table 6). The low incidence of nodular lymphomas (7.3%) is evident and significant. Stages III and IV constituted 72.6% of all cases of NHL (Table 5). The total absence of Burkitt's lymphoma, mycosis fungoides, and Sézary syndrome is notable.

TABLE 11. *Leukemia subtypes,*
Cancer Institute, Madras, 1970–1980

Types[a]	Total	Adult	Pediatric
ALL	111	52	59
	(48.1%)		
AML	53	41	12
	(22.9%)		
CML	65	61	4
	(28.1%)		
CLL	2	2	—
	(0.9%)		
Total	231	156	75

[a]ALL = acute lymphatic leukemia; AML = acute myeloid leukemia, including monocytic and myelomonocytic; CML = chronic myeloid leukemia; CLL = chronic lymphatic leukemia.

The results of treatment in NHL are far from satisfactory. Careful staging procedures, introduction of extended radiation, and multidrug cytotoxic therapy have had little impact on the prognostic outlook for NHL (Table 10).

LEUKEMIAS

Acute leukemias constituted 71% and chronic leukemias 29% of all leukemias. Acute lymphatic leukemia (ALL) is by far the most common type, accounting for 67.7% of all acute leukemias. The frequency of chronic lymphatic leukemia (CLL) is significantly low (0.9%) (Table 11).

The peak age incidence in ALL was five to 10 years. This is at variance with the two- to five-year age peak seen in Caucasian races. The male-female ratio was 2.6:1 and the pediatric-adult ratio was 1.1:1 (Tables 12 and 13). No correlation with regard to region, ethnic factors, socioeconomic status, religion, rural-urban distribution, or dietary habits was noted.

More than 75% of patients with ALL were seen in an advanced stage and in a very poor general condition; 36.9% were moribund and died within 24 hours to a week after admission. Forty-six percent of patients had hepatosplenomegaly. Despite other high-risk parameters, incidence of mediastinal adenopathy was low

TABLE 12. *Age-sex distribution of acute lymphatic leukemia, Cancer Institute, Madras, 1979–1980*

Sex	Total	Adult	Pediatric
Male	80	37	43
Female	31	15	16
Total	111	52	59
		(46.8%)	(53.2%)

TABLE 13. *Age and sex incidence of leukemia, Cancer Institute, Madras*

Age group (years)	Sex		
	Male	Female	Total
0–4	15	4	19
5–10	19	9	28
11–14	9	3	12
15–24	9	3	12
25–34	10	4	14
35–44	10	4	14
45–54	4	—	4
55+	4	4	8
Total	80	31	111

(Table 14). A large percentage of patients were in the high-risk category and presented with a high white cell count, a large number of blasts, gross anemia, and severe thrombocytopenia (Table 15).

Pediatric ALL

The therapeutic policy for pediatric ALL at our Institute consists of remission induction with two drugs (vincristine and steroid) in standard-risk cases and with three drugs (vincristine, adriamycin, and steroid) in high-risk cases. As soon as M1 is achieved, patients are started on L-asparaginase and intrathecal methotrexate followed by cerebral radiation (2,400 rads in two and a half weeks). Maintenance therapy consists of monthly consolidation using the drugs that achieved remission,

TABLE 14. *Clinical presentation, acute lymphatic leukemia, Cancer Institute, Madras*

Presentation	Number of cases
Moribund	41
Lymphadenopathy	48
Lymphadenopathy and mediastinal adenopathy	8
Mediastinal adenopathy only	8
Hepatosplenomegaly	51
Central nervous system disease	8
Testicular involvement	2

TABLE 15. *Hematologic presentation, acute lymphatic leukemia, Cancer Institute, Madras*

Presentation	Number of patients	Percentage
Hemoglobin less than 60%		62.2
Total leukocyte count over 50,000/mm³		37.7
Blasts over 50%		47.2
Platelets less than 50,000/mm³		53.8
White cell count at first presentation		
Less than 3,000/cmm	11	10.4
3–10,000/cmm	23	21.7
10–25,000/cmm	20	18.9
25–50,000/cmm	12	11.3
50–100,000/cmm	11	10.4
Over 100,000/cmm	29	27.4
Blast count at presentation		
Less than 10%	6	5.7
10–25%	24	22.6
25–50%	26	24.5
50–80%	30	28.3
Over 80%	20	18.9

TABLE 16. *Results of treatment of pediatric acute lymphatic leukemia*

Period	Unfit for treatment or declined treatment (number of patients)	Accepted for treatment		
		Total	M1 achieved	M1 not achieved
1970–1975	11	8	3 (37.5%)	5 (62.5%)
1975–1980	16	24	22 (91.7%)	2 (8.3%)
Total	27 (45.8%)	32 (54.2%)	25	7

along with oral 6-mercaptopurine (6MP) and methotrexate. Marrow is monitored carefully, and therapy is continued for 24 to 36 months, whenever possible.

Our therapeutic experience with ALL in children is summarized in Table 16. In 1970–1975, eight patients were accepted for treatment, the average survival was eight to 10 months, and none of the patients is now surviving. Seven of 22 cases in the 1975–1980 period are in remission, ranging from 19 to 68 months. Of these, six are two to five years old and one is a 13-year-old boy. Two children treated in 1977 who were in continuous complete remission relapsed after 43 months and 50 months, respectively, one in the marrow and the other in the marrow and testis. Both have been reinduced and are now in remission.

CONCLUSIONS

The fact that malignant lymphomas and leukemias constitute the second most common malignancy in children made them a subject of study. A dramatic change in the outlook in HD is evident in our treatment results, although the progress in NHL has been slight. In NHL, the high proportion of poor-prognosis histologic types with advanced disease is the problem. In ALL, the challenge is advanced disease occurring in an unfavorable age group. The factors involved in the low frequency of CLL, nodular sclerosis Hodgkin's, and nodular lymphomas need to be studied. Studies on environmental or other etiologic factors and host factors that may be responsible for the differences in incidence of these types in different population groups are likely to be useful.

REFERENCES

1. Carbone, P. P., Kaplan, H. S., Musshoff, K., Smithers, D. W., and Tubiana, M. (1971): Report of the committee on Hodgkin's disease staging. *Cancer Res.*, 31:1860–1861.
2. Correa, P., and O'Conor, G. T. (1973): Geographic pathology of lymphoreticular tumors. Summary of survey from the Geographic Pathology Committee of the International Union Against Cancer. *JNCI*, 50:1609–1617.
3. Kaplan, H. S. (1966): Role of intensive radiotherapy in the management of Hodgkin's disease. *Cancer*, 19:356–367.
4. Lukes, R. J., Craver, L. F., Hall, T. C., Rappaport, H., and Rubin, P. (1966): Report of the Nomenclature Committee. *Cancer Res.*, 26:1311.
5. McElwain, T. J., and Smith, I. E. (1979): Hodgkin's disease: Present concepts and advances in management. In: *Topics in Paediatrics, Vol. 1: Haematology and Oncology*, edited by M. Jones, pp. 84–99. Pitman Medical, London.
6. Shanta, V., Sastri, D. V. L. N., Sagar, T. G., Sasikala, K., and Krishnamurthi, S. (1982): A review of Hodgkin's disease at the Cancer Institute, Madras. *Clin. Oncol.*, 8:5–15.

*Pathogenesis of Leukemias and Lymphomas:
Environmental Influences*, edited by
I. T. Magrath, G. T. O'Conor, and B. Ramot.
Raven Press, New York © 1984.

Spectrum of Lymphoid Malignancies with Particular Reference to Plasma Cell Dyscrasias in Chandigarh, India

*S. Sehgal, *U. Datta, **D. R. Gulati, †A. Grover, and †B. D. Gupta

*Departments of *Immunopathology, **Neurosurgery, and †Radiotherapy, Postgraduate Institute of Medical Education and Research, Chandigarh-160012, India*

Multiple myeloma, a term coined by Rustizky in 1873, is now recognized to be caused by neoplastic proliferation of a single clone of B cells. Its historical evolution and morphological, clinical, and immunological characteristics have been summarized in an excellent monograph by Snapper and Kahn (26). There are, however, inevitable differences in the average incidence, age of onset, sex predilection, clinical manifestations, and immunological subtypes in different geographic areas. This chapter communicates the experience of 200 patients with immunochemically categorized M-component disease in Northern India.

PATIENTS AND METHODS

The study was conducted at the Nehru Hospital, Chandigarh. Nearly 250 patients with plasma cell dyscrasias were encountered over a period of 13 years. The diagnosis of multiple myeloma was confirmed by criteria laid down by Osserman and Takatsuki (22), namely, (a) lytic lesion or severe osteoporosis of bones, (b) plasma cell proliferation in the marrow without an identifiable antigenic stimulus, and (c) elaboration of serum or urinary M components. Patients fulfilling at least two of the three criteria were designated as having myeloma. Immunochemical typing was done in 200 of the 250 patients.

A skeletal survey, bone marrow examination, and/or excision biopsy of the tumor was done in all cases. The sera were screened for M components by paper electrophoresis and immunoelectrophoresis. Urine examination was performed in 170 patients. Urine was routinely concentrated and subjected to electrophoresis and immunoelectrophoresis for confirmation of the light chain class.

RESULTS

It is difficult to give a precise incidence of myelomatosis in this geographic area, because Nehru Hospital is primarily a referral center. The population of Chandigarh in 1968, when the study was started, was barely 150,000. During the next 12 years, it steadily rose to 450,000, while the total number of patients in all age groups coming to the hospital steadily increased from 200,000 to 500,000 per year. In general, 25 to 30% of the patients are referred from the surrounding states of Punjab, Haryana, and Himachal Pradesh because of the better diagnostic and therapeutic facilities available at the Institute. The percentage of acutely ill patients among those referred from outside Chandigarh is generally greater than that among patients coming from Chandigarh itself.

Age and Sex

Of the 200 patients in the study, 136 were males and 64 were females (Fig. 1). The mean age at the time of diagnosis was 51.2 ($\pm$11.4) years. Thirty-five patients were under 40, and 14 with M-component disease were 30 or younger. Ten of those 14 patients could be clearly designated as having myeloma. The youngest was a male 21 years old, admitted to the dermatology service with severe staphylococcal pyoderma. He rapidly developed rib tumors while under observation in the ward. Electrophoresis revealed an M-spike with an IgA-kappa paraprotein. The other four patients under 30 had lymphoreticular malignancies variously diagnosed as immunoblastic lymphoma, alpha chain disease, plasma cell lymphoma, and non-Hodgkin's lymphoma (Table 1).

Presenting Features

Most patients presented with the usual clinical features of anemia, severe bone pains, pathological fractures, fever, bone tumors, or soft tissue masses. Neurological

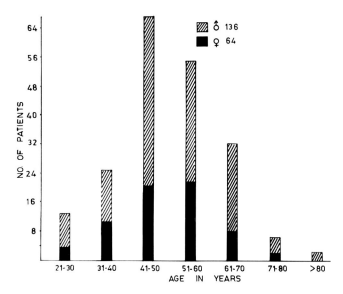

FIG. 1. Age and sex incidence in myelomatosis and other plasma cell dyscrasias, Nehru Hospital, Chandigarh.

TABLE 1. *Plasma cell dyscrasias in 14 patients 30 years old and younger*

No.	Age	Sex	M Comp.	BJ[a,b]	TP gm%[b,c]	Gobulin (g)[b]	Mobility	Type	Symptoms
1	21	M	+++[d]	+	11.00	9	Gamma	A kappa	Pyoderma, pains
2	27	M	+	++	7.61	4	Gamma	Lambda	Bone pains, anemia
3	25	M	+	ND	7.4	3.5	Beta	G kappa	Paraplegia
4	26	M	−[e]	+++	6.49	ND	Gamma	Kappa	Pallor, pains
5	29	F	−	−	7.86	3	—	—	Epilepsy
6	28	F	++	−	ND	ND	Gamma	G kappa	Bone pains
7	28	M	+	++	6.6	3.5	Gamma	Lambda	Lumps, fever
8	30	M	++	−	8.2	4.4	Beta-2	A lambda	Pains, anemia
9	25	M	−	+	6.2	4.2	Alpha-2	Kappa	Paraplegia ?[f] caries spine
10	28	F	++	−	7.7	ND	Gamma	G kappa	Pains, weight loss
Nonmyeloma cases									
11	26	M	++	++	ND	ND	Beta	M kappa	—
12	20	M	+	Alpha chain +	7.5	3.6	Beta-2	Alpha chain	Intestinal obstruction
13	30	M	+++	ND	10.5	ND	Gamma	M kappa	—
14	22	M	++	ND	8.3	ND	Beta	Kappa	—

[a]Bence Jones protein.
[b]ND = not determined.
[c]Total proteins in gm%.
[d]+ to +++ = intensity of M bands.
[e]− = no M bands.
[f] = suspected caries spine but actually myeloma.

manifestations were the main presenting feature in 34 patients. These manifestations included paraplegia caused by extradural spinal tumors in the majority, retroorbital tumor in one, and neuropathy and autonomic disturbances in three (17). Three patients presented with epilepsy. At the time of diagnosis, two did not reveal M components in the serum. One patient with light chain disease presented with an oral plasma cell tumor. One patient presented with tonsillar amyloid. Amyloidosis, however, was the main presenting feature in only eight cases. Other unusual presenting features included proptosis, ear polyp, epistaxis, congestive cardiac failure, and intestinal obstruction. Patients with neurological deficits presented relatively early during the course of the disease, because the strategic site of the tumor produced alarming symptoms. Moderate to severe renal impairment was encountered in 30 patients.

Staging

Most patients reported in an advanced stage of the disease except for those with neurological disturbances, who presented much earlier. Only about 10% of the patients presented in Stage I. Anemia was present in the majority. Total proteins varied from 4.5 to 14.6 gm%. The mean value in IgG myelomatosis was 8.6 gm%, whereas in light chain disease it was 7.5 gm%. Hypoalbuminemia was a fairly constant feature. Thirty-four patients had either hypogammaglobulinemia or a very faint M band. Of these, 30 were patients with light chain disease. Sixty of the M components had beta mobility, four had alpha-2 mobility, and the rest were either fast- or slow-moving gamma bands. The highest erythrocyte sedimentation rate—150 mm in the first hour—was observed in a patient with IgG-kappa myelomatosis with a massive M component. M components of more than 7 and 5 g were present in 20% of patients with IgG and 30% of patients with IgA myelomatosis, respectively. In spite of the advanced disease encountered in this series, hypercalcemia was not a conspicuous feature. In 118 of the 175 urine samples examined (67%), Bence Jones proteins were positive.

Immunochemical Typing

The immunological heterogeneity of M components in the 200 patients is depicted in Table 2 and compared with findings in other published series. In our cases, IgG was detected in 44% of the patients, light chain disease in 25%, and IgA in 19.5%. In addition, eight cases had IgM paraprotein (one with Waldenström's syndrome), and seven had IgD M component.

Next to IgG myelomatosis, light chain disease formed the largest group. The mean age of patients with light chain disease was not statistically different from the average age of other patients. One patient with light chain disease presented with an ear polyp that was reported as a plasmacytoma, and urine examination revealed renal damage with heavy Bence Jones proteinuria (Figs. 2 and 3); she died of pulmonary mucormycosis and renal failure.

TABLE 2. *Percentage of various M components in published series*

Series	Total no.	G	A	M	BJ[a]	D	Nonsecretory
Hobbs et al. (14)	212	53	25	?	19	1	—
Brackenridge and Lynch (8)	202	58	29	?	12	1.2	—
Belpomme et al. (5)	102	59	21	—	10	1	7
Bachmann (3)	554	57.4	19.6	17	3.2	0.5	1
Zawadzki and Edwards (32)	200	53	28	3.5	12.5	?	?
Osserman and Takatsuki (22)	262	54	23	?	22	—	2
Present chapter[b]	200	44	19.5	3.5	25	3.5	1

[a]Bence Jones protein.
[b]Alpha chain disease = 3, Waldenstrom's disease = 1, No M components = 2.

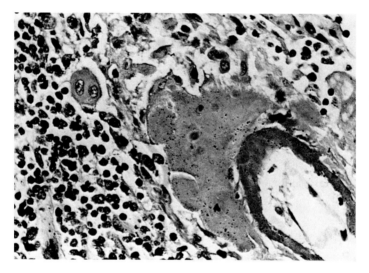

FIG. 2. Aural polyp from a patient with light chain disease. Histology revealed a plasma cell tumor with massive amyloid deposits (haematoxylin and eosin stain).

The details of patients with IgD myelomatosis are given in Table 3. One patient presented with a large bone tumor suspected of being an osteogenic sarcoma. It was not possible initially to screen all patients with light chain disease for IgD, and it is likely that a few cases were missed. The mean age of patients with IgD myelomatosis was 54 years, and all of six cases tested for Bence Jones proteins were positive. Three had frank amyloidosis. The M components, as expected, were only modest ones and moved faster than in cases with IgG or IgM disease.

Follow-up was poor on the whole—only a few of the better educated patients could be followed for long periods. All of the six patients that survived for five to nine years had IgG paraproteins without Bence Jones proteins. One patient, who

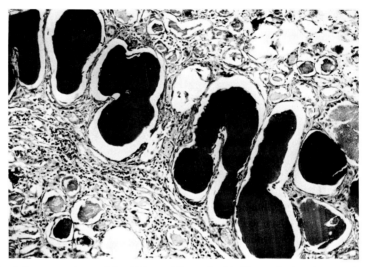

FIG. 3. Autopsy specimen of the kidney of the patient in Figure 2, showing massive Bence Jones protein casts.

TABLE 3. *Details of seven patients with IgD myelomatosis*

Age	Sex	M comp.[a]	BJ[b]	Mobility	TP[c] (g/m%)	Symptoms	Type
50	M	+ + [h]	+ + +	Gamma	8.5	Bone tumor	D kappa
50	M	+	+ +	Beta	7.7	Pains, fever, anemia	D lambda
51	M	+	+	Beta	7.5	CHF[d], amyloid	D kappa
60	F	+	+ +	Beta	7.7	Paraplegia, CRF[e], anemia	D lambda
58	M	− [i]	+ +	Alpha-2	6.37	Amyloid disease	D lambda
58	F	+ + +	+	Gamma	5.6	Epistaxia, pain, ESR[f] 72	D lambda
53	M	+ + +	ND[g]	Gamma	7.5	—	D lambda
Summary	5:2	5/6	6/6		7.3		2K, 5L

[a]Monoclonal peak on serum protein electrophoresis.
[b]Bence Jones protein.
[c]Total protein.
[d]Congestive heart failure.
[e]Congestive renal failure.
[f]Erythrocyte sedimentation rate.
[g]Not determined.
[h]+ to + + + = intensity of M bands.
[i]− = no M band.

has now been followed for eight years, showed Bence Jones escape phenomenon after eight years of therapy. One of the two patients with nonsecretory myeloma started passing lambda light chains before death. One patient with alpha chain disease and a history of severe malabsorption presented with intestinal obstruction on two occasions. The morphology of the first resected specimen showed a classical plasma cell infiltration (Fig. 4), whereas the second specimen showed immuno-blastic proliferation originally interpreted as Hodgkin's disease (Fig. 5). He reported to the hospital three years later with a cervical lymph node showing unclassifiable lymphoma (Fig. 6).

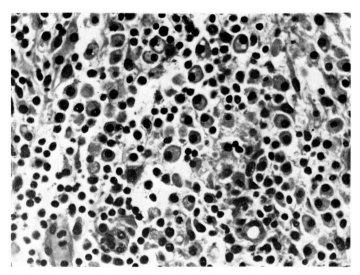

FIG. 4. Typical plasma cell proliferation in the lamina propria of a patient with alpha chain disease.

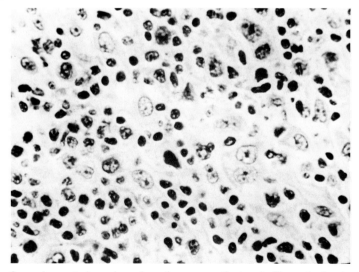

FIG. 5. Second resected specimen from the same patient as in Figure 4, showing immuno-blastic proliferation.

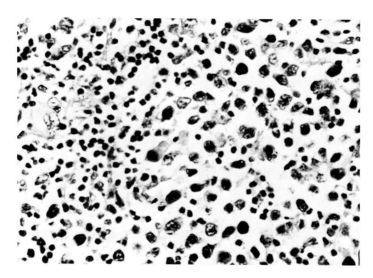

FIG. 6. Cervical lymph node neoplasia in the same patient as in Figures 4 and 5 after two years, showing a rather bizarre morphology not easily categorized (haematoxylin and eosin stain).

DISCUSSION

This study shows a marked preponderance of males with plasma cell dyscrasias. The disease occurs at a younger age in India. Belpomme et al. (5) reported less than 9% of patients below 50 years old, and Osby et al. (21) reported a figure of 8%. In the present series, 35 patients were below 40 years of age, and nearly half the patients were 50 years old or younger. The SEER Registry figures for 1973 to 1977 from the United States (31) indicate that myeloma is rare below 40 years; the incidence is only 0.006% (17 in 2,582), compared to 17.5% (35 in 200) in the present series. This finding is clearly not simply the result of a different age structure in the Indian population. Banerjee et al. (4) have observed that intracranial tumors, particularly gliomas, also occur a decade earlier in India than reported from the West.

The incidence of light chain disease and IgD M components is higher in our cases than in most reported series. The mean normal levels of IgD in Indians are also high. The mean level of total proteins (8.5 g) in this series is lower than the figures reported in the literature. Hart et al. (13) observed the highest total serum protein concentrations of 18, 19.8, and 12.6 g/100 ml in cases of IgG, IgA, and IgM monoclonal gammopathies, respectively. In their series, monoclonal peaks were more often encountered when the levels of total proteins exceeded 11 g/100 ml.

Hypercalcemia, in spite of the advanced stage of the disease, was never a striking feature, which might be attributable to low calcium reserve or tubular dysfunction because of a high incidence of Bence Jones proteinuria. The other clinical presentations do not differ significantly from those reported from the West except that the spinal lesions are quite frequent.

OTHER LYMPHOMAS

In all, 18,000 patients with various malignant tumors were treated at the radiotherapy unit in Chandigarh from 1971 to 1982. Malignant lymphoma was diagnosed in 815 patients (4.44%).

A review and analysis of 742 of these cases revealed Hodgkin's disease in 276 (37%). There was a marked male preponderance; females accounted for barely 16% of the 276 patients. Forty-five patients (16.3%) were below 10 years of age, and 15 patients were five years old or younger. The details of age distribution are depicted in Fig. 7.

In an earlier study (July 1964 to December 1972), Vashisht and Aikat (30) also reported a male-female ratio of 6:1 in 119 patients with Hodgkin's lymphoma (HL). These authors observed a bimodal age distribution, with the first peak between 10 and 20 years and a second peak between 40 and 50 years. Ten percent of the patients were less than 10 years old, and no patient was younger than five years old. In a more recent study, however, Goswami and Banerjee (11) documented 72 patients with HL below the age of 15 years; the youngest in their series was a three-year-old child. Such a shift in age distribution could partly be the result of the special therapeutic expertise available in the current decade, yet a genuine shift to the left cannot be ruled out. The histological data of the two published series, however,

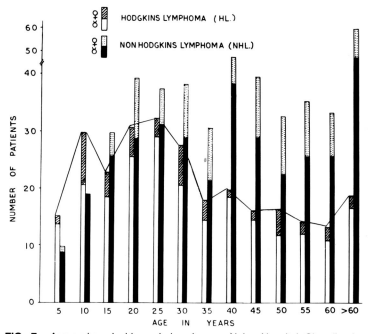

FIG. 7. Age and sex incidence in lymphomas, Nehru Hospital, Chandigarh.

show a fair degree of uniformity (Table 4). In children, mixed cellularity and lymphocyte depletion were the histological subtypes in 65% of the cases, whereas nodular sclerosis was the diagnosis in only 11% of the patients. Thus, the nodular sclerosing variety of Hodgkin's disease is infrequent in India, and mixed cellularity and lymphocyte depletion types form the bulk of HL subtypes in both adults and children.

Extranodal HL was recored in 8 to 10% of the patients; the gastrointestinal tract was most frequently involved. Of 10 cases reported by Vashisht and Aikat (29), seven were in the gastrointestinal tract, two in the lungs, and one in the bone. The incidence of extranodal non-Hodgkin's lymphoma (NHL) is higher than that of extranodal HL. Cf 70 patients with extranodal lymphomas studied by Vashisht and Aikat (29), 57 (81.4%) were NHL and the remaining 13 (18.6%) were HL. In the small intestine, extranodal lymphomas constituted 42% of all malignancies, with a mean age of 28 years and a male-female ratio of 7:2. Thirty percent of all extranodal lymphomas originated in the gastrointestinal tract. Poorly differentiated tumors (e.g., lymphocyte depletion type of HL, histiocytic lymphomas, or "stem cell lymphomas") originated more frequently at extranodal sites (29).

The age and sex distribution of NHL is depicted in Figure 7. In most published series from India, data on NHL are based on old classifications, and no large-scale studies identifying the immunological cell types (T cells, B cells, or histiocytes) are available at the moment. Burkitt's lymphoma is diagnosed approximately once every year (2). Unfortunately, no Epstein-Barr virus studies have been conducted.

LEUKEMIAS

Several large-scale studies of leukemias in India have been published (Table 5). In one study (18), leukemias accounted for 7.5% of all malignancies. Males are affected twice as frequently as females. In all these studies, chronic myeloid leukemia (CML) is the most common of all leukemias, accounting for 31 to 83% of all cases, in contrast to the figures reported from the United States, where CML is

TABLE 4. *Histological subtypes[a] in Hodgkin's disease*

Authors	LP (%)	MC (%)	LD (%)	NS (%)	Total number
Keller et al. (15)	4	38	5	53	176
Gough (12)	20	29	36	15	96
Correa and O'Conor (10)	16	50	22	12	102
Selzer et al. (25)	14	35	25	26	122
Vashisht and Aikat (30)[d]	4	54	27	15	100
Goswami and Banerjee (11)[b,d]	12.5	48.6	16.7	11.1[c]	72
Lennert and Mohn (19)	27.8	30.5	7.0	34.7	72

[a]LP = lymphocyte predominance, MC = mixed cellularity, LD = lymphocyte depletion, NS = nodular sclerosis.
[b] Patients in this study were less than 15 years old.
[c] Rest unclassifiable.
[d] Indian series.

TABLE 5. *Relative frequency of various leukemias[a] in different series*

Authors	Total no. of cases	ALL (%)	AML (%)	CML (%)	CLL (%)
Boggs et al. (7) (United States)	565	31.5	25.5	19.5	23.5
Kushwaha et al. (18) (Lucknow)	392	8.1	31.6	56.1	4.2
Vasavada et el. (28) (Indore)	100	3.0	8.0	82.0	7.0
Chatterjee et al. (9) (Calcutta)	544	20.2	32.5	35.9	5.5
Bhatia et al. (6) (Uttar Pradesh)	258	13.0		83.0	4.0
Talwalkar (27) (Bombay)	316	10.0	4.6	68.9	14.2
Menzes and Malik (20) (Goa)	66	51.5	7.5	34.8	6.0
Krishna Dass (16) (Kerala)	543	45.4	11.3	31.8	11.5
Advani et al. (1) (Lucknow)	1126	30	13	40	9
Prakash et al. (23) (Pondicherry)	278	35.0	29.4	30.8	3.2
Rani et al. (24) (Delhi)	490	19.3	29.7	45.4	6

[a]ALL = acute lymphatic leukemia; AML = acute myeloid leukemia; CML = chronic myeloid leukemia; CLL = chronic lymphatic leukemia.

much less frequent. The relative frequency of acute lymphatic leukemia shows a wide regional variation. Figures from the southwest regions are generally higher (45 to 50%) than those from the north central region (3 to 8.1%). The precise reason for such differences is not clear, and further studies are required. Chronic lymphatic leukemia is not unknown but is much less frequent than in the West; it ranges from 3.2 to 14% of all leukemias.

Kushwaha et al. (18) have reported a maximum incidence of leukemia between February and August. Advani et al. (1) documented that 80% of all cases of acute lymphoblastic leukemia occur in children under the age of 10 years.

Clearly a better characterization of the types of leukemia in the population served by the Nehru Hospital in Chandigarh would be of interest for comparison with other areas in India and abroad and would permit observations of changes over time.

ACKNOWLEDGMENTS

We are grateful to Neelam Pasricha for technical assistance, to the many physicians and surgeons who allowed us access to their patients, and to Professor B. N. Datta, Chairman of the Department of Pathology, for his invaluable help.

REFERENCES

1. Advani, S. H., Jussawalla, D. J., Nagaraj, D., and Gangadharan, P. (1979): Leukemias at Lucknow: A study of 200 cases. *Indian J. Cancer*, 16:8–17.
2. Aikat, B. K., Pathak, I. C., and Dutta, B. N. (1973): Burkitt's lymphoma. *Indian J. Cancer*, 3:128–142.
3. Bachmann, R. (1965): The diagnostic significance of the serum concentration of pathological proteins (M-components). *Acta Med. Scand.*, 198:801–808.
4. Banerjee, A. K., Samanta, H. K., and Aikat, B. K. (1972): Intracranial space occupying lesions— An analysis of 200 cases. *Indian J. Pathol. Bacteriol.*, 15:83–92.
5. Belpomme, D., Simon, F., Pouillart, P., Amor, B., Feuilhade de Chauvin, F., Belpomme, A., Menkes, C., Delrieu, A., Depierre, R., Le Mevel, B., Serrou, B., Fries, D., Delbarre, F., and

Mathé, G. (1978): Prognostic factors and treatment of multiple myeloma: Interest of a cyclic sequential chemohormonotherapy combining cyclophosphamide, melphalan, and prednisone. *Recent Results Cancer Res.*, 65:28–40.

6. Bhatia, B. B., Paul, D., and Singh, D. (1957): Life history of leukaemia in the state of Uttar Pradesh. *J. Assoc. Physicians India*, 5:171–175.

7. Boggs, D. R., Wintrobe, M. M., and Cartwright, G. E. (1962): The acute leukemias: Analysis of 322 cases and review of the literature. *Medicine*, 41:163–225.

8. Brackenridge, C. J., and Lynch, W. J. (1967): Some observations on myeloma and macroglobulinemia. *Med. J. Aust.*, 54:493.

9. Chatterjee, J. B., Ghosh, S., and Ray, R. N. (1962): Incidence of leukaemia—An analysis of 544 cases studied in Calcutta. *J. Assoc. Physicians India*, 10:673–676.

10. Correa, P., and O'Conor, G. T. (1971): Epidemiologic patterns of Hodkin's disease. *Int. J. Cancer*, 8:192–201.

11. Goswami, K. C., and Banerjee, C. K. (1982): Hodgkin's disease in children: histopathological classification in relation to age and sex. *Indian J. Cancer*, 19:24–27.

12. Gough, J. (1970): Hodgkin's diseases: A correlation of histopathology with survival. *Int. J. Cancer*, 5:273–281.

13. Hart, J. S., Lawrence, M. C., Ritzmann, S. E., and Levin, W. C. (1965): II. Hyper- and hypoproteinemias. 1. Hyperproteinemia. Correlation of elevated total serum protein values and their responsible globulin fractions with various polyclonal and monoclonal gammopathies. A study of 173 sera. *Tex. Rep. Biol. Med.*, 23:445–457.

14. Hobbs, J. R., Slot, G. M. J., Campbell, C. H., Clein, G. P., Scott, J. T., Crowther, D., and Swan, H. T. (1966): Six cases of gamma-D myelomatosis. *Lancet*, 2:614–661.

15. Keller, A. R., Kaplan, H. S., Lukes, R. J., and Rappaport, H. (1968): Correlation of histopathology with other prognostic indications in Hodgkin's disease. *Cancer*, 22:487–499.

16. Krishna Dass, K. V., Aboobacker, C. M., and Omana, M. (1974): Clinical presentation of leukemia in children in South Kerala. *Indian Pediatr.*, 11:431–438.

17. Kumar, B. R., Chopra, J. S., Sapru, R. P., Chugh, K. S., and Sehgal, S. (1977): Uncommon neurological manifestations of multiple myeloma. *Neurol. India*, 25:170–175.

18. Kushwaha, M. R. S., Bagchi, M., and Mehrotra, R. M. L. (1978): Leukaemias at Lucknow—A study of 200 cases. *Indian J. Cancer*, 15:28–34.

19. Lennert, K, and Mohn, N. (1974): Histological classification: Histologische Klassifizierung und Vorkommen des M. Hodgkin. *Internist*, 15:57–65.

20. Menzes, S., and Malik, G. B. (1977): Myeloma proteins and antibodies. *Ind. J. Path. Microb.*, 20:83–89.

21. Ösby, E., Carlmark, B., and Reizenstein, P. (1978): Staging of myeloma. A preliminary study of staging factors and treatment in different stages. *Recent Results Cancer Res.*, 65:21–27.

22. Osserman, E. F., and Takatsuki, K. (1963): Plasma cell myeloma: Gamma globulin synthesis and structure. A review of biochemical and clinical data, with the description of a newly-recognized and related syndrome, "$H^{\gamma-2}$-chain (Franklin's) disease." *Medicine*, 42:357–384.

23. Prakash, S., Ramamurthi, Gopalan, R., and Aurora, A. L. (1981): Leukemias at Pondicherry. *Indian J. Cancer*, 18:1–6.

24. Rani, S., Beohar, P. C., Mohanti, T. K., and Mathur, M. D. (1982): Leukemic pattern in Delhi—A ten year study of 490 cases. *Indian J. Cancer*, 19:81–86.

25. Selzer, G., Kahn, L. B., and Sealy, R. (1972): Hodgkin's disease: clinicopathological study of 122 patients. *Cancer*, 29:1090–1100.

26. Snapper, T., and Kahn, A., editors (1971): *Myelomatosis: Fundamentals and Clinical Features.* S. Karger, Basel.

27. Talwalkar, G. V. (1961): Leukaemia incidence in 316 cases. *J. Assoc. Physicians India*, 9:351–358.

28. Vasavada, P. S., Akbar, A., and Mukherjee, D. P. (1962): Clinical studies in leukaemia. A review of 100 cases in symposium in leukaemia. *J. Assoc. Physicians India*, 10:677–682.

29. Vashisht, S., and Aikat, B. K. (1973): Extranodal malignant lymphomas. *Indian J. Pathol. Bacteriol.*, 17:9–26.

30. Vashisht, S., and Aikat, B. K. (1973): Hodgkin's disease—retrospective study of 119 cases. *Indian J. Cancer*, 10:263–279.

31. Young, J. L., Jr., Percy, C. L., and Asire, A. J., editors (1981): *Surveillance, Epidemiology, and End Results: Incidence and Mortality Data, 1973–1977*. Nat. Cancer Inst. Monogr. 57, National Cancer Institute, Bethesda, MD.
32. Zawadzki, Z. A., and Edwards, G. A. (1967): M-components in immunoproliferative disorders. Electrophoretic and immunologic analysis of 200 cases. *Am. J. Clin. Pathol.*, 48:418–430.

*Pathogenesis of Leukemias and Lymphomas:
Environmental Influences*, edited by
I. T. Magrath, G. T. O'Conor, and B. Ramot.
Raven Press, New York © 1984.

A Survey of Lymphoid Malignancies at University Hospital, Kuala Lumpur, Malaysia

*J. Bosco, **R. Cherian, †H. P. Lin, and ‡T. Pang

*Departments of *Medicine, **Pathology, †Paediatrics, and ‡Medical Microbiology, University Hospital, University of Malaya, Kuala Lumpur, Malaysia*

Epidemiological studies of leukemias and lymphomas show differences in the incidence of different subtypes among various racial and socioeconomic groups. Demographically, Malaysia is a middle-income country with a multiracial population made up of three ethnic groups, Malays (55%), Chinese (35%), and Indians (10%). Therefore, it is particularly suitable for such studies. We present here a preliminary, descriptive epidemiological survey of lymphoid malignancies at the University Hospital, Kuala Lumpur, since January 1980.

METHODS

The study population consisted of patients with either acute lymphoblastic leukemia (ALL) or malignant lymphoma seen at the University Hospital, a major referral center. Because a hospital-based study such as this may be biased by selective use of hospital services by a particular race, all cases discharged from the hospital during 1980, 1981, and early 1982 (for all diagnoses, including lymphoid malignancies), were analyzed (Table 1) through a computer-based medical record system. The total number of patients with hematological malignancies was obtained similarly (Table 2).

Bone marrow and histopathological slides with diagnosis of ALL or malignant lymphoma over the study period were reviewed. The non-Hodgkin's lymphomas were classified according to the Rappaport classification. Cells from the bone marrow and peripheral blood of patients with ALL were also characterized for different cell surface antigen expression (Table 3).

RESULTS

Approximately 60.1% of the 283 hematological malignancies seen during the study period were of lymphoid origin. The male-female ratio for all lymphoid malignancies was 1.6:1 and the leukemia-lymphoma ratio was approximately 2:1. The highest fre-

TABLE 1. *Lymphoid neoplasms[a] by ethnic group compared with all patients, University Hospital, Kuala Lumpur, 1980–Dec. 1981*

Ethnic group	All patients		Patients with lymphoid neoplasms	
	Number	Percentage	Number	Percentage
Malays	17,162	29.9	34	27.6
Chinese	23,620	41.2	69	56.2
Indians[b]	15,930	27.8	18	14.6
Others[c]	654	1.1	2	1.6
Total	57,366	100	123	100

[a]Lymphoid neoplasms include all acute lymphoblastic leukemias, non-Hodgkin's lymphomas, and Hodgkin's lymphomas but exclude multiple myelomas.

[b]Includes Sri Lankans and Pakistanis.

[c]Includes Caucasians, Eurasians, Arabs, Japanese, and Aborigines of Malaysia.

TABLE 2. *Hematological malignancies diagnosed in all age and ethnic groups, University Hospital, Kuala Lumpur, January 1980 to May 1982*

Diagnosis	No. cases
Acute lymphoblastic leukemia	97
Acute myeloblastic leukemia	18
Acute myelomonocytic leukemia	19
Acute undifferentiated leukemia	5
Acute promyelocytic leukemia	6
Erythroleukemia	4
Non-Hodgkin's lymphoma	
Diffuse[a]	47
Nodular	2
Hodgkin's lymphoma	22
Malignant histiocytosis	10
Multiple myeloma	22
Chronic myeloid leukemia	23
Myeloproliferative disorders[b]	7
Chronic lymphocytic leukemia	1
Total	283

[a]Includes Burkitt-like lymphomas and one case of mycosis fungoides.

[b]Includes myelofibrosis and polycythemia rubra vera.

quency of these malignancies occurred among the Chinese (56.2%), perhaps a slightly higher percentage in relation to their hospital utilization rate (41.2%).

Non-Hodgkin's Lymphoma

Only 4.1% of non-Hodgkin's lymphomas were of the nodular variety. The large majority (approximately 90%) of the diffuse lymphomas were of the histiocytic or

TABLE 3. *Characterization of cell surface markers in acute lymphoblastic leukemia and lymphoma-leukemias*

Study	No. patients tested	Surface marker expression			
		cALL	T	B	Null
1[a]	18	NT[c]	6	—	12
2[b]	14	7	4	—	3
Total	32	7	10	—	15

[a]Limited study carried out before 1982. Only two markers were investigated: sheep erythrocyte (E) rosettes and surface membrane immunoglobulin.
[b]Study begun in 1982 as part of the International ALL Subgroup Survey (coordinated by Dr. M. F. Greaves, Imperial Cancer Institute, London). Cells were analyzed for E rosettes, TdT, and 12 other surface markers using monoclonal antibodies and immunofluorescent visualization.
[c]Not tested.

poorly differentiated type. There were three cases of Burkitt-like lymphoma and only one case of chronic lymphocytic leukemia (CLL). There was no strong association with any particular age, sex, or racial group.

Acute Lymphoblastic Leukemia

Ninety-seven cases of ALL were seen in the same period. Peak frequency was at three years of age (Fig. 1). The male-female ratio was 1.9:1. There was no difference among the three racial groups. Immunological studies carried out in 1980 and 1981 indicated a majority of null ALL (non-T, non-B, the presence or absence of common ALL antigen being unconfirmed), although several cases of T-cell lymphoma-leukemia were detected in older children and adolescents, 90% of them male, with clinical features of a mediastinal mass, hepatosplenomegaly, lymphadenopathy, and high white cell count. Preliminary data from a more thorough study begun in 1982 have so far indicated 50% cALL, 29% T-ALL, and 21% null ALL. Overall, 31% of the cases typed were in the T-cell category (Table 3).

DISCUSSION

The leukemia-lymphoma ratio of 2:1 in this study is slightly below that in industrialized or developed countries but above that in some low-income countries, and is perhaps consistent with the incidence in middle-income countries. It would be interesting to compare the frequency of these disease groups over the next 10 years in a specific area within the country marked for development, such as the eastern states of Malaysia, where marked socioeconomic changes are anticipated. Such a comparison might be useful in testing the hypothesis that socioeconomic changes alter the leukemia-lymphoma ratio (3).

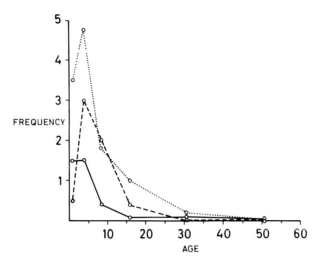

FIG. 1. Frequency polygon of age distribution in acute lymphoblastic leukemia, University Hospital, Kuala Lumpur. Dotted line, Chinese; dashed line, Malay; solid line, Indian. Age given in years.

The nonexistence of nodular or follicular lymphomas in the spectrum of non-Hodgkin's lymphomas is an intriguing feature of this study. The prevalence of diffuse-type lymphomas was also noted in the majority of patients with stage I disease as well as among sections of the community with great concern for health care. An extremely low incidence of CLL has been observed before in Singapore, a neighboring country to Malaysia (5). A survey within the University Hospital shows only four cases of CLL in the last 14 years.

Our study also shows the peak incidence of ALL between two and five years of age. This is similar to that found in a number of countries, including, more recently, Japan and China (1,2). A retrospective analysis to see if there has been any change in this age peak incidence would be interesting, because it has been suggested that this feature may refect socioeconomic status and industrial development. The apparently increased incidence of T-ALL warrants further and more detailed studies, because it has been postulated that a group of T-cell malignancies may be related to geographical and environmental factors (4) and that increased incidence of T-cell disease may also be related to socioeconomic status (3).

In summary, this preliminary survey of lymphoid malignancies in a Malaysian teaching hospital shows a leukemia-lymphoma ratio of 2:1, a high proportion of T-ALL, and a virtual absence of nodular lymphomas and CLL. Further epidemiological, immunological, biochemical, and genetic studies are indicated.

ACKNOWLEDGMENTS

Our sincere thanks to Dr. John Arokiasamy of the Department of Social and Preventive Medicine, University of Malaya, for his help and guidance, and to Mrs.

F. S. Wong for typing the manuscript. We are also indebted to Dr. M. F. Greaves, Coordinator of the International ALL Subgroup Survey, for providing the reagents for immunological characterization.

REFERENCES

1. Kawashima, K., Suzuki, H., Yamada, K., Kato, Y., Watanabe, E., Morishima, Y., Takeyama, H., and Kobayashi, M. (1980): Long-term survival in acute leukemia in Japan. A study of 304 cases. *Cancer*, 45:2181–2187.
2. Li, F. P., Jin, F., Tu, C. T., and Gao, Y. (1980): Incidence of childhood leukaemia in Shanghai. *Int. J. Cancer*, 25:701–703.
3. Ramot, B., and Magrath, I. (1982): Hypothesis: The environment is a major determinant of the immunological sub-type of lymphoma and acute lymphoblastic leukaemia in children. *Br. J. Haematol.*, 50:183–189.
4. Uchiyama, T., Yodoi, J., Sagawa, K., Takatsuki, K., and Uchino, H. (1977): Adult T-cell leukemia: Clinical and hematological features of 16 cases. *Blood*, 50:481–492.
5. Wells, R., and Lau, K. S. (1960): Incidence of leukaemia in Singapore, and rarity of chronic lymphocytic leukaemia in Chinese. *Br. Med. J.*, 1:759–763.

Pathogenesis of Leukemias and Lymphomas:
Environmental Influences, edited by
I. T. Magrath, G. T. O'Conor, and B. Ramot.
Raven Press, New York © 1984.

Lymphoid Neoplasia in Singapore

R. Suri, K. F. Lui, I. Sng, C. J. Oon, S. H. Chan, L. Chan,
Y. K. Kueh, Y. O. Tan, C. L. Tan, and Y. W. Ong

*University Department of Medicine, National University of Singapore and
Singapore General Hospital, Singapore 0316*

Singapore has an urban population of 2.41 million people, with a mixed, mainly immigrant, racial structure. Chinese make up 76.9% of the population, followed by Malays (14.6%), Indians (6.4%), and others (2.1%) (5). Malignant lymphoproliferative diseases in Singapore have not been investigated using immunological markers, but we began such a study in early 1981. The objective of this study was to determine the types of lymphoid neoplasia seen in Singapore and to make comparisons with the patterns seen in other parts of the world. We also studied racial and intrapopulation socioeconomic differences to identify special differences, if any. Earlier studies were limited to analysis of clinical data, morphology, and some cytochemistry. More recently, immunological subtyping (T- and B-cell surface markers) and terminal deoxynucleotidyl transferase estimation were introduced. We give here the preliminary results of the ongoing survey for 29 patients with various malignant lymphoproliferative diseases.

PATIENTS, MATERIALS, AND METHODS

Patients with malignant lymphoproliferative disease were all referred to the Singapore General Hospital, where the present study was undertaken. Detailed histories were taken, and all patients were carefully assessed for extent of disease. The basic work-up consisted of complete blood counts, liver function tests, serum uric acid, serum lactate dehydrogenase, renal function tests, serum calcium, serum phosphate, chest X-ray, and a radioisotope (Tc^{99}) liver scan. All patients had bone marrow aspiration and a trephine marrow biospy. In addition to standard May-Grünwald Giemsa staining of the films, special stains (periodic acid-Schiff, Sudan black, peroxidase, non-specific esterases, and acid phosphatase) were used as indicated. In the absence of bone marrow involvement or extranodal disease, the work-up included lymphangiogram or computerized axial tomography abdominal scans and, if indicated, exploratory laparotomy. Staging followed the recommendations of the 1971 Ann Arbor Conference.

Lymph Nodes

Paraffin sections of lymph nodes (stained with hematoxylin and eosin) were given a detailed histological examination and lymphomas were classified according to the modified Rappaport classification (1975) (3,8).

Peripheral Blood Mononuclear Cells

Cell surface marker studies of the neoplastic cells were done for patients with a leukemic phase of disease. Mononuclear cell suspensions from peripheral blood were isolated from these patients by density gradient sedimentation using Ficoll-Hypaque (2). The T-cell and B-cell nature of the cells was assessed by their ability to form rosettes with sheep red blood cells (E rosettes) and by the presence of surface immunoglobulin (sIg), respectively (12). The assessment of the ability of the cells to form E rosettes was confirmed using monoclonal antibody (OKT 3, PAN; Ortho). A microlymphocytotoxicity tray containing 10 different monoclonal antibodies against various cell surface antigens (e.g., 1a, T lymphocyte, B cell, T-ALL) was also used (1).

Socioeconomic Grouping

The patients were grouped into socioeconomic levels based largely on occupation: upper socioeconomic level (professionals and business managers), middle level (skilled workers), and lower level (unskilled workers).

RESULTS

Twenty-nine patients with malignant lymphoproliferative disease have been studied. Their ages range from four years to 67 years. Four patients had acute lymphoblastic leukemia (ALL), three of the "null" cell type and one of the T-cell type. Twenty-four patients had non-Hodgkin's lymphoma (NHL) (five nodular and 19 diffuse). Three patients had the typical cellular detail on lymph node biopsy of lymphoblastic lymphoma. One patient had chronic lymphocytic leukemia (CLL) (B-cell type). The relevant data on these patients are displayed in Tables 1 to 3.

The results showed no apparent racial preponderance in this small group. Twenty patients were from the lower socioeconomic group, five from the middle, and four from the upper.

PREVIOUS STUDIES

Wells and Lau (14) analyzed 168 Singapore Chinese patients with leukemia seen between the years 1948 and 1958. Only three patients (2%) with CLL were seen.

During 1960–1969, 377 malignant lymphomas were diagnosed histologically in Singapore (10). Reticulum cell sarcoma (35.8% of all lymphomas) was the most common type, followed by lymphosarcoma (33.6%) and then Hodgkin's disease (20.4%). Burkitt's lymphoma was rarely seen (2.7%). The age-standardized rates

TABLE 1. *Data on patients with non-Hodgkin's lymphoma, Singapore General Hospital*

Disease state[a]	No. patients	Age range (years)	Race[b]	Leukemic phase[c]	Gut involvement[c]	Clinical features/immunology
Nodular (follicular)						
Lymphocytic PD	3	37–64	Chin (1), Mal (1), Oth (1)	0	+ (1)	
Mixed cellularity	2	54, 65	Chin (2)	0	+ (1)	
Large-cell ("histiocytic")	0	—	—	—	—	
Diffuse						
Lymphocytic WD	2	34, 58	Chin (2)	0	+ (1)	LP[d]/B cell (strong surface Ig)
Intermediate	0	—	—	—	—	
PD	3	22–60	Chin (2), Ind (1)	+ (2)	+ (1)	
Mixed cellularity	1	55	Chin	0	0	
Large-cell ("histiocytic")	6	23–57	Chin (6)	+ (1)	+ (2)	LP/B cell (strong surface Ig); heavy chain disease (1)
Lymphoblastic	3	20–50	Chin (2), Mal (1)	+ (2)	0	Typical cellular detail; irregular convoluted nuclei, fine chromatin, one to three nucleoli, high mitotic index
Undifferentiated						
Burkitt's	0	—	—	—	—	
Non-Burkitt's	1	31	Chin	0	+ (1)	
Miscellaneous						
Lennert's	1	56	Chin	0	0	Oropharynx involved
Sézary	1	63	Chin	+	0	T cells 49%, B cells 18%; EM[e]: cerebriform cells; skin biopsy: Pautrier's abscesses +
Cutaneous "T" cell	1	47	Chin	+	0	T cells 74%, B cells 5%; monoclonal anti-T-positive; (PAN); lymphoid cells cleaved

[a]PD = poorly differentiated, WD = well differentiated.
[b]Chin = Chinese, Mal = Malays, Ind = Indians, Oth = others. Numbers in parentheses refer to number of patients.
[c]+ = Involved, 0 = not involved. Numbers in parentheses refer to number of patients.
[d]LP = leukemic phase.
[e]EM = electron microscopy.

TABLE 2. *Data on patients with abdominal lymphoma at presentation, Singapore General Hospital*

Patient no.	Age (years)	Sex	Race[a]	Presentation	Histology[b]	Location of gut involvement	Extent of involvement:[c]					Primary or secondary abdominal lymphoma	Serum immunoglobulin
							Lymph nodes		CXR[d]	Liver/ spleen	Peripheral blood/bone marrow		
							Superficial	Mesenteric					
1	48	F	Chin	Abdominal pain/mass	Diffuse ("histiocytic") (heavy plasmacytic component)	Diffuse small intestine	0	+	N[e]	0	0	1°	Alpha heavy chain paraprotein present
2	54	M	Chin	Abdominal mass/distension	Nodular MC	Jejunum	0	+	N	0	0	1°	Raised IgM (polyclonal)
3	30	M	Chin	Intestinal obstruction	Diffuse PD lymphocytic	Ileum (12 cm)	0	+	N	+	+	?	N
4	67	M	Mal	Abdominal pain/distension	Nodular PD lymphocytic	Diffuse small intestine	0	+	N	0	0	1°	N
5	23	F	Chin	Abdominal mass	Diffuse ("histiocytic")	Stomach	0	0	N	0	0	1°	N
6	58	M	Chin	Intestinal obstruction/perforation	Diffuse WD lymphocytic	Ileum	0	+	N	0	0	1°	N
7	31	M	Chin	Abdominal mass	Undifferentiated non-Burkitt's	Appendix	0	+	N	0	+	?	N

[a]Chin = Chinese, Mal = Malay.
[b]MC = mixed cellularity, PD = poorly differentiated, WD = well differentiated.
[c]+ = Involved, 0 = not involved.
[d]CXR = chest X-ray.
[e]= normal.

TABLE 3. Data on patients with T-ALL/lymphoblastic lymphoma[a]

| Patient no. | Age (years) | Sex | Race[b] | Extent of involvement[c] | | | | | Peripheral blood mononuclear cells | | | |
				CNS	Mediastinal mass	Chest wall soft growth	Marrow	"Leukemic" phase	E rosettes (%)	Surface Ig (%)	Acid PO$_4$ase[d]	Monoclonal[d] anti-T (PAN)
1	20	M	Chin	0	+	+	+	0	51	30	ND	ND
2	50	M	Chin	0	+	0	+	+	21[e]	10[e]	Focal positive	ND
3	25	M	Mal	0	+	+	+	+	14[e]	1[e]	Focal positive	+
4	19	M	Chin	+	+	0	+	+	46[e]	5[e]	ND	ND

[a]Convoluted cell type.
[b]Chin = Chinese, Mal = Malay.
[c]+ = Involved, 0 = not involved.
[d]ND = not determined.
[e]Neoplastic cells.

per 100,000 persons per annum for the years 1968–1972 from the Singapore Cancer Registry for Singapore Chinese for lymphosarcoma and reticulosarcoma were males 3.0, females 1.4, and for Hodgkin's disease, males 0.8, females 0.2. There were two peaks (five to 10 years and 55 to 70 years) in the incidence of Hodgkin's disease. A recent study (January 1976 to December 1980) (6) addressing mainly chemotherapy reported 27 patients with Hodgkin's disease and 70 patients with advanced NHL. Histological subtyping of the patients with Hodgkin's disease showed 40% with nodular sclerosis, 30% with mixed cellularity, 15% with lymphocyte predominance and 15% with lymphocyte depletion. Of the 27 patients, 18 were males and nine were females; their ages ranged from 10 to 88 years (mean age 45 years), and 26% were more than 60 years old. The main subtypes for NHL were diffuse poorly differentiated lymphocytic (35%), diffuse "histiocytic" (29%), well-differentiated lymphocytic (12%), and lymphoblastic lymphoma (10%).

Twenty-two patients with ALL (two-thirds of all leukemias) were seen in Singapore General Hospital's Department of Pediatrics (age 12 and under) from late 1973 to 1976 (15). Sixteen were males and six were females. The age of onset of the disease was mainly below the age of five years (13 patients); five patients were five to six years old at onset, and only four patients were six to 12 years old at onset. Only two of the 22 patients presented with total white blood cell counts above 60,000/mm^3; 18 had presenting counts below 30,000/mm^3. Although no immunological typing was done, most of the patients probably had the "null" childhood ALL phenotype, because 82% achieved complete remission with Pinkel's total therapy regime. During the same period, the same department saw 11 patients (less than 12 years old) with acute myeloid leukemia (one-third of all acute leukemias).

DISCUSSION

NHL in Singapore is similar in many aspects to that reported elsewhere. Although it is not a common neoplasm in Singapore, its incidence is "average" compared to most other countries, whereas the incidence of Hodgkin's disease is decidedly lower in Singapore (10). The commonest histological subtype is the large-cell lymphoma. Diffuse NHL is more common than nodular NHL (4:1), perhaps because of the late presentation of many of our patients or the young age structure of the population.

We identify a group of patients with gut lymphoma, which appears to be a common presentation in Singapore (Tables 1 and 2). The sites of the lesions were small intestine (five), stomach (one), and appendix (one). The gut lymphomas have a broad range of cytological types (diffuse five, nodular two). Dawson et al. (4) established five criteria for the diagnosis of primary lymphoma of the intestine. We have included an additional criterion, the absence of bone marrow involvement as demonstrated by a bone marrow trephine biopsy. Five of the seven patients with gut involvement fulfilled these criteria. One patient had alpha heavy chain disease (the so-called Mediterranean lymphoma). This disease previously has been described mainly among non-European Jews and Arabs in the Middle East (7,9). It has been proposed that gut parasitic antigenic stimulation of the gut lymphoid system acts as the trigger for this disease (7). Singapore, however, has a low gut parasitic infestation rate, and therefore the environmental antigenic influence there may be nonparasitic.

Our study also identified the presence of the lymphoblastic lymphoma (convoluted cell type)/T-ALL in Singapore. The patients present with the typical features and complications of the disease. All four patients reported (Table 3) had a mediastinal mass, and in addition two had soft anterior chest wall growths during the course of the disease and one patient developed this while being treated. The impression of clinicians that this presentation is fairly common among adolescents and young adults in Singapore needs to be confirmed.

CLL is uncommon in Singapore, as in the other countries in the Far East (13,14). The reason for this is not clear. It is not because of underreporting of patients. It may be a reflection, again, of the young Singapore population—the average age is 27.9 years, and only 7.2% of the population is 60 years old or above (5). CLL common in middle-aged women, as reported in Nigeria, is not our experience. The subacute/chronic adult T-cell variant common in regions of Japan (11) has yet to be identified in Singapore. So far, ALL in Singapore shows no differences in immunological subtype from studies elsewhere. The number of patients, however, is too small to draw any conclusions. Further studies, including those to determine the role of environmental factors, will be done on the malignant lymphoproliferative diseases in Singapore, because differences from other countries have been noted in this preliminary study.

ACKNOWLEDGMENTS

This study was supported by a generous grant from the Singapore Turf Club. We thank Esther Kew for typing the manuscript.

REFERENCES

1. Billing, R., Terasaki, P., Segiels, L., and Foon, K. (1983): *J. Immunol. Methods (in press).*
2. Boyum, A. (1968): Separation of leucocytes from blood and bone marrow. *Scand. J. Clin. Lab. Invest.*, 21 (Suppl. 97):77–106.
3. Braylon, R. C., Jaffe, E. C., and Berard, C. W. (1975): Malignant lymphoma: Current classification and new observations. *Pathol. Annu.*, 10:213–270.
4. Dawson, I. M., Cornes, J. S., and Morson, B. C. (1961): Primary malignant lymphoid tumours of the intestinal tract. *Br. J. Surg.*, 49:80–89.
5. Information Division, Ministry of Culture, Singapore (1982): *Singapore '81 (Yearbook)*, pp. 168–169. Ministry of Culture, Singapore.
6. Ong, Y. W., and Goh, C. N. (1981): Chemotherapy of malignant lymphoma. *Ann. Acad. Med. Singapore*, 10:281–287.
7. Ramot, B., and Many, A. (1972): Primary intestinal lymphoma: Clinical manifestations and possible effect of environmental factors. *Recent Results Cancer Res.*, 39:193–199.
8. Rappaport, H., and Braylon, R. C. (1975): Changing concepts in the classification of malignant neoplasms of the hematopoietic system. In: *The Reticuloendothelial System. International Academy of Pathology, Monograph 16*, pp. 1–19. Williams & Wilkins, Baltimore.
9. Seligman, M., Danon, F., Hurez, D., Mihaesco, E., and Preud'homme, J.-L. (1968): Alpha-chain disease: A new immunoglobulin abnormality. *Science*, 162:1396–1397.
10. Tan, K. K., and Shanmugaratnam, K. (1973): Incidence and histologic classification of malignant lymphoma in Singapore. *JNCI*, 50:1681–1683.

11. Uchiyama, T., Yodoi, J., Sagawa, K., Takatsuki, K., and Uchino, H. (1977): Adult T-cell leukemia: Clinical and hematologic features of 16 cases. *Blood*, 50:481–492.
12. Weiner, M. S., Bianco, C., and Nuiseneveig, V. (1973): Enhanced binding of neuramidase treated sheep erythrocytes to human T lymphocytes. *Blood*, 42.939–946.
13. Weiss, N. S. (1979): Geographical variation in the incidence of the leukemias and lymphomas. *Natl. Cancer Inst. Monogr.*, 53:139–142.
14. Wells, R., and Lau, K. S. (1960): Incidence of leukaemia in Singapore, and rarity of chronic lymphocytic leukaemia in Chinese. *Br. Med. J.*, 1:759–763.
15. Wong, H. B., Chan, M., and Vellayappan, K. (1977): Treatment and outcome of acute lymphoblastic leukemia in children. *J. Singapore Paediatr. Soc.*, 19(2):71–78.

Pathogenesis of Leukemias and Lymphomas:
Environmental Influences, edited by
I. T. Magrath, G. T. O'Conor, and B. Ramot.
Raven Press, New York © 1984.

Spectrum of Malignant Lymphomas in Japan, with Special Reference to Adult T-Cell Leukemia-Lymphoma and Its Epidemiology

*Taizan Suchi and **Kazuo Tajima

*Department of Pathology and Clinical Laboratories, Aichi Cancer Center Hospital, and
**Division of Epidemiology, Aichi Cancer Center Research Institute, Tashiro-cho,
Chikusa-ku, Nagoya 464, Japan*

FEATURES OF LYMPHOMA INCIDENCES IN JAPAN

The mortality rate of malignant lymphomas in Japan—3.45 for males and 1.71 for females per 100,000 population by the 1978 statistics (16)—is not high but has shown a steady increase in recent decades. The relative incidences of different subtypes have been shown to be considerably different from those in Western countries, notably the much lower incidences of Hodgkin's disease and follicular lymphomas on the one hand and the much higher incidences of diffuse, large-celled lymphomas (reticulum cell sarcoma) on the other hand (Tables 1 and 2). Considering the low overall mortality rate of lymphomas, the lower incidence of Hodgkin's disease and follicular lymphomas becomes even more significant.

The age-standardized incidence rates in various countries (22) show that Hodgkin's disease in Japan is only one-fifth that in the United States—0.8 versus 4.0 per 100,000 male population. Hodgkin's disease in Japan also differs from that in Western countries in that the proportion of the nodular sclerosis subtype is lower (Table 2). The paucity of chronic lymphocytic leukemia (CLL) in Japan—2% of all leukemia in adults versus 30% in the United States (5)—should also be noted.

ADULT T-CELL LEUKEMIA-LYMPHOMA

With the advent of the immunological age of lymphoma study, a peculiar form of peripheral T-cell leukemia was found and termed "adult T-cell leukemia" (ATL) (18). More than 300 cases have been documented since then, and detailed investigations of many of the cases, as well as a nationwide survey (21), have thoroughly clarified the characteristic features of ATL (3,6,10). It soon was revealed that cases with almost identical features except for the absence of a leukemic picture have also been frequently encountered [Adult T-cell leukemia-lymphoma (ATLL)]. These cases have previously been classified under other histological rubrics.

TABLE 1. *Relative incidence of subtypes of non-Hodgkin's lymphomas in Japan*

Rappaport classification	Study	
	Tajima et al. (14) (%)	Nanba et al. (9) (%)
Follicular	12.6	9.2
Diffuse*a*		
WDL	—	6.3
PDL	18.0	23.2
L&H	17.1	8.5
H	51.4	45.1
Undifferentiated	0.9	7.7
Total	87.4	90.8
(number of cases)	(111)	(142)

*a*WDL = well-differentiated lymphocytic, PDL = poorly differentiated lymphocytic, L&H = mixed, lymphocytic and histiocytic, H = histiocytic.

TABLE 2. *Relative incidence of Hodgkin's disease and its subtypes in Japan*

Subtype*a*	Study	
	Tejima and Watanabe (20) 1962–1977	Tajima and Suchi (13) 1969–1972
Hodgkin's disease	56 (12%)*b*	92 (9.5%)*b*
LP	8 (14.3%)	15 (16.3%)
MC	26 (46.4%)	43 (46.7%)
LD	8 (14.3%)	12 (13.0%)
NS	14 (25.0%)	22 (23.9%)

*a*LP = lymphocyte predominance, MC = mixed cellularity, LD = lymphocyte depletion, NS = nodular sclerosis.
*b*Number of cases of Hodgkin's disease and percentage of Hodgkin's disease among all lymphoma cases in the respective series.

ATLL affects the adult population (22 to 80, mean 52.6 years); male-female ratio ranges from 1.5:1 to 1.0:1 in various series. Besides lymphadenopathy (68 to 94%), hepatomegaly (50 to 78%), and splenomegaly (42 to 51%), the patients frequently exhibit cutaneous involvement ranging from erythematous patches to papules and nodules but do not have thymic masses. Hypercalcemia is found in 30 to 40% of the patients, often with resulting renal failure, and cellular immunity is also impaired, manifested by negative purified protein derivative (PPD) reactions and increased susceptibility to various infectious agents. The patients may be leukemic, subleukemic, or aleukemic, and the leukemic cells in peripheral blood smears are characteristic in appearance in that their nuclei exhibit rosette-like lobulations or deep irregular indentations. The percentage of tumor cells in the bone marrow is usually not very high, and patients lack anemia and thrombocytopenia of significant degree. Most patients die within one year; the median survival reported in one series was 4.7 months (3).

A number of receptor and surface antigen studies of the neoplastic cells indicate that the cells are of peripheral T-cell nature [E$^+$, sIg$^-$, HTLA$^+$ (human T lymphocyte antigen), THYSA$^-$ (thymocyte specific antigen)], with positive Ia-like antigen in some. Application of monoclonal antibodies of OK series (Ortho Pharmaceutical Corp.) to the cells revealed that they are positive to OKT 3, 4, and 10 and negative to 6 and 8, indicating that they are phenotypically of peripheral helper-inducer subset, but they exhibited suppressor activity on B-cell differentiation *in vitro* (19). In a cytogenetic study (19), an abnormality of 14q$^+$ was found in four of seven cases, and Miyoshi et al. (7) recently revealed that the additional chromatin was donated by chromosome 12 in one case and Y in another. Other abnormalities such as a t(1;7) and a 9q$^-$ were also detected.

The histological appearance of the lymph nodes is also characteristic (12). Typically, they show a mixed-cell appearance ranging from small lymphocyte to multinucleated giant cells, in which most of the nuclei are markedly convoluted regardless of their sizes. Giant cells resembling or indistinguishable from Reed-Sternberg cells are encountered fairly often (malignant lymphoma, pleomorphic type) (12).

The most striking fact about this disease is its geographic distribution. Birthplaces of the patients are heavily concentrated in coastal areas of Kyushu (the southwesternmost of the four major islands of Japan), in nearby small islands, and in Okinawa and are also scattered in other areas, mostly along the Pacific coast of the other major islands (Fig. 1) (21). This pattern of distribution naturally stimulated epidemiological and etiological investigations. A type-C retrovirus named ATLV (4) was found in a cell line (MT1) established from one of the ATL cases and later in the cells of a number of other cases. The virus seems to be identical to HTLV (11) previously found in the United States in cell lines from a case of "cutaneous T-cell lymphoma," which retrospectively appears to be a case of the form of ATLL endemic in the Caribbean region (2).

SPECTRUM OF LYMPHOMAS BY IMMUNOLOGICAL CHARACTERS

Non-Hodgkin's lymphomas with T-cell characteristics are relatively more frequent even in the nonendemic part of Japan than in Europe and the United States (21). This indicates that the peripheral T-cell lymphomas other than ATLL are also relatively common, especially in the nonendemic areas, but there is still no universally agreed upon histological classification of these lymphomas.

As an example of the lymphoma spectrum in the nonendemic areas of Japan, the numbers of cases encountered at the Aichi Cancer Center during the past three years are shown in Table 3, according to histological type and immunological characters revealed by marker studies. Note that the numbers in parentheses represent natives of an endemic area who moved to the Aichi Prefecture in their later lives. All except one T-CLL and one cutaneous lymphoma showed typical features of ATLL. In this series, T-cell lymphomas account for 38% of the total (34% if the endemic-area natives are excluded). Table 3 also shows that follicular lympho-

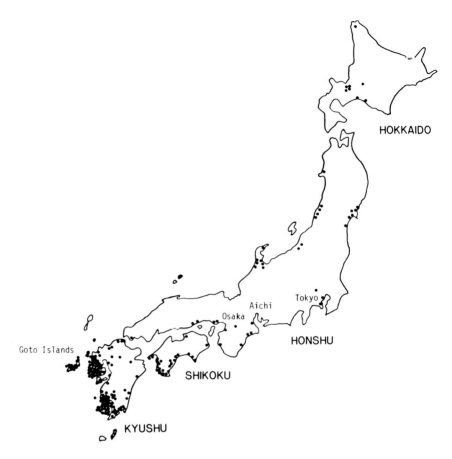

FIG. 1. Birthplaces of 192 patients with adult T-cell leukemia (16). (T- and B-cell Malignancy Study Group, ref. 21).

mas account for only about one-tenth of the non-Hodgkin's lymphoma and that the reticulum cell sarcomas, which in previous studies have been the predominant type of lymphoma in Japan, are mainly large-cell lymphomas with B-cell characteristics including B-immunoblastic lymphoma.

Because the standardized mortality ratio of malignant lymphomas is 200 to 300 in the endemic prefectures (all Japan is 100) (16) and because about three-fourths of lymphomas are of T-cell nature in these districts, it is logical to assume that the increased lymphoma mortality in the higher risk districts is accounted for almost entirely by the prevalence of this very special endemic disease.

EPIDEMIOLOGICAL FEATURES OF ATLL

As already mentioned, ATLL has a defined and localized geographic distribution within Japan. The endemic areas are remote, rural districts in coastal regions, mostly

TABLE 3. *Immunological characteristics and histological types of non-Hodgkin's lymphomas, Aichi Cancer Center, 1979–1981*

Histological type	B	T[a]	U[b]
Follicular lymphoma	13		
Diffuse lymphoma			
Small-cell	5	1 (1)	0
Medium-sized	11	4	2
Mixed-cell	9	2 (1)	0
Large-cell	24	8 (1)	6
Immunoblastic	8	0	0
Pleomorphic	0	9 (4)	0
Lymphoblastic	0	8	3
Burkitt's	3	0	0
Miscellaneous T-lymphomas, including Lennert's		17	0
Cutaneous T		4 (1)	0
Others	2		2
Total	75	53 (8)	13
(percentage)	(53%)	(38%)	(9%)

[a]Numbers in parentheses are of natives of endemic area.
[b]Undetermined.

with warmer climates and abundant rainfall. These places have no endemic infectious diseases at present, but in the past and until the post-World-War-II period, several infectious and parasitic diseases, notably filariasis, were endemic (15).

Other epidemiological features of the disease that have been described so far include peak incidence of clinical onset in the summer; familial clustering; an age distribution limited to adults, with a male-female ratio of 1.3:1, which is lower than most lymphomas; and an occupational association with primary industry, especially agriculture (21). It also has been found that most patients with ATLL, in endemic as well as nonendemic areas, have an antibody against the virus-associated antigen (ATLA) in their serum. Moreover, 10 to 25% of healthy adult inhabitants in the endemic areas also have the antibody in their serum (4). It was later established that the etiologically associated retrovirus (ATLV) can be demonstrated in the peripheral leukocytes of the antibody-positive individuals (8).

EPIDEMIOLOGICAL OBSERVATIONS ON HEALTHY CARRIERS

With co-workers, we recently made some observations on healthy carriers in the endemic area in order to elucidate the mode of transmission of the virus and/or factors influencing its transmission (17). We studied the frequency distribution of anti-ATLA-positive healthy carriers among the inhabitants of the highly endemic Goto Isiand off Nagasaki and have recorded their age, sex, and marital status. The results are summarized in Figs. 2 and 3. Some of the patterns of the distribution of these seropositive adults in family pedigrees are shown in Fig. 4.

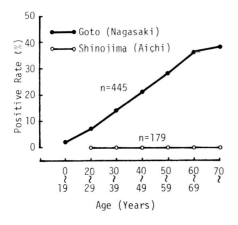

FIG. 2. Age-specific rates of anti-ATLA positivity among inhabitants of Goto (endemic) and Shinojima (non-endemic).

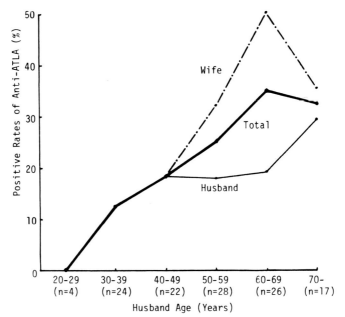

FIG. 3. Age- and sex-specific rates of anti-ATLA positivity in married couples in Goto.

The proportion of antibody-positive individuals increases steadily with age in the Goto inhabitants, whereas not a single person was found to be seropositive in the nonendemic island of Shinojima in Aichi Prefecture (Fig. 2). When the age-specific rates in the Goto inhabitants are analyzed by sex, positive serology in the male population increases only slightly after the age of 40, while that of the female population continues to rise (Fig. 3) (17).

The distribution patterns of antibody-positive carriers in family pedigrees (Fig. 4) definitely shows family clustering, suggesting parent-to-child transmission and

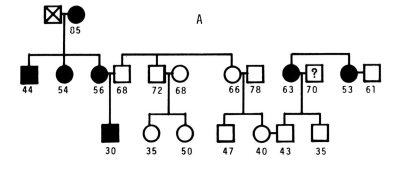

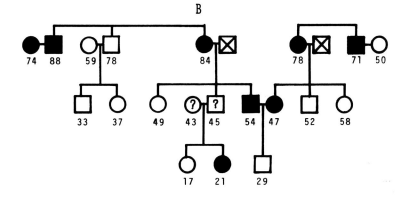

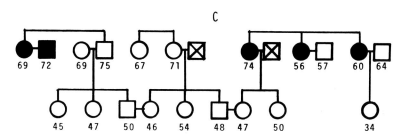

FIG. 4. Three family pedigrees (A–C), showing positive and negative anti-ATLA in family members and relatives. The numbers indicate the age of each individual. Open squares = negative males; open circles = negative females; filled squares = positive males; filled circles = positive females; squares with cross marks = dead males not tested; circles with cross marks = dead females not tested; squares with question marks = living males not tested; circles with question marks = living females not tested.

possibly some transmission among siblings. In many of the couples, both husband and wife are positive or only the wife is positive.

When age-specific seropositive rates of married couples alone are calculated in each sex separately, the divergence of the two curves is quite apparent (Fig. 3); it suggests that women may be more susceptible to infection, including via the spouse, than men. No seropositive child has been found in a family in which both parents are negative. It should be added that the histocompatibility locus antigen (HLA) study in these populations yielded no association of seropositivity with any specific HLA type, although the Goto inhabitants as a whole show frequencies in some HLA types that are quite different from those of the general population of the Japanese mainland (1).

A number of hypotheses about the possible route and mode of transmission of the virus may be formulated from these studies, but much remains to be learned to clarify the matter completely. This virus does not appear to be very contagious and is transmitted only to those in intimate contact with carriers. Parent (especially mother)-to-child and husband-to-wife pathways are very probable routes of transmission. Whether the virus is transmitted directly or indirectly via some vector is another problem to be investigated, but the environment appears to play, in some way, a very important role, in view of the fact that the disease is confined to certain specific regions of the country. The male-female divergence also may suggest a hormonal influence on susceptibility. The search for other factors affecting the development of the disease may prove to be as crucial as investigations of the virus itself to the development of measures to eradicate the disease.

ACKNOWLEDGMENTS

We wish to express our gratitude to Dr. S. Tominaga, Division of Epidemiology, Aichi Cancer Center, for his valuable suggestions and advice. This work was supported in part by a Grant-in-Aid for Cancer Research from the Ministry of Education and Culture (56010010) and from the Ministry of Health and Welfare (56 S-1).

REFERENCES

1. Akaza, T., Suchi, T., and Takagi, H. (1983): HLA study on inhabitants in Goto Islands, Nagasaki. *J. Jpn. Soc. Blood Transfusion*, 29:48–49. *(in Japanese)*.
2. Catovsky, D., Greaves, M. F., Rose, M., Galton, D. A. G., Goolden, A. W. G., McCluskey, D. R., White, J. M., Lampert, I., Bourikas, G., Ireland, R., Brownell, A. I., Bridges, J. M., Blattner, A. R., and Gallo, R. C. (1982): Adult T-cell lymphoma-leukaemia in Blacks from the West Indies. *Lancet*, 1:639–643.
3. Hanaoka, M. (1981): Clinical pathology of adult T cell leukemia. *Acta Haematol. Jpn.*, 44:1420–1430.
4. Hinuma, T., Nagata, K., Hanaoka, M., Nakai, M., Matsumoto, T., Kinoshita, K., Shirakawa, S., and Miyoshi, I. (1981): Adult T-cell leukemia: Antigen in an ATL cell line and detection of antibodies to the antigen in human sera. *Proc. Natl. Acad. Sci. USA*, 78:6478–6480.
5. Kimura, K. (1977): The report of hematologic neoplasms registration in Japan, No. 2 (1974,1975). Joint Committee for Hematologic Neoplasms in Japan, Tokyo. *(in Japanese)*.
6. Kinoshita, K., Kamihira, S., Yamada, Y., Amagasaki, T., and Ikeda, S. (1981): Clinical, hematological and pathological features of T-cell leukemia-lymphoma in the Nagasaki district. *Acta Haematol. Jpn.*, 44:1431–1443.
7. Miyoshi, I., Miyamoto, K., Sumida, M., Nishihara, R., Lai, M., Yoshimoto, S., Sato, J., and Kimura, I. (1981): Chromosome 14q+ in adult T-cell leukemia. *Cancer Genet. Cytogenet.*, 3:251–259.
8. Miyoshi, I., Taguchi, H., Fujishita, M., Niiya, K., Kitagawa, T., Ohtsuki, Y., and Akagi, T.

(1982): Asymptomatic type C virus carriers in the family of an adult T-cell leukemia patient. *Gann*, 73:339–340.

9. Nanba, K., Berard, C. W., Itagaki, T., Akimoto, T., Hara, H., and Iijima, S. (1973): Is reticulum cell sarcoma really frequent in Japan? An analysis of 331 cases of lymph-node biopsies (1962–1972). *J. Jpn. Soc. RES*, 13:96. *(in Japanese)*.

10. Nomura, K., and Matsumoto, M. (1981): Clinical features of adult T-cell leukemia in Kagoshima, the southernmost district in Japan—Comparison with T-cell lymphoma. *Acta Haematol. Jpn.*, 44:1444–1457.

11. Poiesz, B. J., Ruschetti, F. W., Gazdar, A. F., Bunn, P. A., Minna, J. D., and Gallo, R. C. (1980): Detection and isolation of type C retrovirus particles from fresh and cultured lymphocytes of a patient with cutaneous T-cell lymphomas. *Proc. Natl. Acad. Sci. USA*, 77:7415–7419.

12. Suchi, T., Tajima, K., Nanba, K., Wakasa, H., Mikata, A., Kikuchi, M., Mori, S., Watanabe, S., Mohri, N., Shamoto, M., Harigaya, K., Itagaki, T., Matsuda, M., Kirino, Y., Takagi, K., and Fukunaga, S. (1979): Some problems on the histopathological diagnosis of non-Hodgkin's malignant lymphoma—A proposal of a new type. *Acta Pathol. Jpn.*, 29:775–776.

13. Tajima, K., and Suchi, T. (1980): Some problems on the histopathological diagnosis of Hodgkin's disease. *J. Jpn. Soc. RES*, 20:149–156. *(in Japanese)*.

14. Tajima, K., Suchi, T., and Koike, K. (1979): Malignant lymphoma—Immunological characters and histological features. *J. Jpn. Soc. RES.*, 19:333–345. *(in Japanese)*.

15. Tajima, K., Tominaga, S., Shimizu, H., and Suchi, T. (1981): A hypothesis on the etiology of adult T-cell leukemia lymphoma. *GANN*, 72:684–691.

16. Tajima, K., Tominaga, S., and Suchi, T. (1983): Clinicoepidemiological analysis of adult T-cell leukemia. *GANN Monogr.*, 28:197–210.

17. Tajima, K., Tominaga, S., Suchi, T., Kawagoe, T., Komoda, H., Hinuma, Y., Oda, T., and Fujita, K. (1982): Epidemiological analysis of the distribution of antibody to adult T-cell leukemia-virus-associated antigen: Possible horizontal transmission of adult T-cell leukemia virus. *Gann*, 73:893–901.

18. Takatsuki, K., Uchiyama, T., Sagawa, K., and Yodoi, J. (1976): Adult T-cell leukemia in Japan. *Topics in Hematology, Proceedings of the 16th International Congress of Hematology*, pp. 73–77. Excerpta Medica, Amsterdam-Oxford.

19. Takatsuki, K., Uchiyama, T., Ueshima, Y., and Hattori, T. (1979): Adult T-cell leukemia: Further clinical observations and cytogenetic and functional studies of leukemic cells. *Jpn. J. Clin. Oncol.*, 9:317–324.

20. Tejima, S., and Watanabe, S. (1979): Hodgkin's disease in Japan. *J. Jpn. Soc. RES*, 19:347–355. *(in Japanese)*.

21. The T- and B-cell Malignancy Study Group (1981): Statistical analysis of immunologic, clinical and histopathologic data on lymphoid malignancies in Japan. *Jpn. J. Clin. Oncol.*, 11:15–38.

22. Waterhouse, J., Muir, C. S., Correa, P., and Powell, J., editors (1976): *Cancer Incidence in Five Continents*, Vol. 3, p. 520. IARC Scientific Publication 15, Lyons, France.

*Pathogenesis of Leukemias and Lymphomas:
Environmental Influences*, edited by
I. T. Magrath, G. T. O'Conor, and B. Ramot.
Raven Press, New York © 1984.

An Overview of Lymphoreticular Malignancies in Peru

*Oscar Misad, **Andres Solidoro, †Luis Quiroz, and
‡Laura Olivares

*Departments of *Pathology and **Medicine, †Clinical Laboratories Service, and
‡Departments of Statistics and Epidemiology, Instituto Nacional de Enfermedades
Neoplasicas, Lima, Peru*

Lymphoreticular malignancies (LRM) represent approximately 11% of all malignancies seen at the Instituto Nacional de Enfermedades Neoplasicas (INEN) of Lima, Peru; they are outnumbered only by cancer of the cervix and cancer of the breast. LRM constitute a large proportion of malignant tumors in children and, along with retinoblastoma, are the most common malignancies seen at INEN in the pediatric age group. Although the disease in most patients is well advanced when first seen, malignant lymphomas in Peru have some interesting characteristics compared to those in the United States and Europe (6,12,14,15). In 1966, for example, Solidoro et al. (15) called attention to the high incidence of Hodgkin's disease (HD) in Peruvian children. Another striking feature is the high incidence of the so-called nasal lymphomas (NL) observed during the last 30 years (5,9,13,16,17). Patients with LRM tend to have a poor prognosis because of the predominance of unfavorable histologic types, and some data suggest that the incidence of these malignancies has increased in recent years. INEN (142 beds) admits a large number of patients with malignant lymphomas and leukemias every year: the 269 new cases in 1978 comprised 161 cases of leukemia, 84 cases of non-Hodgkin's lymphomas (NHL), and 24 cases of HD.

We describe here some aspects of LRM in Peru as seen at INEN, the only cancer hospital in the country. Although immunologic techniques were not applied to this material, we hope that classification based on histology alone will serve as the basis for future studies that might be of epidemiologic or etiologic significance.

MATERIALS AND METHODS

The case material reviewed (Table 1) covers a period of 10 years (January 1971 to December 1980) for leukemias and lymphomas and a period of 28 years (1952 to 1980) for other related malignant lymphoid conditions. All cases of LRM from the INEN files for the periods under consideration were reviewed and classified according to histologic type and the age and sex of the patients. Approximately

85

TABLE 1. *Leukemias, malignant lymphomas, and related conditions*

Histologic type	Number of cases
Lymphomas	
Non-Hodgkin's disease[a]	641
Hodgkin's disease[a]	251
Nasal lymphoma[b]	70
Mycosis fungoides[b]	32
Others[b]	24
Total lymphomas	1,018
Leukemias	930
Total	1,948

[a]1971–1980.
[b]1952 1980.

10% of the cases had to be discarded because the original diagnosis was incorrect or because insufficient material was available for review. This report is based on the remaining 1,948 cases of LRM—930 cases of leukemia and 1,018 cases of solid lymphomas. Only acute leukemias have been considered, and they have been classified according to the French–American–British (FAB) classification (3,10). The NHL have been classified according to the Rappaport classification with minor modifications. The Rye system was used to classify HD. The category "others" in Table 1 includes malignant histiocytosis (12 cases), plasmacytoma (six cases), granulocytic sarcoma (three cases), cutaneous reticulosis (two cases), and Sézary syndrome (one case).

Paraffin sections were prepared in the standard manner and stained with hematoxylin and eosin. Peripheral blood and bone marrow samples were prepared according to standard procedures. Histochemical typing of acute leukemias included the use of myeloperoxidase, periodic acid-Schiff, and neutral lipid stains. Acid phosphatase and esterase reactions were used when indicated. No immunologic marker techniques were used in this study.

RESULTS

Non-Hodgkin's Lymphomas

The findings on NHL (January 1971 to December 1980) are summarized in Tables 2 to 6. Although NHL are seen at all ages, they occur predominantly in adults. A slight preponderance of female patients was present in children, but the overall male-female ratio was 1:1. The diffuse to nodular ratio of 13:1 shows the marked predominance of diffuse over nodular histology. Among the small number of nodular lymphomas, poorly differentiated lymphocytic was the most common histologic type. Table 5 shows the frequency of nodal versus extranodal NHL and the correlation with histologic type; for both groups, diffuse histiocytic lymphoma appears

TABLE 2. *Non-Hodgkin's lymphomas: histologic classification of 641 cases, Lima, Peru, 1971–1980*

Histologic type	Number of cases	Percentage	Nodular/diffuse[b]
Lymphocytic[a]	171	26.9	30/141
Histiocytic	388	60.8	14/374
Mixed	16	2.5	3/13
Lymphoblastic	10	1.1	0/10
Burkitt's	16	2.5	0/16
Composite	1	0.2	—
Unclassified	39	6.0	—
Total	641	100.0	47/554

[a]Includes well-differentiated lymphocytic and poorly differentiated lymphocytic.
[b]Nodular Non-Hodgkin's lymphomas: 92.1%.
Diffuse Non-Hodgkin's lymphomas: 7.8%.

to be the most common variety. In approximately two-thirds of all cases, lymph nodes were primarily involved, and in 10.9%, primary presentation, whether nodal or extranodal, was not established. Burkitt's lymphoma was much more frequently seen in an extranodal location. The histologic type by primary site of extranodal lymphomas is shown in Table 6. The gastrointestinal tract accounts for approximately 40% of all extranodal lymphomas, followed by Waldeyer's ring, the nasal cavity, and the paranasal sinuses. Two-thirds of all extranodal NHL are of the diffuse histiocytic type; 23 cases (12.2%) could not be classified histologically.

Hodgkin's Disease

The findings on HD are summarized in Table 7. In all, 475 cases were analyzed, because for this disease the series was extended to embrace a 28-year period (1952–1980). Nodular sclerosis was the most common histologic type of HD, accounting for more than half of the cases. We have included in this type cases with minimal sclerosis associated with lacunar cells presenting as small aggregates—the so-called cellular phase of nodular sclerosing HD. The lymphocyte-predominance and lymphocyte-depletion types were relatively uncommon in our material. The relative frequency of histologic types in children and adults is also compared in Table 7, and it can be seen that these two age groups do not differ significantly in histology. Note that nodular sclerosing HD is the most common variety in both children and adults.

Acute Leukemia

Tables 8 to 10 show the findings in 930 cases of acute leukemia (AL). The distribution of cases by sex and relative frequency of cytologic types is shown in Table 8. The categories with the most patients were L1, L2, M1, and M2. The lymphoid categories L1, L2, and L3 represented 66.6% of all cases; in other words,

TABLE 3. *Non-Hodgkin's lymphomas: age distribution by histologic type, 641 cases, Lima, Peru, 1971–1980*

Histologic type[a]	Ukn[b]	≤4	≤9	≤14	≤19	≤24	≤29	≤34	≤39	≤44	≤49	≤54	≤59	≤64	≤69	≤74	≤79	≤84	Total
WDL, diffuse	—	—	—	1	1	—	1	1	—	1	1	4	4	4	3	1	1	—	23
MWDL, diffuse	—	—	—	—	1	—	—	—	—	2	2	2	1	1	—	2	—	—	11
PDL, nodular	—	—	—	—	—	2	1	2	2	5	4	1	—	5	3	4	1	—	30
PDL, diffuse	—	5	6	6	7	5	9	3	2	7	10	6	12	11	5	11	—	2	107
Histiocytic, nodular	—	—	—	—	—	—	—	2	—	1	4	3	1	—	—	—	3	—	14
Histiocytic, diffuse	2	—	6	4	13	15	22	14	26	25	35	50	36	29	36	21	25	15	374
Mixed nodular	—	—	—	—	—	—	—	1	—	—	—	1	1	—	—	—	—	—	3
Mixed diffuse	—	—	—	—	—	2	—	—	—	—	3	1	3	2	—	2	—	—	13
Lymphoblastic	—	4	2	1	2	1	—	—	—	—	—	—	—	—	—	—	—	—	10
Burkitt's	—	6	7	3	—	—	—	—	—	—	—	—	—	—	—	—	—	—	16
Composite	—	—	—	—	—	—	—	—	—	—	—	—	—	1	—	—	—	—	1
Unclassified	—	8	3	3	3	1	1	1	2	4	4	—	2	3	2	—	2	—	39
Total	2	23	24	18	27	26	34	24	32	45	63	68	60	56	49	41	32	17	641

[a] WDL = well-differentiated lymphocytic, MWDL = moderately well-differentiated lymphocytic, PDL = poorly differentiated lymphocytic.
[b] Unknown.

TABLE 4. *Non-Hodgkin's lymphomas: distribution of 641 cases by age and sex, Lima, Peru, 1971–1980*

Age (years)	Males	Females	Total	Percentage
0–4	16	7	23	3.6
5–9	18	6	24	3.7
10–14	11	7	18	2.8
15–19	14	13	27	4.2
20–24	10	16	26	4.0
25–29	11	23	34	5.3
30–34	16	8	24	3.7
35–39	15	17	32	5.0
40–44	24	21	45	7.0
45–49	28	35	63	9.8
50–54	37	31	68	10.6
55–59	23	37	60	9.4
60–64	25	31	56	8.7
65–69	24	25	49	7.6
70–74	23	18	41	6.4
75–79	11	21	32	5.0
80 +	8	9	17	2.7
Unknown			2	0.3
Total	314	325	641	99.9

TABLE 5. *Non-Hodgkin's lymphomas: nodal versus extranodal by histologic type, 641 cases, Lima, Peru, 1971–1980*

Histologic type	Nodal	Extranodal	Site undetermined
Lymphocytic[a]	115	24	32
Histiocytic	232	128	28
Mixed	14	1	1
Lymphoblastic	6	2	2
Burkitt's	3	10	3
Others and unclassified	13	23	4
Total	383 (59.7%)	188 (29.3%)	70 (10.9%)

[a]Includes well-differentiated lymphocytic and poorly differentiated lymphocytic.

two-thirds of all leukemias corresponded to acute lymphoid leukemia (ALL). Table 8 also shows that female patients outnumbered male patients slightly, with a male-female ratio of 0.9:1. One hundred and ten cases (11.8%) could not be classified in any of the subcategories of AL.

The age distribution of all the AL patients is shown in Table 9. More than two-thirds of the cases occurred in children, and less than 5% occurred after the sixth decade of life. Peak incidence is at the age of about four years, followed by a gradual and steady decrease with age.

TABLE 6. *Extranodal non-Hodgkin's lymphomas: histologic type[a] by primary site, Lima, Peru, 1971–1980*

Primary site	WDLD	PDLN	PDLD	MD	HN	HiD	Burkitt's	Lymphoblastic	Unclassified	Total
Small intestine	—	—	3	—	1	31	4	—	1	40
Waldeyer's ring	—	1	6	—	1	20	—	—	12	40
Nasal cavity, sinuses, and larynx	—	1	3	—	—	27	—	—	3	34
Stomach	—	—	2	1	2	12	—	—	5	22
Bones and soft tissues	—	—	2	—	—	16	—	—	2	20
Colon and rectum	—	—	2	—	—	11	—	—	—	13
Facial bones	—	—	1	—	—	1	5	—	—	7
Skin and subcutaneous tissues	1	—	1	—	—	4	—	—	—	6
Miscellaneous sites	1	—	—	—	—	2	1	2	—	6
Total	2	2	20	1	4	124	10	2	23	188

[a]WDLD = well differentiated lymphocytic, diffuse; PDLN = poorly differentiated lymphocytic, nodular; PDLD = poorly differentiated lymphocytic, diffuse; MD = mixed diffuse; HN = histiocytic nodular; HiD = hystiocytic, diffuse.

TABLE 7. *Hodgkin's disease: relative frequency of histologic types in children and adults, 475 cases, Lima, Peru, 1952–1980*

	Children		Adults		Total	
Histologic type	Number	Percentage	Number	Percentage	Number	Percentage
Lymphocyte predominance	25	11.5	19	7.4	44	9.3
Mixed cellularity	66	30.2	73	28.4	139	29.3
Lymphocyte depletion	12	5.5	23	8.9	35	7.3
Nodular sclerosis	111	50.9	140	54.5	251	52.8
Unclassified	4	1.8	2	0.8	6	1.3
Total	218	99.9	257	100.0	475	100.0

TABLE 8. *Acute leukemias: distribution of 930 cases by sex and relative frequency of cytologic subtypes, Lima, Peru, 1971–1980*

Cytology	Male	Female	Total	Percentage
L1	225	269	494	53.2
L2	63	60	123	13.2
L3	—	2	2	0.2
M1	58	55	113	12.2
M2	27	16	43	4.6
M3	1	3	4	0.4
M4	13	9	22	2.4
M5	6	10	16	1.7
M6	3	—	3	0.3
Unclassified	58	52	110	11.8
Total	454	476	930	100.0

TABLE 9. *Acute leukemias: age distribution of 930 cases, Lima, Peru, 1971–1980*

Age (years)	Number of cases	Percentage
0–14	624	67.1
15–29	160	17.1
30–44	60	6.4
45–59	48	5.2
60–74	22	2.4
75+	16	1.7
Total	930	99.9

TABLE 10. Acute leukemias: age distribution by cytologic type, 930 cases, Lima, Peru, 1971–1980[a]

Cytology	Age (years)																Total
	≤4	≤9	≤14	≤19	≤24	≤29	≤34	≤39	≤44	≤49	≤54	≤59	≤64	≤69	≤74	75+	
L1	167	130	91	39	10	8	5	3	1	1	7	3	3	2	1	5	476
L2	21	19	27	13	6	9	3	7	3	3	4	1	1	3	—	3	123
L3	2	—	—	—	—	—	—	—	—	—	—	—	—	—	—	—	2
M1	17	25	18	16	5	2	4	3	5	5	3	3	2	1	2	2	113
M2	5	6	7	3	5	4	2	2	2	2	—	3	—	—	—	2	43
M3	—	—	1	—	1	—	—	—	1	—	1	—	—	—	—	—	4
M4	2	1	4	—	2	—	—	—	1	—	3	3	2	2	1	1	22
M5	6	4	1	1	—	1	—	—	—	2	—	—	—	—	—	—	15
M6	2	—	—	1	—	—	—	—	—	—	—	—	—	—	—	—	3
Unclassified	25	21	21	14	6	3	2	6	3	2	2	—	—	1	1	3	110
Total	247	206	170	87	35	27	16	21	16	15	20	13	8	9	5	16	911

[a]Age unknown, in 19 cases.

Table 10 shows the age distribution of leukemias by cytologic type; 457 cases, or approximately 50% of all AL, were lymphoid and occurred in children (zero to 14 years old), whereas only 99 cases of myeloid subtypes, or 10% of all AL, occurred in this age group.

Table 11 summarizes the most important findings on leukemia and lymphoma in both children and adults. Although 67.1% of all leukemias appear before 15 years of age, only 10.1% of NHL are seen in this age group, whereas 45.9% of HD occurred in children. The male-female ratio for both leukemia and lymphoma is approximately 1:1. For HD, however, there is a definite predominance of males over females, especially in children. The male preponderance is even higher in the first years of life; in our series, all patients less than three years old were males.

Nasal Lymphoma

Weiss (16) in 1954 called attention to the high incidence in Peru of a special type of LRM that in the majority of cases arises in the nose, either on the skin of the nasal pyramid or in the mucosa of the nasal cavity, and that involves the paranasal sinuses, soft palate, and pharynx. In some patients, it may extend into the larynx. The disease progresses slowly and may remain localized for long periods. Sometimes it may extend into the base of the brain and may kill the patient rapidly or may spread into the lymph nodes and become a generalized disease. The cell type involved in this process has not been clearly established, but the tumors are believed to be of lymphoid origin. They do not have the usual characteristics of other NHL, and necrosis is a prominent feature. Nasal lymphoma represents approximately 8% of all LRM in Peru. It has been observed at all ages with a slight preponderance of male over female patients. This disease offers interesting features not only in its clinicopathologic presentation but also in its geographic distribution. Most of the patients come from the coastal part of the country, especially from Piura, a city in the northern part of Peru, and from the central region around Lima. We are now reviewing our series of NL; a thorough clinicopathologic study will be presented separately.

DISCUSSION

LRM are relatively common in Peru as seen at INEN in Lima. The material that has been analyzed at INEN seems to be highly representative, because the hospital is a referral institution for neoplastic diseases for the entire country and, according to some estimates, takes care of approximately half of all known malignancies that occur in Peru. However, although our material provides a representative sample of the incidence and distribution of LRM in Peru, the population served by the hospital lives predominantly in the coastal part of the country, which includes the more developed areas and has better communications, less poverty, and greater industrialization. The patients coming to INEN are predominantly mestizos, which designates the native Peruvian background combined with the cultural effects of an encroaching industrial environment.

TABLE 11. *Leukemias and lymphomas: number and percentage of cases and sex ratio in children and adults, Lima, Peru*

Age group	Leukemia			Non-Hodgkin's lymphomas			Hodgkin's lymphoma		
	Cases	Percentage	M:F	Cases	Percentage	M:F	Cases	Percentage	M:F
Children	624	67.1	1.0	65	10.1	2.1	116	45.9	4.4
Adults	306	32.9	0.9	576	89.9	1.0	139	54.1	1.9
All ages	930	100.0	1.0	641	100.0	1.0	255	100.0	2.3

We must emphasize the fact that our material has been analyzed on a morphologic basis only. Further insights may be gained as we begin to include immunologic characterization, but even without this, our findings may contribute to the knowledge of the distribution of the subtypes of LRM around the world. Our major findings relate to HD, NHL, and NL.

The high incidence of HD in children in Peru has been recognized for nearly 20 years. This is not peculiar to Peru. HD in children is a relatively common disease in developing countries, as has been reported from Brazil (8), Colombia (7), Lebanon (2), and some parts of Africa (4). The less favorable histologic types of HD [mixed cellularity (MC) and lymphocyte depletion (LD)] also occur more frequently in these countries. Interestingly enough, the histology of HD in Peru shares to some extent the pattern described in the United States and Europe, with a high incidence of nodular sclerosis type. The incidence in children and the morphology are therefore discordant when compared with other countries. Even within Peru, the distribution of histologic types seems to show some differences. In 1973, Albujar (1) reported from Trujillo, a city on the Peruvian coast 600 km north of Lima, that as much as 85% of HD consisted of the histologic types associated with a poor prognosis (MC 30%, LD 55%). Although the number of cases presented in that report was very small, the result may be epidemiologically important.

The prognosis of patients with NHL in the material of INEN is very poor, not only because of well-advanced disease at consultation but also because of the marked predominance of unfavorable histologic types: 92% of NHL had a diffuse histology and nearly 60% of them were diffuse histiocytic lymphomas. Nodular lymphomas accounted for only 7.8% of all cases. The rarity of nodular lymphomas seems to be a feature of LRM in Peru and perhaps could be explained, at least in part, by the fact that most patients present with advanced disease when first seen. Some of these cases may have started as nodular lymphomas, later developing into diffuse lymphomas as a result of the natural progression of the disease. Nodular lymphomas, however, are rare not only in Peru but also in Japan, Brazil, India, and in U.S. Blacks (1 to 5% of all malignant lymphomas). Our findings regarding the high incidence of histiocytic lymphoma are similar to those reported from Japan (75% of all lymphomas), where histiocytic lymphoma is the most common malignant lymphoma. Burkitt's lymphoma and intestinal lymphoma are relatively rare in our material.

Overall, LRM are quite frequent in Peruvian children and account for approximately half of all LRM seen at INEN. Among children of 0–14 years in this study, there were 624 cases of AL, 65 cases of NHL, and 217 cases of HD, out of a total of 906 cases. The major difference between our studies and studies in the United States and Europe is our finding of relatively high frequency of poorly differentiated lymphocytic lymphoma in Peruvian children. This finding requires further investigation.

These findings must be tempered by the fact that, because approximately 45% of the Peruvian population is less than 15 years old, population-based studies will be necessary to determine the real incidence of these malignancies. In spite of this difference in population structure between Peru and the United States and Europe, AL does seem to be truly rare in Peruvian adults. In industrialized nations, the major form of adult AL is acute myeloid leukemia (AML). Whereas the ratio of ALL to AML in Peruvian children is similar to that in the United States, however, the marked lack of AML in older individuals in Peru is striking. The age distribution of ALL, however, is very similar to that in industrialized nations. Further epidemiologic and immunologic studies will be awaited with interest.

One interesting group in Peru is the native population that still lives in the high mountains of the Andes. This is the second most populated area of the country, accounting for approximately 5 million people with very limited medical facilities and of very low socioeconomic status. In this region, there are some communities whose way of living and habits have not changed significantly through the centuries. They have only sporadic contact with other groups, and their environment has therefore been stable for a very long time. The only study regarding LRM among these native groups is one report in 1964 by Krüger and Arias-Stella (11). They described a series of 20 cases of malignant tumors from Cerro de Pasco, a mining city more than 11,000 feet above sea level, in which there were two cases of what was called reticulum cell sarcoma of peripheral lymph nodes. Interestingly enough, most of the cases reported in that series were cancer of the cervix and cancer of the stomach.

In summary, this study demonstrates that LRM in Peru have some unusual features that should be further investigated. We hope that this study will serve as a basis for comparison with other countries and will stimulate continuing studies in Peru.

ACKNOWLEDGMENTS

We thank Dr. A. Wachtel, Dr. L. Casanova, Mrs. E. Suares, and Y. Herrera for their collaboration and Miss G. Prieto for typing the manuscript.

REFERENCES

1. Albujar, P. (1973): Hodgkin's disease in Trujillo, Peru. *Cancer*, 31:1520–1522.
2. Azzam, S. A. (1966): High incidence of Hodgkin's disease in children in Lebanon. *Cancer Res.*, 26:1202–1207.
3. Bennett, J. M., Catovsky, D., Daniel, M.-T., Flandrin, G., Galton, D. A. G., Gralnick, H. R., and Sultan, C. (1976): Proposals for the classification of the acute leukaemias. French-American-British (FAB) Co-operative Group. *Br. J. Haematol.*, 33:451–458.
4. Burn, C., Davies, J. N., Dodge, O. G., Briggita, C. N. (1971): Hodgkin's disease in English and African children. *JNCI*, 46:37–41.
5. Caller, A., and Puron, R. (1970): Linfoma endonasal de Weiss. Presentacion de dos casos. *Rev. Med. Hospital Central del Empleado*, 10:58–64.
6. Chang, A. (1967): Enfermedad de Hodgkin: Histopatologic. *Acta Cancerologica*, 6:30–41.
7. Correa, P., and Llanos, G. (1966): Morbidity and mortality from cancer in Cali, Colombia. *JNCI*, 36:717–745.
8. Dalldorf, G., Carvalho, R. P. S., and Jamra, M., Frost, P., Erlich, D., and Marigo, C. (1969): The lymphomas of Brazilian children. *JAMA*, 208:1365–1368.
9. Fernandez, L. E. (1965): Linfoma de la piramide nasal, presentacion de tres casos. *An. Fac. Med. (Lima)*, 48:90–103.
10. Gralnick, H. R., Galton, D. A. G., Catovsky, D., Sultan, C., and Bennett, J. M. (1977): Classification of acute leukemia. *Ann. Intern. Med.*, 87:740–753.

11. Krüger, H., and Arias-Stella, J. (1964): Malignant tumors in high-altitude people. *Cancer*, 17:1340–1347.
12. Misad, O., Galvez, J., and Albujar, P. (1973): Lymphoreticular tumors in Peru. *JNCI*, 50:1663–1668.
13. Romero, L., and Meth, V. (1969): Linfoma endonasal de Weiss. *Revista Sociedad Peruana Dermatología*, 3:1–21.
14. Solidoro, A. (1967): Linfoma maligno. Analisis de 668 casos atendidos en el Instituto Nacional de Enfermedades Neoplasicas. *Acta Cancerologica*, 6:5–22.
15. Solidoro, A., Guzmán, C., and Chang, A. (1966): Relative increased incidence of childhood Hodgkin's disease in Peru. *Cancer Res.*, 26:1204–1208.
16. Weiss, P. (1954): Casos de linfosarcoma de la naríz. *Actas Dermosifiliogr.*, 4:1–4.
17. Weiss, P., and Takano, J. (1962): Linfomas (reticulo-sarcomas) nasales. *Dermatología Revista Mejicana*, 6:34–42.

Pathogenesis of Leukemias and Lymphomas: Environmental Influences, edited by I. T. Magrath, G. T. O'Conor, and B. Ramot. Raven Press, New York © 1984.

Distribution of Lymphomas and Leukemias at University Hospital of the West Indies, Jamaica

*W. N. Gibbs, *W. S. Lofters, *B. Hanchard, *Marie Campbell, and **O. S. Morgan

*Departments of *Pathology and **Medicine, University of the West Indies, Kingston 7, Jamaica*

Information about the distribution of lymphomas and leukemias in Jamaica is available from the records of the Jamaica Cancer Registry. This information is based on data collected by the Registry staff on patients diagnosed in the Corporate area, the conurbation in the southeast of the island, consisting of Kingston and the surrounding areas of St. Andrew. Some of the classification schemes used by the Registry are outdated—for example, the classification of non-Hodgkin's lymphomas (NHL)—and others have changed over the years. In addition, the criteria for establishing or excluding diagnoses have varied from time to time because of the large number of anatomical pathologists and hematopathologists involved.

The distribution of lymphomas and leukemias reported in this chapter is based on data on patients presenting to the hematology service of the University Hospital of the West Indies (UHWI) between January 1, 1970 and June 30, 1979. Selection bias cannot be entirely eliminated from data based on admissions to one institution, but the bias is probably small for UHWI, a 500-bed public institution serving patients of all ages (including children), socioeconomic levels, and ethnic origins. Another advantage is the fact that the diagnoses at UHWI are made by a small number of anatomical pathologists and hematopathologists using well-defined criteria.

MATERIALS AND METHODS

The recommendations of the Rye Conference (8) were followed for histopathological classification of Hodgkin's disease (HD). The Rappaport classification (9) was used for NHL.

Diagnosis and classification of leukemias were based on hematological features, including the morphology of Wright's-stained blood and bone marrow films and, where appropriate, cytochemical methods: periodic acid-Schiff, myeloperoxidase, Sudan black B, nonspecific esterases, and leukocyte alkaline phosphatase (5). The criteria recommended by the French-American-British (FAB) cooperative group (1)

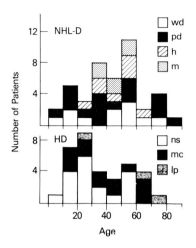

FIG. 1. Age distribution of diffuse non-Hodgkin's lymphomas (NHL-D) **(top)** and Hodgkin's disease (HD) **(bottom)**. wd = well differentiated, pd = poorly differentiated, h = "histiocytic," m = mixed cell, ns = nodular sclerosing, mc = mixed cellularity, and lp = lymphocyte predominance.

TABLE 1. *Histological subtypes of lymphomas, University Hospital of the West Indies, Jamaica, 1970–1979*

Subtype	Male	Female
Non-Hodgkin's lymphomas	24	24
Diffuse:		
Well differentiated	7	5
Poorly differentiated	8	9
"Histiocytic"	5	3
Mixed cell	3	3
Undifferentiated	0	2
Nodular		
Well differentiated	1	0
Mixed	0	2
Hodgkin's disease	21	13
Lymphocyte predominance	1	2
Nodular sclerosing	11	7
Mixed cellularity	9	4
Lymphocyte depletion	0	0

were followed for classifying acute nonlymphoblastic leukemias, but in this chapter the term "acute myeloblastic leukemia" includes M1 and M2 of the FAB cooperative group; i.e., myeloblastic leukemia with and without maturation.

RESULTS AND DISCUSSION

In Table 1, 48 cases of NHL and 34 cases of HD seen at UHWI are listed according to histological type and sex of the patient. Nodularity was detected in only 3 (6%) of the 48 patients with NHL. The proportion of such patients in series reported in the United States is 30 to 50% (6,7). The reasons for this difference

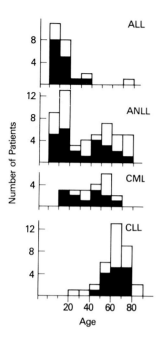

FIG. 2. Age and sex distribution of leukemia cases by type. ALL = acute lymphoblastic leukemia, ANLL = acute nonlymphoblastic leukemia, CML = chronic myeloid leukemia, and CLL = chronic lymphocytic leukemia. *Closed bars* represent males; *open bars* represent females.

are unknown. One possibility is that the patients at UHWI present at a later stage of disease. Many of our patients had symptoms attributable to their disease at least 6 months before the diagnosis was made, and it has been shown that the histological pattern usually changes from nodular to diffuse as the disease progresses (10). Data are insufficient to examine this possibility or to explore a relationship with ethnic origin or the environment.

Our series includes a high proportion of patients with diffuse poorly differentiated or well-differentiated lymphocytic lymphoma and three patients less than 20 years old who had diffuse well-differentiated lymphocytic lymphoma (DWDL) (Fig. 1). DWDL is rare in the young age groups, and the possibility that these patients had lymphocyte-predominant HD must be considered. DWDL was diagnosed in the 12 patients in this series only after a careful search failed to reveal typical or mononuclear variants of the Reed-Sternberg cell.

Nodular sclerosis (NS) is the most common histological subtype of HD at UHWI. Jamaica is a developing country, and we would have expected most patients to have mixed cellular disease (4). The proportion of children with HD is also lower than expected in a developing country (Fig. 1), and the preponderance of NS HD in young adults is the pattern usually found in developed countries.

Table 2 lists all leukemia cases registered at UHWI during the period covered by this review according to type of leukemia and sex of the patient. Nearly all of the patients who had acute lymphoblastic leukemia (ALL) were less than 15 years old (Fig. 2): four were less than five years old; five were between five and 10 years

TABLE 2. *Leukemia types, University Hospital of the West Indies, Jamaica, 1970–1979*

Type	Male	Female
Acute lymphoblastic	15	8
Acute nonlymphoblastic	25	29
Myeloblastic	20	20
Promyelocytic	0	1
Myelomonocytic	0	4
Monocytic	4	3
"Erythroleukemia"	1	1
"Smoldering acute leukemia"	2	1
Chronic myeloid leukemia	12[a]	9
Chronic lymphocytic leukemia	15	19
Hairy cell leukemia	5	0

[a]Includes one patient who presented in blast crisis.

old; and three were between 10 and 15 years old. In predominantly White populations, the peak incidence is usually earlier, at three years of age (2). Acute nonlymphoblastic leukemia (ANLL) occurred at all ages (Fig. 2), but the proportion of children was unusually high. This could be because of a higher frequency of patients presenting at UHWI with ANLL or a lower frequency of patients presenting with ALL, or both. Most ANLL patients had acute myeloblastic leukemia (Table 2).

In most series describing patients with chronic lymphocytic leukemia (CLL), the ratio of males to females is approximately 2:1. Women outnumbered men at UHWI (Table 2), but the age distribution (Fig. 2) is similar to that described in other series (2). Chronic myeloid leukemia occurred in all age groups but was most common in patients more than 30 years old (Fig. 2).

Surface marker studies are now being done at UHWI to improve the classification of ALL and NHL. We hope to combine these studies with epidemiological studies involving all of Jamaica to find out if the distribution of ALL subtypes really differs in predominantly White and Black populations and to examine the relationships between this distribution and the poorer prognosis of ALL in Black children.

Epidemiological and surface marker studies of NHL would be useful in clarifying the relationship between the human T-cell lymphoma virus (HTLV) and the lymphoma/leukemia syndrome described recently in Caribbean patients (3). Antibody to HTLV so far has been detected in seven Jamaican patients. One who has ALL, was diagnosed elsewhere and was in remission when referred to UHWI. Three had lymphoma/leukemia syndromes, and preliminary data suggest that the neoplastic cells in one were T lymphocytes. The other three patients have CLL.

REFERENCES

1. Bennett, J. M., Catovsky, D., Daniel, M.-T., Flandrin, G., Galton, D. A. G., Gralnick, H. R., and Sultan, C. (1976): Proposals for the classification of the acute leukaemias. *Br. J. Haematol.*, 33:451–458.

2. Boggs, D. R., Wintrobe, M. M., and Cartwright, G. E. (1962): The acute leukemias. Analysis of 322 cases and review of the literature. *Medicine*, 41:163–225.
3. Catovsky, D., Greaves, M. F., Rose, M., Galton, D. A. G., Goolden, A. W. G., McCluskey, D. R., White, J. M., Lampert, I., Bourikas, G., Ireland, R., Brownell, A. I., Bridges, J. M., Blattner, W. A., and Gallo, R. C. (1982): Adult T-cell lymphoma-leukaemia in Blacks from the West Indies. *Lancet*, 1:639–643.
4. Correa, P., and O'Conor, G. T. (1971): Epidemiologic patterns of Hodgkin's disease. *Int. J. Cancer*, 8:192–201.
5. Dacie, J. V., and Lewis, S. M. (1975): *Practical Haematology*, 5th edition. Churchill Livingstone, Edinburgh.
6. Garvin, A. J., Simon, R., Young, R. C., DeVita, V. T., and Berard, C. W. (1980): The Rappaport classification of non-Hodgkin's lymphomas. *Semin. Oncol.*, 7:234–243.
7. Jones, S. E., Fuks, Z., Bull, M., Kadin, M. E., Dorfman, R. F., Kaplan, H. S., Rosenberg, S. A., and Kim, H. (1973): Non-Hodgkin's lymphomas. IV. Clinicopathologic correlation in 405 cases. *Cancer*, 31:806–823.
8. Lukes, R. J., Craver, L. F., Hall, J. C., Rappaport, H., and Ruben, P. (1978): Report of the Nomenclature Committee. *Cancer Res.*, 26:1311.
9. Rappaport, H. (1966): *Tumors of the Hematopoietic System*. Armed Forces Institute of Pathology, Washington, D.C.
10. Risdall, R., Hoppe, R. T., and Warnke, R. (1979): Non-Hodgkin's lymphoma. A study of the evolution of the disease based upon 92 autopsied cases. *Cancer*, 44:529–542.

Pathogenesis of Leukemias and Lymphomas:
Environmental Influences, edited by
I. T. Magrath, G. T. O'Conor, and B. Ramot.
Raven Press, New York © 1984.

Diagnostic Features of Adult T-cell Lymphoma-Leukemia

*D. Catovsky, *M. O'Brien, **C. O'Brien, **I. Lampert,
*A. Crockard, *S. E. Johnson, †G. E. Francis, ††J. Sharp,
and *D. A. G. Galton

*Medical Research Council Leukaemia Unit and **Department of Histopathology, Royal
Postgraduate Medical School; †Department of Haematology, Royal Free Hospital;
and ††Department of Haematology, Kings College Hospital Medical School,
London, United Kingdom

We recently described a group of Black patients, born in the Caribbean, suffering from a distinct T-cell lymphoproliferative disorder called adult T-cell lymphoma-leukemia (ATLL). On clinical and morphological grounds, it is possible to distinguish ATLL from other T-cell neoplasias with a mature T-membrane phenotype (3). The cells in ATLL have a degree of pleomorphism and nuclear irregularities that have been associated in the past with the term "lymphosarcoma cell leukemia" (4). Because of the association of ATLL with a new human retrovirus, HTLV (13; see also M. S. Reitz et al., *this volume*), and the similarity to a T-cell lymphoma-leukemia seen in southern Japan (7,8,16,18,20; T. Suchi and K. Tajima, *this volume*), it is important to establish the unique diagnostic features of ATLL so that its precise incidence and epidemiology can be worked out properly.

MATERIALS AND METHODS

Material from eight patients with ATLL was studied. Six of the cases have been reported elsewhere (2). Of the other two, one was described separately in relation to the neurological aspects of hypercalcemia (14), and the other was previously studied at Hammersmith Hospital but was not included in the early series (2). All the patients were Black and were born in the West Indies and the Caribbean basin (Fig. 1). Seven had hypercalcemia as one of the main laboratory findings; the white blood cell count (WBC) ranged between 20 and 67×10^9/liter with a predominance of abnormal lymphoid cells.

The following studies were conducted: (a) morphological analysis of the neoplastic cells by light microscopy (in May Grünwald-Giemsa stained blood films) and by electron microscopy (peripheral blood in six cases, lymph nodes in two), using techniques previously described (4); (b) cytochemistry (in five cases) by means

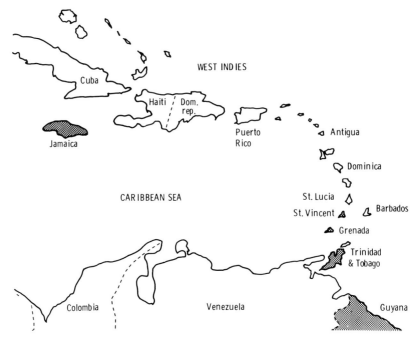

FIG. 1. The Caribbean region, showing the birth places *(shadowed areas)* of five of the eight patients described in this chapter. The other three were also born in this region, but the precise locations are not known.

of the periodic acid-Schiff (PAS) reaction and techniques for four acid hydrolases; and (c) histopathology of the lymph nodes (in seven cases).

RESULTS

Morphology

Light Microscopy

The cells in all cases had a high nuclear cytoplasmic ratio and, characteristically, an irregular nuclear outline (Fig. 2). They varied from medium-sized lymphocytes to large blasts; in blood films, the latter cells were infrequent. The nuclear irregularities were variable in each case; some cells had a highly convoluted nucleus, and in a few, multiple nuclear lobes were seen. Most cells in each case formed E rosettes (Fig. 2E).

Ultrastructure

In almost every case, three types of lymphoid cells were seen: 70 to 75% of the cell population were medium-sized with irregular nucleus; 10 to 20% were small, also with nuclear irregularities; and 5 to 10% were large blasts with little chromatin

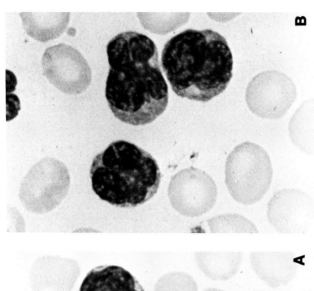

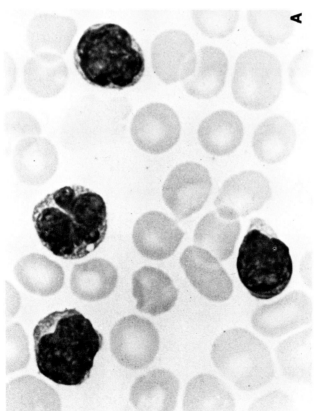

FIG. 2 A and B. *(See legend, p. 109)*

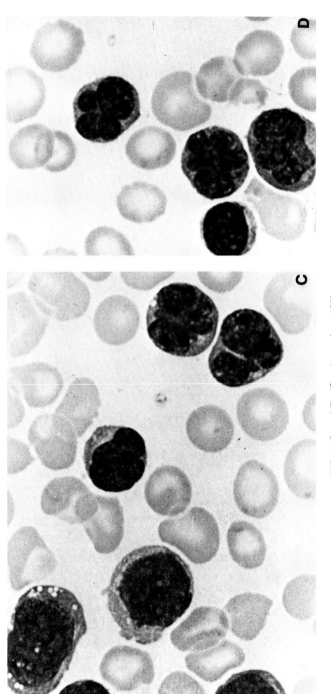

FIG. 2 C and D. *(See legend, p. 109)*

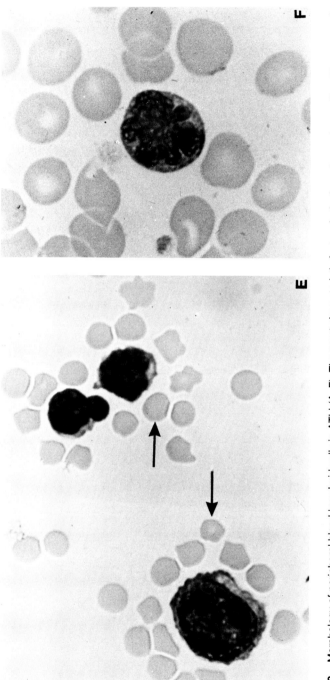

FIG. 2. Morphology of peripheral blood lymphoid cells in ATLL(A–F). The most characteristic feature is the irregular nuclear outline. **E** corresponds to a cytocentrifuge-prepared slide of E-rosettes, showing small and large cells binding sheep red blood cell (*arrows*).

condensation and a more regular nuclear outline. In one case, only small and medium-sized cells were present and, in another, medium-sized and large cells predominated. The nuclear irregularities seen ranged from slight indentations to horseshoe-shaped forms, convolutions, and lobulations with two to four distinct lobes. A "cerebriform" nucleus (Sézary-like) was seen in 4 to 15% of cells from three of the six patients studied (Fig. 3B). Most cells showed discrete intranuclear clumps of chromatin condensation and a distinct, compact nucleolus. The blast cells had less chromatin condensation and a larger nucleolus (Fig. 4A). The cytoplasm showed a small but well-developed Golgi apparatus in 50% of cells (Fig. 4A). Lysosomal granules varied in number, size, and electron density and were often seen in clusters (Fig. 4B). Perinuclear bundles of microfibrils were prominent in three cases. Short strands of endoplasmic reticulum were visible in most cells. Parallel tubular arrays were seen in a minority of cells from one patient. (Fig. 3A).

Cytochemistry

The PAS reaction was negative in the cells of two cases and positive in one with discrete granules and large blocks. The acid phosphatase reaction was positive in 80 to 100% of the lymphoid cells of the five cases tested. The reaction was strong, however, in only one; in the others, it was weak to moderately positive in diffuse or granular form and was tartrate-sensitive. The alpha-naphythyl acetate esterase ANAE reaction was positive, with single or several discrete granules in more than 85% of cells. β-glucuronidase and β-glucosaminidase were also positive in almost all the cells of the two cases tested.

LYMPH NODE HISTOLOGY

Lymph nodes showed preservation of the capsule and peripheral sinuses in most cases, with distortion rather than destruction of internal architecture in some. In two, lymphoid follicles were present, one with prominent germinal centers. A cellular infiltrate, expanding and apparently arising from the paracortical T zone, was present, pushing apart and in some cases displacing the B zones. This cellular infiltrate was limited to the paracortical area in the node with prominent germinal centers, resembling T-zone lymphoma (11). A marked proliferation of small vessels was seen accompanying the infiltrate in five of seven cases examined (Fig. 5A).

The neoplastic infiltrate was made up of two cell types: a small cell, up to twice the size of a normal lymphocyte, with an irregular, convoluted nucleus and coarsely clumped chromatin, and a large cell with abundant amphophilic cytoplasm and a round or oval nucleus, sometimes slightly irregular, a fine chromatin pattern, and a prominent nucleolus. The relative proportion of these cells varied from case to case. In four, they were present in equal proportions, giving a pleomorphic ap-

FIG. 3. Electron micrographs of ATLL cells. **A:** Note the presence of parallel tubular arrays *(arrows)*, which were seen in a minority of cells in one case. **B:** A highly convoluted cell, indistinguishable from a Sézary cell. These cells were seen in small proportions in three patients. Lead citrate and uranyl acetate stain; × 13,000.

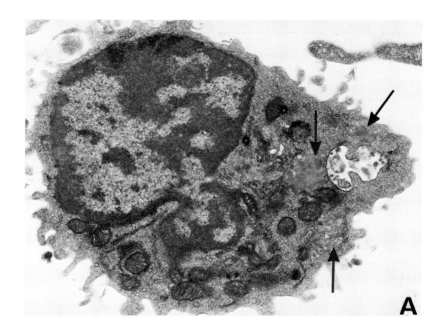

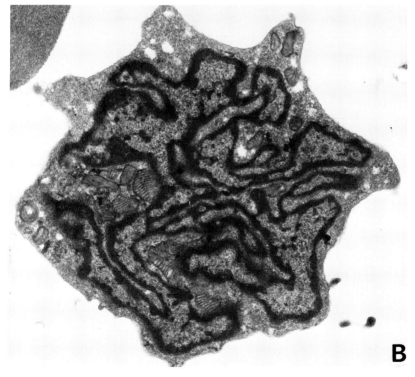

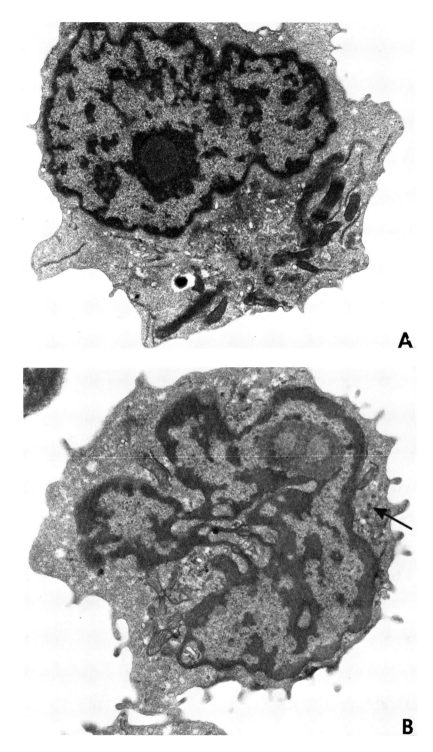

FIG. 4. Electron micrographs of immature lymphoid cells from two patients. Both show irregular nuclear outline, marked in **B,** a prominent nucleolus, and peripheral and intranuclear chromatin condensation. The Golgi apparatus is well developed in **A;** small, membrane-bound granules are seen clustered in **B** *(arrow).* Lead citrate and uranyl acetate stain; ×13,000.

pearance; in two, the predominance of one type gave a nearly monomorphic appearance. One of these two cases had a uniform infiltrate of the large-cell type, resembling a large-cell, immunoblastic lymphoma; this case had the highest mitotic rate. Multinucleated tumor cells were not a feature of any of the cases studied.

DISCUSSION

ATLL is a distinct clinicopathological entity that, in our series, was present exclusively in adult Blacks of West Indian origin (2). Analysis of these and other similar patients reported in the literature (1,6) shows the following common clinical features: Black race; hypercalcemia, despite the absence of osteolytic lesions in the majority; lymphadenopathy; and, less frequently, hepatosplenomegaly and skin lesions. The mean WBC was 42×10^9/liter with more than 60% of pleomorphic lymphoid cells with nuclear irregularities. The overall survival was short, with a median of only four months. ATLL has now been identified in Whites from the Pacific Northwest of the United States (9). The diagnostic features of this disease suggest that ATLL in our series is indistinguishable from the "adult T-cell leukemia" prevalent in rural and coastal areas of Kyushu and southern Shikoku in Japan (7,16,18).

The cytochemical findings were similar to those of other mature T-cell lymphoproliferature disorders (3) and of ATLL in Japan (21). However, the acid phosphatase in the cells from our cases was tartrate-sensitive, whereas in the study by Usui et al. (21), they were reported to be tartrate-resistant. We have seen resistance to tartaric acid inhibition previously in other mature T-cell leukemias (4). There are two detailed reports of the ultrastructure of ATLL cells in Japanese patients (5,15). The features were the same as in the cases described here, namely; convoluted nucleus, speckled chromatin pattern, and lysosomal granules in clusters. Parallel tubular arrays were seen in the cells of one case (15). Eimoto et al. (5), in a study of 18 cases, described the same variation in size and nuclear irregularities as seen in our series.

The histology of the lymph nodes shows a diffuse and pleomorphic cell infiltrate with small and large cells and a proliferation of postcapillary venules also described in Japanese patients (5,7). The histopathology of ATLL does not fit exactly in any of the current classification schemes. The lymph nodes have several of the features seen in T-zone lymphoma (11) and in peripheral T-cell lymphoma (22), but when large cells predominate (as in one case in this series), the appearance is that of diffuse, large-cell, T-immunoblastic lymphoma. The type with multilobulated large cells (5) was not represented in our series. The three key features of ATLL (7) are cell pleomorphism with nuclear irregularities and size heterogeneity; diffuse involvement, usually from the paracortical zones and rarely (one case in this series) with the infiltrate limited to that area; and the proliferation of postcapillary venules.

The analysis of skin involvement is of interest in relation to the cutaneous T-cell lymphomas (Sézary syndrome and mycosis fungoides). In two of our cases the infiltrate was predominartly dermal, as in the majority of ATLL in Japan (7).

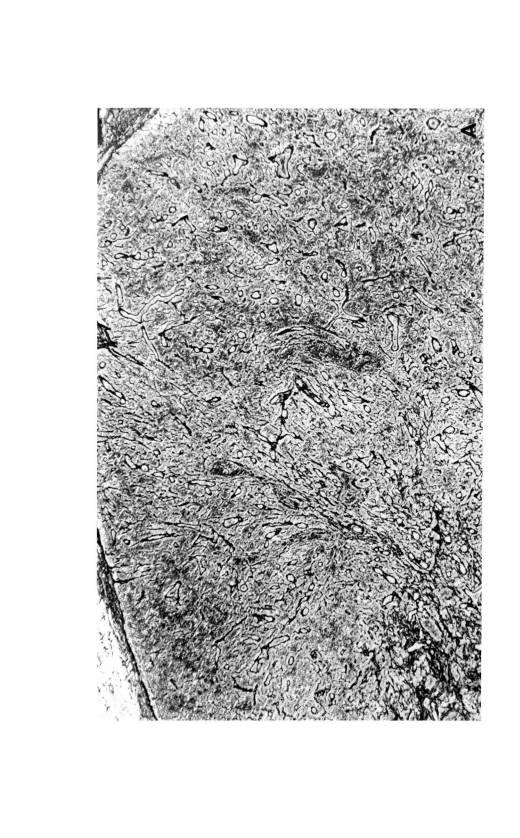

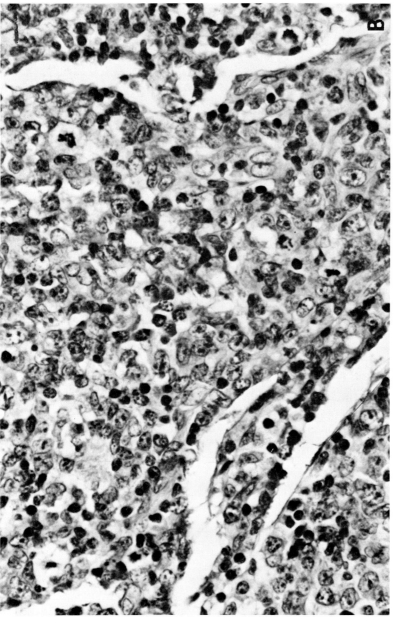

FIG. 5. Histological sections of a lymph node from ATLL. **A:** Note the characteristic proliferation of postcapillary venules (×60). **B:** Higher magnification, showing the diffuse pleomorphic cellular infiltrate with small and large, irregularly shaped lymphoid cells (×400).

However, some epidermotropism occurs, and even Pautrier's microabscesses have been reported, both in Japanese cases (7,12) and in Black patients (6) with ATLL.

Cell marker studies frequently show a mature T-helper phenotype (OKT 4 +, OKT 6 − , TdT −) (2), as in other mature T-cell disorders, such as Sézary syndrome and T-prolymphocytic leukemia (3,10), as well as ATLL in Japanese cases (8,20). Markers atypical for mature T-lymphoid cells (OKT 3 − or OKT 4 − and OKT 8 −) were demonstrated in one of our cases (2), some Japanese ATLL (20), and three American cases (9). Functional studies on Japanese patients have shown that ATLL cells act as suppressors *in vitro* (8,17), despite a "helper" phenotype (8). Similar findings were observed in an American Black with ATLL (1). This suggests that, unlike Sézary cells (10), ATLL cells may belong to a minor subset within the OKT 4 + population that has suppressor function (19).

The methods we have described should help to establish clear and objective criteria for the diagnosis of ATLL and thus to permit the assembly of epidemiological information on the true incidence of the disease, its pathogenesis, and its relation to other T-cell disorders.

REFERENCES

1. Burns, J. B., Antel, J. P., Haren, J. M., and Hopper, J. E. (1981): Human T-cell lymphoma with suppressor effects on the mixed lymphocyte reaction (MLR). II. Functional *in vitro* lymphocyte analysis. *Blood*, 57:642–648.
2. Catovsky, D., Greaves, M. F., Rose, M., Galton, D. A. G., Goolden, A. W. G., McCluskey, D. R., White, J. M., Lampert, I., Bourikas, G., Ireland, R., Brownell, A. I., Bridges, J. M., Blattner, W. A., and Gallo, R. C. (1982): Adult T-cell lymphoma-leukaemia in Blacks from the West Indies. *Lancet*, 1:639–643.
3. Catovsky, D., Linch, D. C., and Beverley, P. C. L. (1982): T-cell disorders in haematological diseases. *Clin. Haematol.*, 11:661–695.
4. Costello, C., Catovsky, D., O'Brien, M., Morilla, R., and Varadi, S. (1980): Chronic T-cell leukemias. I. Morphology, cytochemistry and ultrastructure. *Leuk. Res.*, 4:463–476.
5. Eimoto, T., Mitsui, T., and Mashahiro, K. (1981): Ultrastructure of adult T-cell leukemia/lymphoma. *Virchows Arch. (Cell Pathol.)*, 38:189–208.
6. Grossman, B., Schechter, G. P., Horton, J. H., Pierce, L., Jaffe, E., and Wahl, L. (1981): Hypercalcemia associated with T-cell lymphoma-leukemia. *Am. J. Clin. Pathol.*, 75:149–155.
7. Hanaoka, M., Sasaki, M., Matsumoto, H., Tankawa, H., Yamabe, H., Tomimoto, K., Tasaka, C., Fujiwara, H., Uchiyama, T. and Takatsuki, K. (1979): Adult T-cell leukemia. Histological classification and characteristics. *Acta Pathol. Jpn.*, 29:723–738.
8. Hattori, T., Uchiyama, T., Toibana, T., Takatsuki, K., and Uchino, H. (1981): Surface phenotype of Japanese adult T-cell leukemia cells characterized by monoclonal antibodies. *Blood*, 58:645–647.
9. Kadin, M. E., and Kamoun, M. (1982): Adult T-cell lymphoma leukaemia in U.S. Whites. *Lancet* 1:1016–1017.
10. Kung, P. C., Berger, C. L., Goldstein, G., LoGerfo, P., and Edelson, R. L. (1981): Cutaneous T-cell lymphoma: characterization by monoclonal antibodies. *Blood*, 57:261–266.
11. Lennert, K. (1978): *Malignant Lymphomas Other Than Hodgkin's Disease*. Springer-Verlag, Berlin.
12. Nakajima, H., Nagatani, T., and Nagai, R. (1979): Histopathological and immunological studies of malignant lymphoma of the skin. *Jpn. J. Clin. Oncol.*, 9:373–386.
13. Poiesz, B. J., Ruscetti, F. W., Reitz, J. S., Kalyanaraman, V. S., and Gallo, R. C. (1981): Isolation of a new type C retrovirus (HTLV) in primary uncultured cells of a patient with Sézary T-cell leukaemia. *Nature*, 294:268–271.
14. Schott, G. D. (1975): Hypercalcaemic stupor as a presentation of lymphosarcoma. *J. Neurol. Neurosurg. Psychiatry*, 38:382–385.

15. Shamoto, M., Murakami, S., and Zenke, T. (1981): Adult T-cell leukemia in Japan: An ultra-structural study. *Cancer*, 47:1804–1811.
16. Shimoyama, M., Minato, K., Saito, H., Kitahara, T., Konda, C., Nakazawa, M., Watanabe, S., Inada, N., Nagatani, T., Deura, K., and Mikata, A. (1979): Comparisons of clinical, morphologic and immunologic characteristics of adult T-cell leukemia-lymphoma and cutaneous T-cell lymphoma. *Jpn. J. Clin. Oncol.*, 9:357–371.
17. Tatsumi, E., Takiuchi, Y., Domae, N., Shirakawa, S., Uchino, H., Baba, M., Yasuhira, K., and Morikawa, S. (1980): Suppressive activity of some leukemic T-cells from adult patients in Japan. *Clin. Immunol. Immunopathol.*, 15:190–199.
18. The T- and B-cell Malignancy Study Group (1981): Statistical analysis of immunologic, clinical and histopathologic data on lymphoid malignancies in Japan. *Jpn. J. Clin. Oncol.*, 11:15–38.
19. Thomas, Y., Rogozinski, L., Irigoyen, O. H., Friedman, S. M., Kung, P. C., Goldstein, G., and Chess, L. (1981): Functional analysis of human T-cell subsets defined by monoclonal antibodies. IV. Induction of suppressor cells within the OKT4+ population. *J. Exp. Med.*, 154:459–467.
20. Tobinai, K., Hirose, M., Yamada, H., Minato, K., and Shimoyana, M. (1982): Cellular origin of human lymphoid malignancies as based on immunologic analysis of membrane differentiation antigens. *Jpn. J. Clin. Oncol.*, 12:73–90.
21. Usui, T., Kita, K., Kimura, K., Uehara, N., Sawada, H., Takatsuki, K., and Uchino, H. (1979): Acid phosphatase and acid α-naphthyl acetate esterase activities in various lymphoid cells. *Jpn. J. Clin. Oncol.*, 9(Suppl.):459–468.
22. Waldron, J. A., Leech, J. H., Glick, A. D., Flexner, J. M., and Collins, R. D. (1977): Malignant lymphoma of peripheral T-lymphocyte origin. *Cancer*, 40:1604–1617.

Pathogenesis of Leukemias and Lymphomas:
Environmental Influences, edited by
I. T. Magrath, G. T. O'Conor, and B. Ramot.
Raven Press, New York © 1984.

Analysis of Immunologic Phenotype of Non-Hodgkin's Lymphomas at the National Cancer Institute

Jeffrey Cossman and Elaine S. Jaffe

Hematopathology Section, Laboratory of Pathology, National Cancer Institute, National Institutes of Health, Bethesda, Maryland 20205

During the past 10 years, our laboratory has undertaken a study of the immunologic phenotypes of malignant lymphomas and related disorders. We have explored the relationship of immunologic phenotype to the classification and clinical behavior of these diseases. These studies have the additional benefit of furthering our understanding of the biology of both the lymphoma cells and their normal, nonneoplastic counterparts, the lymphocytes. A variety of laboratory techniques have been applied to viable cells in suspension and to frozen tissue sections. The recent introduction of monoclonal antibodies directed at the cell surface membrane determinants of lymphocytes, coupled with sensitive fluorescence analysis on the fluorescence-activated cell sorter, has proved to be a powerful tool that allows us to determine the phenotype of the non-Hodgkin's lymphomas in great detail. Armed with this technology, virtually all non-Hodgkin's lymphomas studied in our laboratory can be classified immunologically into T-cell, B-cell, and, rarely, true histiocytic categories.

The entire range of both childhood and adult non-Hodgkin's lymphomas is seen at the National Cancer Institute (NCI). The histologic distribution of 473 patients seen at NCI over a 22-year period was determined in a study by Garvin et al. (2) using the Rappaport classification (Table 1).

Non-Hodgkin's lymphomas with a relatively indolent (low-grade) clinical course are most nodular (follicular) lymphomas, diffuse lymphomas of well-differentiated lymphocytic (DWDL) type, and most cases of diffuse, poorly differentiated lymphocytic (DPDL) lymphomas. Nodular lymphomas have been shown to be of B-cell type by virtue of their expression of monoclonal surface membrane immunoglobulin (sIg), i.e., restriction to one light chain type, and surface complement receptors in nearly every case studied (64 of 65). The DWDL lymphomas are nearly always of B-cell type (37 of 38), and these bear monoclonal sIg, complement receptors of the C3d type (1), and an antigen (p65) found on mature T cells and thymocytes, identified by the monoclonal antibodies T101, Lyt2, and Leu1 (10 of 10 cases studied). This antigen also occurs on the leukemic cells from most cases

markedly convoluted. All cases of Burkitt's lymphoma studied in our laboratory have had B-cell markers (5).

These studies have shown that the immunologic phenotype can be determined in nearly every case of non-Hodgkin's lymphoma. Peripheral T-cell lymphomas were found to be relatively common and represented approximately 40% of diffuse, aggressive non-Hodgkin's lymphomas. By phenotypic analysis, T-cell lymphoblastic lymphomas appear to be somewhat more mature than T-cell acute lymphoblastic leukemias but are less mature than peripheral T-cell lymphomas. Finally, not all lymphoblastic lymphomas are of T-cell type, and pre-B forms of this disorder have been identified.

REFERENCES

1. Cossman, J., and Jaffe, E. S. (1981): Distribution of complement receptor subtypes in non-Hodgkin's lymphomas of B cell origin. *Blood*, 58:20–26.
2. Garvin, A. J., Simon, R., Young, R. C., DeVita, V. T., and Berard, C. W. (1980): The Rappaport classification of non-Hodgkin's lymphomas: A closer look using other proposed classifications. *Semin. Oncol.*, 7:234–243.
3. Jaffe, E. S., and Berard, C. W. (1978): Lymphoblastic lymphoma, a term rekindled with new precision. *Ann. Intern. Med.*, 89:415–417.
4. Jaffe, E. S., Strauchen, J. A., and Berard, C. W. (1982): Predictability of immunologic phenotype by morphologic criteria in diffuse aggressive non-Hodgkin's lymphomas. *Am. J. Clin. Pathol.*, 77:46–49.
5. Mann, R. B., Jaffe, E. S., Braylan, R. C., Nanba, K., Frank, M. M., Ziegler, J. L., and Berard, C. W. (1976): Non-endemic Burkitt's lymphoma: A B cell tumor related to germinal centers. *N. Engl. J. Med.*, 295:685–691.
6. Nathwani, B. N., Kim, H., and Rappaport, H. (1976): Malignant lymphoma, lymphoblastic. *Cancer*, 38:964–983.
7. Ritz, J., Pesando, J. M., Notis-McConarty, J., Lazarus, H., and Schlossman, S. H. (1980): A monoclonal antibody to human acute lymphoblastic leukemia antigen. *Nature*, 283:583–585.
8. Royston, I., Majda, J. A., Baird, S. M., Meserve, B. L., and Griffiths, J. C. (1980): Human T cell antigens defined by monoclonal antibodies: The 65,000 dalton antigen of T cells (T66) is also found on chronic lymphocytic leukemia cells bearing surface immunoglobulin. *J. Immunol.*, 125:725–731.

Pathogenesis of Leukemias and Lymphomas:
Environmental Influences, edited by
I. T. Magrath, G. T. O'Conor, and B. Ramot.
Raven Press, New York © 1984.

Geographical Variations in the Occurrence of Leukemias and Lymphomas: Summary and Comments

Gregory T. O'Conor

Office of International Affairs, National Cancer Institute, National Institutes of Health,
Bethesda, Maryland 20205

The principal objective of the first section of this volume is to provide a general overview of the geographical pathology of malignant lymphomas and leukemias in order to highlight international or regional differences that might be related to environmental factors. Such information is intended to provide a basis for planning and implementing future collaborative etiological and clinical studies.

Many of the chapters in this first section briefly review available data relating to the incidence or relative frequency of lymphomas and leukemias in different regions. The reports vary greatly in number of cases, classification system employed, and points of emphasis. This variation is, of course, expected because the authors were not instructed to report data in any fixed format, but rather to present the material currently available to them and to emphasize those aspects that appeared to be of special interest. In some instances, the data were derived from population-based registries: in others, the material reviewed represents the experience of a specific hospital or institution. Immunological markers have not been employed in most laboratories, so classification is usually based only on morphological interpretation. The detailed information from the U.S. National Cancer Institute presented by Cossman and Jaffe (Chapter 13) provides a useful data base for comparative purposes.

El-Bolkainy et al. (Chapter 2) report data from the National Cancer Institute of Cairo University, where a large number of cases of lymphoma (200 per year) and leukemia (60 per year) are seen. As a group, lymphoreticular tumors represent the third most common cancer after bladder and breast, but accurate estimates of incidence rates are not available in Egypt. Hodgkin's disease constitutes more than 70% of the lymphomas seen in children, and the mixed cellularity type is predominant. The vast majority of non-Hodgkin's lymphomas (NHL) were classified as diffuse and of the poorly differentiated lymphocytic type. In a small subset in which limited marker studies were carried out, more than 90% of NHL were characterized as of B-cell origin. Extranodal lymphomas, particularly with a gastrointestinal primary, are common. Acute lymphocytic leukemia (ALL) in children is the most common of the leukemias. Again, on the basis of a small subset tested for E rosettes and surface immunoglobulin, the great majority are thought to be non-T, non-B. This suggests that the Western pattern of ALL with an early age peak may prevail in Egypt, but further studies with monoclonal antibodies are clearly necessary.

Data from West Africa, which focus on leukemia, are presented by Williams et al. (Chapter 3). Based on review of material from the population-based tumor registry and the University Hospital in Ibadan, Nigeria, during two time periods, the authors suggest that the incidence of ALL has been significantly increasing and at a much higher rate than acute myeloid leukemia (AML). Further, the major increase occurred in young children. An attempt was made to relate this phenomenon to socioeconomic factors, but the numbers here are small, and the suggested trends require confirmation. Most cases of ALL are of the "poor risk" type, but immunological typing has not been done in the past. The disease is considered relatively rare in children in Nigeria, where Burkitt's tumor is highly endemic and is by far the most common tumor in patients under the age of 15. AML with chloroma, and generally occurring with the same age distribution as Burkitt's tumor, is mentioned as another malignancy occurring with unusual frequency in Nigeria. Finally, two types of chronic lymphocytic leukemia (CLL) are identified. One seen in older individuals, but with a male predominance, is not different from that seen in the West. A second type is prevalent in middle-aged and younger women. It is often associated with immunodeficiency, sometimes with pregnancy, and it appears to run a more benign course than CLL in older persons.

The pattern of lymphomas and leukemias in East Africa is described by Owor (Chapter 4), based on data from the Kampala Cancer Registry, Uganda. Here too, Burkitt's tumor is still the most common lymphoma, but the total number of cases may have decreased some in recent years. This decrease is difficult to assess because of recent political upheavals in Uganda. The relative frequency of Burkitt's tumor, Hodgkin's disease, other lymphomas, and leukemias has not changed significantly over the last 20 years, and the pattern of other developing countries is maintained—that is, a paucity of ALL and CLL and a predominance of diffuse lymphomas. As in Nigeria, ALL may be increasing in incidence; further, CLL in young and middle-aged women also occurs in Uganda.

In one of two reports from India, Shanta et al. (Chapter 5) review material from the Cancer Institute of Madras. Lymphomas and leukemias are relatively uncommon, constituting only 2.7% of all malignancies treated at the Institute. They are, however, common in children and rank second in relative frequency after retinoblastoma. Information relating to age and sex distribution, presentation, histologic type, and socioeconomic status and religion are presented. In Hodgkin's disease, the mixed cellularity type is prevalent and nodular sclerosis is rare. Most NHL are diffuse, and no cases of Burkitt's tumor are seen.

Seghal et al. (Chapter 6) focus mainly on multiple myeloma and other plasma cell dyscrasias seen in Chandigarh in northern India. Seghal has studied over 200 cases seen at the Nehru Hospital over a 13-year period. Her data suggest that these diseases may occur at a much younger age than in Western countries and that patients present at a more advanced stage. No other unusual aspects were documented, apart from an increased frequency of IgD myeloma consistent with the higher serum IgD levels of Indians. The data on other lymphomas and leukemias are limited but do indicate that, as in other developing countries, Hodgkin's disease occurs more frequently in children and that there is a deficiency of the nodular sclerosis type. With NHL, an extranodal presentation is common. Chronic myeloid leukemia is by far the commonest leukemia, but in India the frequency of acute leukemias varies dramatically from region to region. CLL is generally rare, but it appears that the form of CLL noted in middle-aged women in Nigeria also occurs in northern India.

Bosco et al. (Chapter 7) provide information on lymphoid malignancies seen at the University Hospital, Kuala Lumpur, Malaysia. This is a particularly interesting area because the inhabitants include three ethnic groups (Malay, Chinese, and Indian) and marked socioeconomic changes are occurring in the eastern part of the country. Diffuse histiocytic or poorly differentiated lymphomas accounted for nearly all lymphomas. Nodular lymphomas, chronic lymphocytic leukemia and Burkitt's lymphoma were rare. Of interest is the presence of an early age peak in acute lymphoblastic leukemia, and the confirmation that "common acute" lymphoblastic leukemia does occur. The overall incidence of T cell acute lymphoblastic leukemia was 31%.

Suri et al. (Chapter 8) describe detailed studies, including immunologic markers, on a series of patients with lymphoproliferative disease recently admitted to the Singapore General Hospital. Lymphomas and leukemias of both B- and T-cell type have been identified, but numbers are yet too small to make any geographical comparisons. Functional studies will be routinely employed in the work-up of all patients in the future. Some general comments on lymphomas and leukemias in Singapore are made, based on the Cancer Registry data. The incidence of Hodgkin's disease is low, NHL are predominantly diffuse, and extranodal presentation is common. Common ALL is relatively rare, but T-cell ALL with mediastinal tumor is often seen in adolescent children and young adults. CLL is rare.

In recent years, the B- and T-cell study group in Japan has provided much new information on leukemias and lymphomas. Suchi and Tajima (Chapter 9) review the published data and discuss in detail some of the epidemiological characteristics of adult T-cell leukemia-lymphoma (ATLL). Hodgkin's disease and nodular NHL are quite uncommon in Japan. Diffuse, large-cell lymphomas are predominant and have usually been called reticulum cell sarcoma. It is now evident that a high proportion of these are T-cell tumors, called adult T-cell leukemia-lymphoma (ATLL), with well-defined clinical and pathological characteristics, and are associated with the recently isolated type C retrovirus, HTLV. ATLL has a definite geographical distribution pattern in Japan. These tumors also occur in the so-called nonendemic areas of Japan, but here most diffuse, large-cell lymphomas are of B-cell type. Suchi and Tajima describe seroepidemiological studies that strongly suggest that the putative virus (HTLV) is horizontally transmitted. Similar or identical HTLV-associated tumors have been described in Blacks from the Caribbean, and Catovsky et al. (Chapter 12) provide detailed histologic and ultrastructural descriptions of the tumor cells.

The Instituto Nacional de Enfermedades Neoplasicas in Lima is the principal institution to which patients with cancer from all of Peru are referred. Most of the population served by the hospital, however, comes from the coastal areas. Misad et al. (Chapter 10) present data on 1,948 cases of lymphoma and leukemia seen during a 10-year period. These diseases constitute a high proportion of malignancies in children and are exceeded only by cancer of the cervix and breast in adults. ALL is the most common type of leukemia, and 67% of all acute leukemias occur before the age of 15. Unlike in the United States, however, there is a slight female preponderance. Hodgkin's disease has a high incidence in children, as in other developing countries, but nodular sclerosis is the predominant histologic type reported in Peru. Misad et al. state that in this category were included cases of the so-called cellular phase of nodular sclerosis. Since this is in distinct contrast to reports from other developing countries, it is a point worthy of further study. In the NHL group, again, the nodular architecture is rarely seen, and extranodal presentation of the diffuse lymphomas is common. In Peru, a lymphoma with unusual morphologic characteristics and presenting in the nose and nasal and paranasal spaces occurs with a high frequency. It is estimated that this nasal lymphoma accounts for up to 8% of all lymphoreticular neoplasms in Peru, and its occurrence appears to be limited to two regions of the country.

Gibbs et al. (Chapter 11) provide information from Jamaica. Although there is an excellent Cancer Registry in Kingston, the data on lymphomas and leukemias suffer from the outdated classification systems used. Therefore, the report is limited to data on patients seen at the Hematology Service of the University Hospital of the West Indies over a period of nine and a half years. There were 48 cases of NHL with a paucity of the nodular type and 34 cases of Hodgkin's disease, most of which were classified as nodular sclerosis or mixed cellularity. This is similar to the Peruvian data, but differs from most other developing countries. The proportion of children with Hodgkin's disease was also lower than expected for a developing country. Twenty-three cases of active lymphoblastic leukemia were studied, and 34 cases of CLL. This also is unusual for a developing country. Most of the ALL cases were in children, and most of the CLL cases were in patients over 60 years old. Immunological marker studies were not done on this case material but, in view of the recent report of several cases of ATLL from the Carribean area, characterized in detail by Catovsky et al. (Chapter 12), such studies will be imperative for the future.

A few general conclusions can be drawn from these reports, which are representative of the best data available on a worldwide basis. NHL are high-incidence tumors in Egypt (and perhaps in other Middle Eastern countries) and are relatively uncommon or even rare in Asia, e.g., India, Japan, and Singapore. The very high frequency of Burkitt's tumor in children accounts for the elevated incidence rates in Black Africa. In Latin America, the picture is less clear in terms of relative incidence, and countries and population groups probably differ greatly.

In all the developing countries, the NHL are predominantly diffuse, the nodular variety being quite remarkable by its rarity. Whether this reflects a more rapid disease progression from nodular to diffuse and/or delay in diagnosis, or whether it represents a deficit in a specific disease entity common in more developed countries remains a matter of speculation requiring further studies. Another aspect of NHL in developing countries is the age distribution (more frequent in children) and the high prevalence of extranodal presentation.

The pattern of Hodgkin's disease likewise differs in the developing countries and in some ways is similar to NHL: increased incidence in children and histologic types carrying an unfavorable prognosis. In India, however, and in Japan, Hodgkin's disease, like NHL, has a low incidence rate, while in Peru and Jamaica the nodular sclerosing type predominates.

In most of the developing countries, an early age peak in ALL is not seen, and CLL, as well as acute leukemia, is uncommon in the elderly. Considerably more work is needed to establish geographical patterns more clearly, but the available data, although incomplete, do suggest important differences. This would seem to be a priority area for new research and an area where special efforts should be made.

Situations of particular interest that are highlighted in this first section of this book include CLL in young or middle-aged women in both East and West Africa and in northern India; ML with chloroma in African children; nasal lymphoma in Peru; and ATLL in Japan. It is quite evident from these reports that there are indeed many important international and interregional differences in the epidemiological and clinical characteristics of lymphoreticular neoplasms. A better definition of the various types of lymphomas and leukemias, using modern laboratory techniques, would undoubtedly serve to better our understanding of those differences that are now recognized and to identify others. This would permit, in turn, the formulation of new and testable etiological hypotheses suitable for collaborative research.

The regions, centers, and/or institutions represented by the authors in this section were well chosen in that they have the clinical material and other resources on which to confidently base future collaborative investigations.

Pathogenesis of Leukemias and Lymphomas:
Environmental Influences, edited by
I. T. Magrath, G. T. O'Conor, and B. Ramot.
Raven Press, New York © 1984.

Subtypes of Acute Lymphoblastic Leukemia: Implications for the Pathogenesis and Epidemiology of Leukemia

Melvyn F. Greaves

Membrane Immunology Laboratory, Imperial Cancer Research Fund,
London WC2A 3PX, England

IDENTIFICATION OF THE MAJOR SUBCLASSES OF ACUTE LYMPHOBLASTIC LEUKEMIA

Since 1975, we have been able to subdivide acute lymphoblastic leukemia (ALL) into four subtypes (6): common (cALL), thymic (T-ALL), B-ALL, and null (or unclassified) ALL. These four subclasses have distinct immunological and enzymatic phenotypes (Table 1). These antigenic markers were previously detected with absorbed heteroantisera (e.g., rabbit) and indirect immunofluorescence; visualization was by microscopy or flow cytometry (6). Since 1980, monoclonal antibodies have come into routine use for cell typing (8,15). This development has been important, because well-standardized reagents can now be made more generally available. Enzyme markers (Table 1) were evaluated by cytochemistry [acid phosphatase (AP)] or enzymatic assay on cell extracts [hexosaminidase isoenzyme, intermediate peak (Hex-I); adenosine deaminase (ADA); terminal deoxynucleotidyl transferase (TdT)]. Since 1979, immunofluorescence assays for nuclear TdT have become routine (1).

In the United Kingdom, the differential diagnosis of ALL subtypes was established in 1975 as part of the Medical Research Council chemotherapy trials for ALL (9). Other centers not participating in these trials have also referred ALL and other leukemia samples to our laboratory; these samples, together with the trials input, have enabled a very large number of leukemias to be evaluated in a single center. Heparinized marrow and blood are sent by first-class mail, railway delivery service, taxi, or other transport systems, and most (approximately 90%) samples from outside London are received within 24 hours. Samples are also frequently stored over weekends at 4°C and are satisfactorily tested by the following week. Whenever enough cells are available, they are stored in a liquid nitrogen cell bank. Slides for TdT are made as soon as possible but stored at −20°C (unfixed) for up to 1 week before being stained as a batch. Over the past 2 years, the sample input into this diagnostic service has averaged 50 per week, with samples coming from

TABLE 1. *Major phenotypes of subclasses of acute lymphoblastic leukemia (ALL)*

	Membrane antigens[h]				Enzymes			
ALL subclass	cALL antigen	HLA-DR (Ia) antigen[a]	T-cell antigens E-rosettes	SmIg[b]	Hex-I[c]	TdT[d]	AP[e]	ADA[f,g]
Common	+	+	−	−	+	+	−	L
T-ALL	−	−	+	−	−	+	+	H
B-ALL	−	+	−	+	−	−	−	L
Null	−	+	−	−	−	+	−	L

[a]Human leukocyte antigen.
[b]Surface membrane immunoglobulin.
[c]Intermediate peak of hexosaminidase isoenzyme.
[d]Terminal deoxynucleotidyl transferase.
[e]Acid phosphatase.
[f]Adenosine deaminase.
[g]L = low,   H = high.
[h]These represent the dominant phenotypes observed in these subclasses; individual markers are not necessarily as exclusive or invariant as indicated by + and − signs. Thus, only 90% of T-ALLs have focal acid phosphatase staining. Some 10% of T-ALL and a higher proportion of thymic lymphomas are cALL-antigen+. A variety of antisera against T-cell antigens have been used, especially with the more recent introduction of monoclonal antibodies. Sheep erythrocyte (E) rosettes are positive (more than 20% of blasts) in approximately 90% of T ALLs. The same phenotype is usually observed in marrow and blood but may alter in relapse (10).

all over the United Kingdom as well as Eire and Denmark. A formal arrangement for feedback on each tested sample is available; also, many physicians telephone for immediate results.

In many, probably most, cases, immunological subtyping makes little if any contribution to patient management besides confirming the hematological diagnosis. However, in a proportion of cases, the precise and objective classification of subtypes does have a clinical impact, e.g., identification of T-ALL for U.K. ALL trials, distinction between ALL and acute myeloid leukemia (AML), and identification of ALL phenotypes within acute undifferentiated leukemia or chronic granulocytic leukemia blast crisis. More recently it has become possible to use particular markers or combinations of markers (14) to detect individual leukemic cells in small numbers (i.e., residual or reemerging disease). For example, anti-TdT and/or anti-cALL can be used to detect extramedullary leukemic cells in the central nervous system or testis, and combinations (i.e., simultaneous or double staining) of anti-thymic monoclonals with TdT can detect T leukemic cells in marrow. Unfortunately, anti-cALL and/or TdT cannot be easily used to monitor marrows in ALL, since these reagents react with normal lymphocyte progenitors in this site (10).

INCIDENCES OF THE ALL SUBCLASSES: ASSOCIATIONS WITH AGE, SEX, AND PROGNOSIS

Tables 2 and 3 show the breakdown of ALL subclasses during two periods— 1975 to 1979 (conventional antisera) and 1980 to December 1981 (monoclonal

TABLE 2. *Acute lymphoblastic leukemia (ALL) subtypes, 1975–1979[a]*

ALL subtype	Number (%)	Male	Female	Male-female ratio
Common	397 (73.2)	223	174	1.3 : 1
T-ALL	73 (13.5)	60	13	4.6 : 1
Null ALL	68 (12.5)	41	27	1.5 : 1
B-ALL	4 (0.7)	4	0	—

[a]Typed with "conventional" antisera and enzymatic TdT. Data from (9). All patients in this study were 20 years old or younger.

TABLE 3. *Acute lymphoblastic leukemia (ALL) subtypes, February 1980–December 1981[a]*

ALL subtype	Number (%)	Male	Female	Male-female ratio
Common	950 (74.9)	534	416	1.28 : 1
T-ALL	145 (11.4)	114	31	3.68 : 1
Null ALL	153 (12.1)	97	56	1.73 : 1
B-ALL	21 (1.7)	16	5	3.20 : 1

[a]Typed with monoclonal antibodies (6). Patients of all ages are included.

antibodies). The results are essentially the same during the two periods despite the change of reagents and some alterations to assay protocols. In addition to the patients listed, approximately 15% of the samples referred were not adequately assessed. In half of those cases, the sample itself was too small or in poor condition; in the other 5 to 7%, no subclassification was possible despite a hematological diagnosis of ALL. Those cases were either non-reactive with all markers except TdT or were even TdT-negative. More recent investigations with anti-T monoclonals indicate that at least some of these previously unallocated cases are probably very immature T-ALLs that lack most T-cell markers, including erythrocyte (E) rosettes. Ten untreated patients typed as cALL of the set of more than 1,200 listed in Table 4 were diagnosed and treated as having AML. All but one case was considered on review to be ALL or a mixed ALL/AML.

Some cases typed immunologically as null ALL (DR$^+$, TdT$^+$) were diagnosed as AML. In a 15-month period of follow-up on such cases (January 1980 to May 1981), 34 such cases were detected from 313 provisionally referred as AML (or simply acute leukemia) and 955 referred as ALL. None of these cases were diagnosed as ALL, and none were cALL-positive. Review of the data indicated that some of these cases were a mixed lymphoid-myeloid population and others were TdT$^+$ cells with myeloid enzymology (13). These curious cases represent a max-

TABLE 4. *Biological features of two subtypes of acute lymphoblastic leukemia*

Biological feature	B-precursor ALL	T-precursor ALL
Dominant phenotype	TdT[+] HLA-DR[+] T[-] B[+] cALL[+] Hex-I[+]	TdT[+] HLA-DR[-] T[+] B[-] cALL[-] Hex-I[-]
Ig genes	mu ± kappa/ lambda rearranged[a]	No or minimal rearrangement
Growth fraction	Low	High
Karyotype	Hyperdiploidy common	Pseudodiploidy common
Likely cellular origin	Bone marrow B lineage progenitor or stem cell	Marrow or thymic (subcapsular) T lineage progenitor or stem cell
Diagnostic subtypes	cALL Pre-B ALL Null ALL	T-ALL
Alternative diagnoses	AUL[b] Ph[1+] ALL[c] NHL (rare)	T-NHL

[a]Approximately one-third of B-precursor ALLs synthesize mu chains and were originally referred to as "pre-B ALL" (11,21). All B-precursor ALLs have rearranged/recombined Variable, Diversity, and Joining (VDJ)-mu heavy chain genes and may in addition have rearranged kappa or lambda light chain genes (5).
[b]Acute undifferentiated leukemia.
[c]Ph[1+] = presence of the Philadelphia chromosome.

imum of 5% of AML. The combination of cALL antigen and TdT provides an unequivocal diagnosis of ALL.

The breakdown of ALL subclasses indicates the rarity of B-ALL, which in any case is probably a misnomer. B-ALL probably represents a disseminated non-Hodgkin's lymphoma (NHL) (6,17) and in children usually has a Burkitt-like/L3 morphology. Note that apart from this association with L3, the immunological subgroups show no correspondence with the French-American-British subtypes, nor is there any strong association with para-aminosalicylic acid staining (9). As reported before in a number of small series of patients, there is a marked preponderance of boys in the T-ALL subgroup (Tables 2 and 3). Whether this interesting bias reflects hormonal effects or X-chromosome-linked immune response defects (see D. Purtilo et al., *this volume*) is unknown.

The four subclasses also show significant associations with initial white cell counts, mediastinal mass and organomegaly, and hemoglobin levels (4,9). As anticipated from these associations, the immunologically defined subtypes show strong prognostic correlations with a rank order of favorable prognosis (i.e., duration of first remission): cALL >null-ALL >T-ALL >B-ALL (6,9). These are overlapping rather than discrete prognostic subgroupings. Within the subgroups (e.g., cALL), clinical response is markedly heterogeneous and is linked strongly to initial white cell count; overall, immunological subtypes have little or no statistically significant prognostic correlation *independent* of white cell count (9). An exception to this latter conclusion may be infrequent cases of "low-count" T-ALL and B-ALL. A model linking immunological subtype growth rate and clinical response has been proposed (7,9).

The relative proportions of the four ALL subclasses given in Tables 2 and 3 disguise a potentially important age association of those leukemias. Figure 1 illustrates the numbers of each subclass detected as a function of patient age, and Fig. 2 shows the relative frequency of the subclasses in relation to age. Clearly, age has a marked impact on ALL subclass distribution. Relative frequency is, however, very misleading; Fig. 3 provides a more appropriate representation of the data in terms of the actual number of cases typed. The typical peak incidence of ALL seen in Europe and the United States is a distinctive feature of cALL, although patients up to the age of 80 can have cALL (Fig. 1). T-ALL is not, as suggested by the relative incidence (Fig. 2), a disease of adolescence but is distributed fairly uniformly between the ages of 2 and 15 (Figs. 1 and 3). T-ALL in adults over 35 is very rare, but six cases were recorded in this series. They had unequivocal T-ALL phenotypes and, in three cases, mediastinal masses. Null ALL has a curious distribution. Although ALL is rare in babies less that 12 months old, when it does occur it is mostly null ALL (Figs. 2 and 3); after this age, null ALL remains at a similar low incidence, although proportionately it appears to increase in older adults (Fig. 3) because of the decrease in incidence of cALL.

Biological Diversity and Natural History of ALL

The striking age associations of ALL subtypes are intriguing although at present difficult to interpret. It is probably significant that ALL (leaving aside B-ALL) as indicated by immunological phenotype is a leukemia of T- and B-cell *progenitors*, i.e., the "pre-T" or "pre-B" differentiation compartments (Table 4). In contrast to childhood-associated ALL, malignancies of *mature* lymphoid cells, e.g., chronic lymphocytic leukemia (CLL), B-NHL, myeloma, and Sézary syndrome, are predominantly diseases of adults. Table 5 lists an analysis of immunological phenotype in 174 consecutive cases of T-cell-lineage malignancy classified clinically and typed by monoclonal antibody studies into subgroups corresponding to stages of intrathymic differentiation or postthymic, mature T-cell subsets (11,19). Note that ALL and childhood T-NHL (convoluted, lymphoblastic lymphoma with a mediastinal mass, or "Sternberg's sarcoma") were exclusively of thymic phenotype, whereas the *adult* leukemias/lymphomas—T-CLL, T-prolymphocytic leukemia, T-cutaneous lymphoma/leukemia, T-NHL (no mediastinal mass), and T-lymphosarcoma cell leukemia (T-LCL), corresponding to Japanese adult T-cell leukemia (ATL) (2)— were exclusively of mature T phenotypes. It is also of considerable interest that

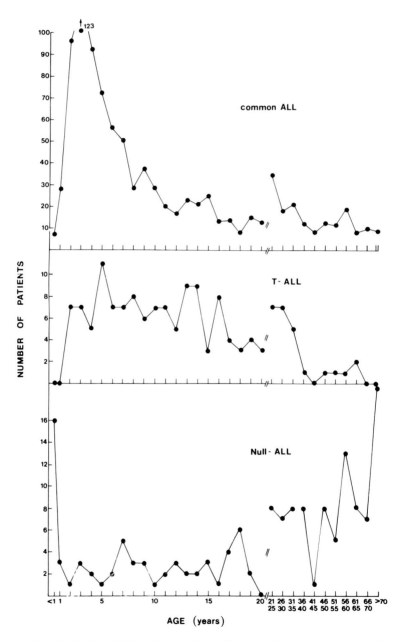

FIG. 1. Age distribution of ALL subtypes. Note differences in vertical scales and break in horizontal scales.

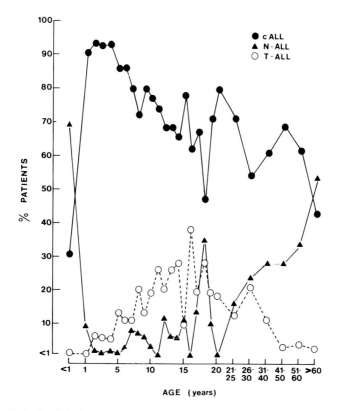

FIG. 2. Relative proportions of ALL subtypes as a function of age.

the group of six patients listed as T-LCL (or ATL) were all Negroid, first-generation immigrants from the Caribbean and, in contrast to the other T-cell leukemias listed, all six had high-titer antibodies to the human retrovirus, human T-cell leukemia virus (HTLV) (18; W. A. Blattner et al. and M. S. Reitz et al., *this volume*). This suggests a striking association between cell type "at risk" of malignancy and age, with precursor or progenitor lymphocytes at risk during early development (when the immune system is "expanding"), and mature, immunocompetent lymphocytes at risk with advancing age. Another perspective on this association views ALL as a clonal defect in development and differentiation of lymphocytes and mature lymphoid malignancies (or myeloma) as reflecting, or being associated with, defective immunoregulatory networks. Note that a similar age association is observed with other cancers. The other common pediatric tumors, such as neuroblastoma, Ewing's sarcoma, Wilms' tumor, and connective tissue sarcomas (18), are exceedingly rare in adults, whereas most epithelial carcinomas are absent or very rare in infants (Fig. 4). Once again the cell types involved in those different malignancies are probably a reflection of proliferating cells at risk during particular periods of growth or prolonged periods of adult life (the latter providing the possibility for a

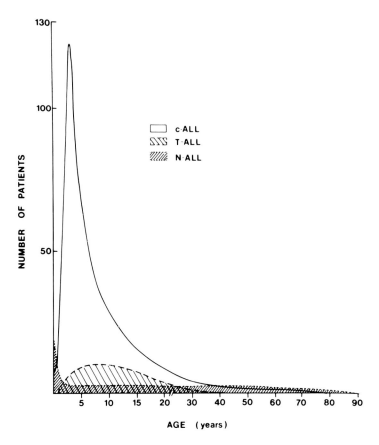

FIG. 3. Comparative age distribution of ALL subtypes: Numerical incidence as a function of age.

sequence of sequential or "multiple-hit" rare events). Obviously the etiological agents and pathogenic mechanisms involved in these two age-associated groups of cancers could be quite distinct.

Leukemic Subtypes, Genetics, and Geography

Extensive immunological investigations of ALL now permit the conclusion that ALL is in fact at least two quite distinct biological and clinical entities representing leukemic counterparts of T-cell (T-ALL) or B-cell (cALL, null ALL) precursors (Table 4) clonally expanded and in apparent maturation arrest. It may be possible to induce further differentiation of ALL cells *in vitro* by compounds such as phorbol ester (3) as described previously with other animal and human leukemia cell lines (20). The objective recognition of this diversity emphasizes the need to reexamine epidemiological links in this and other leukemias. The remarkable link between

TABLE 5. *Phenotypic heterogeneity of T-cell leukemia (numbers of patients)*

T-lineage subgroup[a]	Diagnostic subgroup						
	ALL	T-NHL(c)[b]	Cutaneous lymphoma[c]	CLL[d]	PLL[e]	LBL[f] NHL	LCL[g]
T precursors							
Early/pre-T(1)	11	0	0	0	0	0	0
Early/pre-T(2)	17	1	0	0	0	0	0
Early/pre-T(3)	73	5	0	0	0	0	0
Cortical thymocyte	6	11	0	0	0	0	0
Mature T							
"Helper/inducer"	0	0	17	5	7	3	4
"Suppressor/ cytotoxic"	0	0	1	6	1	2	0
Uncertain	0	0	0	0	2	0	2
Total	107	17	18	11	10	5	6

[a]Identified by a series of monoclonal antibodies plus E rosettes and TdT (10).
[b]Thymic non-Hodgkin's lymphoma in children.
[c]Diagnosed as mycosis fungoides or Sézary syndrome in a leukemic phase.
[d]T-chronic lymphocytic leukemia.
[e]T-prolymphocytic leukemia.
[f]Lymphoblastic lymphoma.
[g]T-lymphosarcoma cell leukemia or adult T-cell leukemia (2).
Modified from Greaves et al. (10).

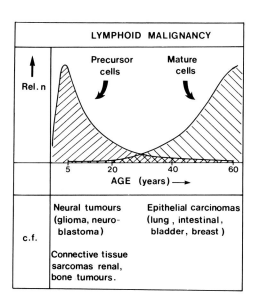

FIG. 4. A summary view of the association of immature and mature lymphoid malignancies with age. c.f., compare with; Rel. n, relative number.

HTLV and mature T-cell leukemia of a particular variety illustrates what specific etiological and epidemiological associations may exist.

Different subtypes of ALL may have distinctly different incidence rates in different parts of the world, reflecting the influence of genetic and/or environmental factors. This has already been hinted at (21; various chapters in this volume). To examine this question systematically, we have established an international collaboration to investigate ALL subtypes in different parts of the world. At present, 11 centers are involved in this study (Fig. 5), in which we have incorporated a standardized panel of monoclonal "typing" antibodies (Table 6) and assay protocols. We anticipate that further centers will join the collaborative group and that these studies will enable us to determine with some accuracy the geographic and ethnic variation in incidence of ALL subtypes.

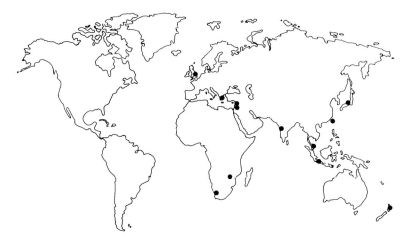

FIG. 5. Leukemic subtyping international survey. *Large dots* show locations of participating centers: London, Athens, Jerusalem and Chaim Sheba (Israel), Johannesburg and Cape Town (South Africa), Bombay (India), Kuala Lumpur (Malaysia), Jakarta (Indonesia), Taipei (Taiwan), Kyoto (Japan), and Auckland (New Zealand).

TABLE 6. *A standardized reagent panel of ALL typing*

		Result		
Reagents	cALL	T-ALL or T-NHL[a]	Null ALL	Mature B leukemia (B-ALL) or disseminated B lymphoma
J-5 anti-cALL	+	− (or +)	−	−
DA-2 anti-HLA-DR	+	−	+	+
WT-1 anti-T ("pan-T")	−	+[b]	−	−
OKT 11 anti-T (anti-E rosette receptor)	−	+[b]	−	−
E (sheep) rosettes	−	+[b]	−	−
Anti-Ig, kappa, lambda light chain	−	−	−	+
Anti-TdT	+	+	+	−

[a]Retest with T-subset monoclonals (cf. OKT 3, 4, 6, 8).
[b]Reactivity in one or more of these three assays required for T-cell typing.

REFERENCES

1. Bollum, F. J. (1979): Terminal deoxynucleotidyl transferase as a hematopoietic cell marker. *Blood*, 54:1203–1215.
2. Catovsky, D., Greaves, M. F., Rose, M., Galton, D. A. G., Goolden, A. W. G., McCluskey, D. R., White, J. M., Lampert, I., Bourikas, G., Ireland, R., Brownell, A. I., Bridges, J. M., Blattner, W. A., and Gallo, R. C. (1982): Adult T-cell lymphoma-leukaemia in Blacks from the West Indies. *Lancet*, 1:639–643.
3. Delia, D., Greaves, M. F., Newman, R. A., Sutherland, D. R., Minowada, J., Kung, P., and Goldstein, G. (1982): Modulation of T leukaemic cell phenotype with phorbol ester. *Int. J. Cancer*, 29:23–31.
4. Dow, L. W., Borella, L., Sen, L., Aur, R. J. A., George, S. L., Mauer, A. M., and Simone, J. V. (1977): Initial prognostic factors and lymphoblast-erythrocyte rosette formation in 109 children with acute lymphoblastic leukemia. *Blood*, 50:671–682.
5. Ford, A., Molgard, H., Greaves, M. F., and Gould, H. (1983): Immunoglobulin gene organisation and expression in haemopoietic stem cell leukemia. *EMBO Journal (in press)*.
6. Greaves, M. F. (1981): Analysis of the clinical and biological significance of lymphoid phenotypes in acute leukemia. *Cancer Res.*, 41:4752–4766.
7. Greaves, M. F. (1981): *Biology of Acute Lymphoblastic Leukaemia*. 16th Annual Guest Lecture. Leukaemia Research Fund, London.
8. Greaves, M. F., Delia, D., Robinson, J., Sutherland, R., and Newman, R. (1981): Exploitation of monoclonal antibodies: A Who's Who of haemopoietic malignancy. *Blood Cells*, 7:257–280.
9. Greaves, M. F., Janossy, G., Peto, J., and Kay, H. (1981): Immunologically defined subclasses of acute lymphoblastic leukaemia in children: Their relationship to presentation features and prognosis. *Br. J. Haematol.*, 48:179–197.
10. Greaves, M. F., Paxton, A., Janossy, G., Pain, C., Johnson, S., and Lister, T. A. (1980): Acute lymphoblastic leukaemia associated antigen. III. Alterations in expression during treatment and in relapse. *Leuk. Res.*, 4:1–14.
11. Greaves, M. F., Rao, J., Hariri, G., Verbi, W., Catovsky, D., Kung, P., and Goldstein, G. (1981): Phenotypic heterogeneity and cellular origins of T cell malignancies. *Leuk. Res.*, 5:281–299.
12. Greaves, M., Verbi, W., Vogler, L., Cooper, M., Ellis, R., Ganeshaguru, K., Hoffbrand, V., Janossy, G., and Bollum, F. J. (1979): Antigenic and enzymatic phenotypes of the pre-B subclass of acute lymphoblastic leukaemia. *Leuk. Res.*, 3:353–362.
13. Jani, P., Verbi, W., Greaves, M. F., Bevan, D., and Bollum, F. (1983): How selective is terminal deoxynucleotidyl transferase for lymphoid lineage leukemias? *Leuk. Res.*, 7:17–29.
14. Janossy, G., Bollum, F. J., Bradstock, K. F., and Ashley, J. (1980): Cellular phenotypes of normal and leukemic hemopoietic cells determined by analysis with selected antibody combinations. *Blood*, 56:430–441.
15. Knapp, W., editor (1981): *Leukemia Markers.*, Academic Press, New York.
16. Korsmeyer, S. J., Hieter, P. A., Ravetch, J. V., Poplack, D. G., Waldmann, T. A., and Leder, P. (1981): Developmental hierarchy of immunoglobulin gene rearrangements in human leukemic pre-B-cells. *Proc. Natl. Acad. Sci. USA*, 78:7096–7100.
17. Magrath, I., and Ziegler, J. L. (1980): Bone marrow involvement in Burkitt's lymphoma and its relationship to acute B-cell leukaemia. *Leuk. Res.*, 4:33–59.
18. Marsden, H. B., and Steward, J. K., editors (1976): *Recent Results in Cancer Research, Vol. 13: Tumours in Children*. Springer-Verlag, New York.
19. Reinherz, E. L., Kung, P. C., Goldstein, G., Levey, R. H., and Schlossman, S. F. (1980): Discrete stages of human intrathymic differentiation: Analysis of normal thymocytes and leukemic lymphoblasts of T-cell lineage. *Proc. Natl. Acad. Sci. USA*, 77:1588–1592.
20. Sachs, L. (1978): Control of normal cell differentiation and the phenotypic reversion of malignancy in myeloid leukaemia. *Nature*, 274:535–539.
21. Sinniah, D., and Peng, L. H. (1981): Malaysian childhood leukemia: A 13 year review at the University Hospital, Kuala Lumpur. *Leuk. Res.*, 5:271–278.
22. Vogler, L. B., Crist, W. M., Bockman, D. E., Pearl, E. R., Lawton, A. R., and Cooper, M. D. (1978): Pre-B-cell leukemia: A new phenotype of childhood lymphoblastic leukaemia. *N. Engl. J. Med.*, 298:872–878.

*Pathogenesis of Leukemias and Lymphomas:
Environmental Influences*, edited by
I. T. Magrath, G. T. O'Conor, and B. Ramot.
Raven Press, New York © 1984.

Observations on Lymphatic Malignancies in Israel

*B. Ramot, *I. Ben-Bassat, and **M. Modan

*Institute of Hematology and **Epidemiology, Chaim Sheba Medical Center,
Tel-Hashomer 52621, and Sackler School of Medicine, Tel-Aviv University, Israel*

INFLUENCE OF ENVIRONMENTAL AND GENETIC FACTORS ON LYMPHATIC MALIGNANCIES

It is well known that the incidence of various malignancies, including leukemias and lymphomas, differs in various populations around the world. There are probably multiple causes for such differences, including both environmental and genetic factors. The role of these factors is exemplified by the differences in the incidence of gastric tumors in Japan and in Japanese living in the United States, the high incidence of esophageal tumors around the Caspian littoral, hepatomas in Orientals, and lung cancer in smokers, to cite just a few of many examples.

In the field of leukemias and lymphomas, it is quite surprising that the incidence rates of childhood leukemia in various populations in the Western world are very close, ranging from 4 to 5 per 100,000. Acute leukemia is the most common childhood malignancy in the Western world, whereas in Africa the most prevalent childhood tumor is Burkitt's lymphoma, which has a similar or even greater incidence than acute lymphoblastic leukemia (ALL) in the West. Acute leukemia is rare in Africa. The age peaks of childhood acute leukemia in various countries show clearly that the peak at 2 to 5 years of age appeared in the 1920s in England, in the 1940s in the United States, and in the 1960s in Japan. This early age peak, which has not yet been observed in Africa, was also absent, until recently, in American Blacks (5) and is not present in T-cell acute leukemia. The most plausible explanation for this observation is that the subtype of childhood leukemia that occurs most frequently in 2- to 5-year olds evolved in part because of industrialization and increased prosperity.

Israel is a country of particular interest for the study of environmental and genetic factors, because its population is heterogeneous in ethnic origin, family size, cultural habits, and socioeconomic status. We present here some observations on lymphatic malignancies in Israel based on our experience at the Chaim Sheba Medical Center.

NON-HODGKIN'S AND BURKITT'S LYMPHOMA IN ISRAEL

A 1963 survey on the subtypes of non-Hodgkin's lymphomas (2) revealed two outstanding features. First, a high prevalence of abdominal presentation in all the histologic subtypes of malignant lymphoma was found in Oriental Jews and Arabs, and second, intestinal lymphoma with malabsorption was observed only in young adults of Arab and Oriental Jewish ancestry. Alpha heavy chain was subsequently detected in the serum of about 25% of these patients. This clinical entity appears to be quite common in Iran, North Africa, the Cape of South Africa, and the Arab countries; however, there are no epidemiologic data on its incidence in any of these countries. Since our description of this clinical entity in the 1960s (7), the incidence of this disease in Israel has decreased markedly, so that only very few patients are seen now. We have no information about whether the high incidence of abdominal presentation of lymphomas, also observed in the 1960s, has similarly decreased. Such a study would be very important because it could clearly demonstrate the effect of environmental factors on the clinical presentation of lymphomas.

One interesting region where the effect of environmental factors can be studied is the Gaza Strip, an area with a population of about 400,000 that has been associated with Israel since 1967. In this region we have observed a dramatic change in the ratio of lymphoma to leukemia in Arab children (5): in 1972–1974, the predominant childhood malignancy was Burkitt's lymphoma and the incidence of acute leukemia was extremely low; the incidence of ALL gradually rose and is now similar to that observed in the Jewish population—4 per 100,000—with a high prevalence of T-cell leukemia (30%) (4). Burkitt's lymphomas of both the African (i.e., associated with jaw tumor) and the sporadic (American) types was observed in this population as well as in the Jewish population. The experience of A. Kimhi, T. Gotlieb-Stematsky, and B. Ramot *(unpublished)* with 25 cases of Burkitt's lymphoma seen at the center during the last eight years is summarized in Table 1. Evolution to Burkitt's cell leukemia occurred in approximately 8% of the patients, and meningeal involvement occurred in approximately 90% of children with jaw and abdominal involvement but in only 12.5% of children with abdominal involvement. Only 50% of the patients in both groups had serum antibodies to the Epstein-Barr (EB) virus; the rest had no detectable antibodies. A preliminary screening study on the acquisition of antibodies to the EB virus in Arab infants of the Gaza Strip in their first two years of life disclosed a trend toward a decrease in seroconversion from 45%

TABLE 1. *Characteristics of 25 Burkitt's lymphoma patients, Chaim Sheba Medical Center*

Characteristic	Abdominal	Abdominal and jaw
Number of patients	16	9
Ethnic group		
Jews/Arabs	5/11	4/5
Occidental/Oriental Jews	3/2	0/4
Male-female ratio	11/5	6/3
Median age	5	3
CNS involvement	2/16	8/9
Burkitt's leukemia	1/16	1/9

in 1974 to 25% in 1981. These results, although performed on a very small sample, are in line with the marked change in socioeconomic status observed in the Gaza Strip during the same period of time.

ACUTE LYMPHOBLASTIC LEUKEMIA IN ISRAEL

Cell marker studies were introduced in 1976 for the subtyping of ALL at our center. E-rosette-forming cells, surface immunoglobulins, activities of adenosine deaminase (ADA) and nucleoside phosphorylase (NP), and more recently, common ALL antigen (cALLA), TdT, and cytoplasmic immunoglobulins have been studied (4). Forty-nine of 52 consecutive patients with ALL seen in the last four years in our center were classified as follows: 16 had T-cell leukemia, 10 had common ALL, five had null cell leukemia, four had pre-B leukemia, and 14 were only partially characterized as non-B, non-T ALL in that Ig and E rosettes were negative but cALLA and T-cell antigens were not tested for.

Analysis of this series revealed the following three distinctive features: (a) a high prevalence of T-cell leukemia (30%) in both the Arab and the Jewish patients; (b) high risk factors in two-thirds of all patients, determined by a high initial white blood cell (WBC) count, unfavorable age, or T-cell characteristics (Table 2); and (c) a seemingly constant incidence of ALL among Jews, in contrast to a clear increase during the last decade in the Gaza Strip Arabs (5). These observations have prompted an ongoing countrywide study to determine if the various ethnic and socioeconomic groups in the country differ with regard to childhood lymphoma and leukemia.

Because the majority of our ALL patients are high-risk patients, additional parameters that could potentially be risk factors were studied. A summary of 57 cases

TABLE 2. *Characteristics of ALL patients, Chaim Sheba Medical Center, Israel*

Characteristic	T-ALL	Non-B, non-T ALL
Number of patients	16	33
Arabs	9	21
Jews	7	12
Children (under 16 years)	12	30
Adults	4	3
Male-female ratio[a]	4.3:1	1.1:1
Mean age[a] (years)	9.4	6.2
Median Initial WBC ($\times 10$/liter)	100	29
Number of patients with WBC ($\times 10$/liter)		
20 or less	3 (19%)	14 (42%)
21–99	4 (25%)	10 (30%)
100 or more	9 (56%)	9 (27%)
ADA activity[b]	44.8 ± 6.3^c	24.3 ± 3.2^c
NP activity[b]	16.2 ± 4.1^d	20.2 ± 3.2^d

[a]Adults (17 years or older) were excluded.
[b]In μmoles/hr/10^8 cells; mean $\pm$ standard error.
[c]$p < 0.0005$.
[d]$p = 0.2$.

of childhood ALL diagnosed and treated in our medical center up to 1978 (6) showed that none of nine Arab patients survived more than two years, where as 45% of Jews survived, indicating that the Arab children were similar in this regard to American Blacks. Therefore, a more aggressive treatment protocol was introduced in our center in 1978 (3). Sixteen patients (10 of them Arabs) with T-cell or other very high-risk ALL were treated under this protocol. All patients attained a complete remission, four succumbed from the disease during the first year, and the rest have remained in continuous remission for six to 53 months. Analysis of the patients by the ADA levels of their leukemic cells revealed that when the patients were subdivided into two groups of ADA activity, i.e., above and below the median value (40 μmoles/hr/10^8 cells), four of seven patients with high ADA activity relapsed and died, whereas all in the low-ADA-activity group are alive and in complete remission. The two groups were very similar in other risk factors except for one additional parameter, the predominance of females in the low-ADA group. This could suggest either that females with high-risk ALL do better, similar to observations in common ALL, or that ADA activity is an independent risk factor. This is not surprising, because high ADA activity is found in immature T cells (1). Studies of this enzyme could be of interest in other acute leukemias, such as the pre-B ALL group, where two of our patients had high ADA activity, similar to that observed in T cells, and the other two had very low activity, similar to that seen in B-cell leukemia. Although most workers now use monoclonal antibodies to characterize leukemic cells, we believe that ADA activity should be included in the battery of markers in order to determine its possible prognostic significance in a large group of patients.

CONCLUSION

Leukemias and lymphomas are multifactorial diseases. Good clinical observations are frequently the impetus for extensive epidemiologic, virologic, immunologic, and other studies. Our findings provide an example of clinical observations leading to the initiation of such studies, and even though no etiologic agent has yet been detected, further exploration might prove more rewarding.

REFERENCES

1. Ben-Bassat, I., Simoni, F., Holtzman, F. and Ramot, B. (1979): Adenosine deaminase activity of normal lymphocytes and leukemic cells. *Isr. J. Med. Sci.*, 15:925–927.
2. Frand, U., and Ramot, B. (1963): Malignant lymphoma: An epidemiological study. *Harefuah*, 55:23.
3. Kende, G., El Najjar, K., Ben-Bassat, I., Neuman, Y., Ballin, A., and Ramot, B. (1983): Results of treatment of high risk childhood acute lymphoblastic leukemia. *Med. Ped. Oncol.*, 11:49–52.
4. Ramot, B., Ben-Bassat, I., Many, A., Kende, G., Neuman, Y., Brok-Simoni, F., Rosenthal, E., and Orgad, S. (1982): Acute lymphoblastic leukemia subtypes in Israel: The Sheba Medical Center experience. *Leukemia Research*, 6:679–683.

5. Ramot, B., and Magrath, I. (1982): Hypothesis: The environment is a major determinant of the immunological sub-type of lymphoma and acute lymphoblastic leukaemia in children. *Br. J. Haematol.*, 50:183–189.
6. Ramot, B., Modan, M., Meerowitz, Y., Potashnick, D., Kende, G., and Berkowicz, M. (1982): Pretreatment prognostic factors and hospitalization time in childhood acute lymphoblastic leukemia. *Isr. J. Med. Sci.* 18:447–455.
7. Ramot, B., Shahin, N., and Bubis, J. J. (1965): Malabsorption syndrome in lymphoma of small intestine: A study of 13 cases. *Isr. J. Med. Sci.*, 1:221–226.

Pathogenesis of Leukemias and Lymphomas:
Environmental Influences, edited by
I. T. Magrath, G. T. O'Conor, and B. Ramot.
Raven Press, New York © 1984.

An Epidemiological Study of Childhood Acute Lymphoblastic Leukemia in the West Midlands of the United Kingdom, Showing Seasonal Variation in T-cell Disease

F. G. H. Hill, K. Al Rubei, and P. A. Trumper

Department of Haematology, The Children's Hospital, Ladywood Middleway, Ladywood, Birmingham B16 8ET, United Kingdom

Although it is apparent that survival of children treated for acute lymphoblastic leukemia (ALL) differs among centers in the same and different countries, whether these differences are related to differences in the disease, the treatment, or host and/or environmental factors has not been shown. An epidemiological study including leukemia phenotype in a mixed racial population might therefore aid in the discrimination of genetic/ethnic and environmental factors contributing to the etiology of childhood ALL.

POPULATION STUDIED

The West Midlands Health Region in the United Kingdom has a pediatric population of mixed ethnic origin of 1.1 million, and the expected incidence of pediatric acute leukemia is approximately 35 to 40 new cases per year. The Children's Hospital in Birmingham acts as the regional pediatric hemato-oncology center. Between January 1976 and December 1980, 130 children with ALL were referred for diagnosis and treatment. Age at presentation, domicile, sex, ethnic origin, and clinical, hematological, and leukemia marker data have been considered in the epidemiological analysis.

ETHNIC FACTORS

Statistics on race/ethnic origin are difficult to obtain, but data on school children aged five to 15 are available for the city of Birmingham. From this information for 1976–1981, the proportion of Caucasian to Asian to Afrocaribbean children has been determined for Birmingham to be 100:14:11. This would be the expected proportion if ALL incidence were the same in each group of children. During the six years of the study, 48 Caucasian, nine Asian, and one Afrocaribbean child from the same population sample were diagnosed as having ALL, in contrast to the expected incidence. It is not clear if there is a true increased incidence among Asian children, but incidence in the Afrocaribbean group is unexpectedly low. The Afrocaribbean child was a girl who presented with a low white cell count but with a mediastinal mass and pleural effusion, and the lymphoblasts were E-rosette-positive. She was treated on UKALL IV intensive and remains in continuous complete remission more than two years after stopping therapy.

Histograms (Fig. 1) show the age and number of Asian and Caucasian children with ALL. The age at presentation and the age of those with different marker phenotypes (data not shown) appear similar, but the number of Asian children is small. In a larger study (2) of Asian children treated in Medical Research Council trials in the United Kingdom, the age at presentation was again similar to Caucasian children. However, this study showed a poorer survival for the Asian children than for matched Caucasian controls.

In our series, 102 of 114 Caucasians, 11 of 15 Asians, and 1 Afrocaribbean had leukemia marker studies at presentation (Table 1). The percentage of cases for each phenotype appeared to be the same for both groups of children (Table 2).

LEUKEMIA MARKER STUDIES

At our own center, E rosettes to detect T cells and SmIg detected by immunofluorescence have been used to classify the leukemic phenotype. Dr. M. F. Greaves determined the common ALL antigen (cALLA) and other markers (e.g., Ia, TdT, and in some cases T cell antigens). Table 1 shows an analysis with respect to number of patients in whom marker studies were performed and a breakdown by

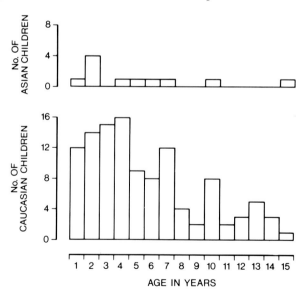

FIG. 1. Age at presentation of Asian and Caucasian children with ALL, January 1976 to December 1981.

TABLE 1. *Number of children with ALL, by phenotype, The Children's Hospital, Birmingham, 1976–1981*

Year	Total	Number with markers	Pre-T	T	Common	Null	Non-T, non-B[a]
1976	15	11	0	6	3	1	1
1977	18	11	0	0	11	0	0
1978	17	16	0	1	14	1	0
1979	20	19	0	2	13	1	3
1980	29	27	1	5	14	2	5
1981	31	30	2	2	19	2	5
Total	130	114	3	16	74	7	14

[a]cALLA status unknown.

TABLE 2. *Sex and lymphoblast phenotype of Asian and Caucasian children with ALL, The Children's Hospital, Birmingham*

Characteristic	Asians	Caucasians
Total	15	114
Male	8	68
Female	7	46
Male-female ratio	1.1 : 1	1.5 : 1
T-ALL (%)	13.3	13.1
Common ALL (%)	60	59.6
Null ALL (%)	—	5.2
Non-T, non-B[a] (%)	6.6	9.6
Unclassified (%)	13.3	11.4

[a]cALLA status unknown.

leukemia phenotype [T (E positive), pre-T (E negative, anti-positive), common, null (non-T, non-B, cALLA-negative), and non-T, non-B (cALLA unknown)].

SEASONAL VARIATION IN LEUKEMIA PHENOTYPE

Because the proportion of T-ALL and common ALL phenotypes was similar in Asian and Caucasian children, data on both groups were analyzed together.

T-cell ALL

The incidence of T-cell disease has varied in each year of the study (Table 1), with an unusual number of cases (6) in July–September 1976 and then no cases in 1977 or the early months of 1978, and with cases only in June and August in 1978 and 1979. But cases occurred in January and February and in July, August, and September in 1980 and in August and November in 1981. When these cases are pooled and analyzed by month of presentation, seasonal variation in T-cell ALL appears to be marked (Fig. 2).

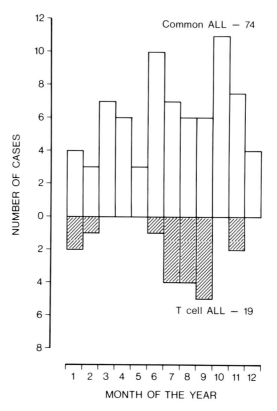

FIG. 2. Month of presentation of T-cell and common ALL, West Midlands cases, January 1976 to December 1981.

Because of the relatively small number of cases (19), data were obtained from other groups for comparison. Dr. Greaves provided the date of diagnosis on 93 children with T-cell ALL (including nine Birmingham cases) from U. K. centers. Although T-cell cases occurred in all months of the year, peak incidence was observed in August, November, and January (Fig. 3). These peaks are similar to those observed with the West Midlands cases.

A further 68 children who presented with mediastinal masses have also been analyzed in relation to date of diagnosis. Other data on these patients have already been published (1). Of these children, 49 had ALL, but marker studies were done on only 15 (13 E-rosette-positive, one null, and one common ALL); 19 had non-Hodgkin's lymphoma (NHL), but marker studies were done on only two cases (one E-rosette-positive, one mixed). Forty-seven percent of the NHL cases subsequently transformed to ALL.

The distribution of these cases by month for three U.K. centers (Birmingham, Liverpool, and Manchester) is shown in Fig. 4. In addition, 4 cases of NHL and one ALL diagnosed at Cardiff in 1977–1978 are shown, but only one other case

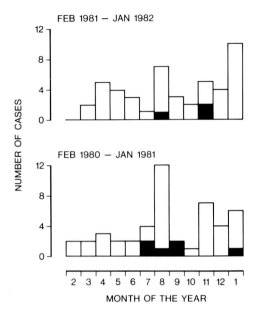

FIG. 3. Distribution of T-cell ALL cases for some U.K. centers by month of presentation. Solid portions represent Birmingham cases. (Data from Dr. M. F. Greaves, Imperial Cancer Research Fund, London.)

with a mediastinal mass occurred from 1969 to 1978. The seasonal pattern of NHL and ALL for the whole group appeared to be similar to that of the Birmingham T-cell cases, but when analyzed for the 3 larger centers, the pattern appears to be different in the different regions of the country (Fig. 4).

Common ALL and Non-T, Non-B (cALLA Status Unknown) ALL

Cases of these phenotypes appeared in all months of the year (Fig. 2), but peak incidence was in June and October, when T-cell cases were either absent or in low numbers. The addition of other non-T, non-B cases (i.e., those for which cALLA status was not known) did not alter this seasonal pattern (Fig. 5).

Two cases of common ALL with mediastinal masses were seen. Interestingly, one was diagnosed in November and the other in January, the months when T-cell cases occur most frequently.

IS THIS SEASONAL VARIATION SIGNIFICANT?

The seasonal presentation of the T-cell ALL cases from Birmingham combined with those from Dr. Greaves (total number 103) varied significantly over the year ($\chi^2_{(11)} = 37.9$; $p < 0.001$), although this effect was almost entirely the result of a higher number of cases in August (21) and in January (17). In contrast, for the common ALL and non-T, non-B (cALLA status unknown) cases (total number 88), no seasonal variation could be demonstrated ($\chi^2_{(11)} = 15.8$; p = not significant).

When combined distributions were considered, there was a difference in the distribution of the two groups of borderline significance ($\chi^2_{(5)} = 17.1$; $p < 0.01$) for

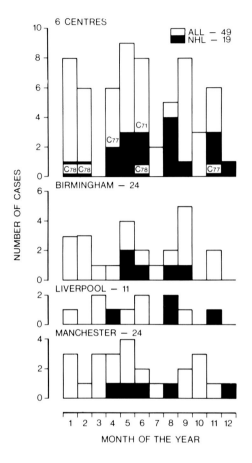

FIG. 4. Mediastinal lymphoblastic mass patients (1) shown by month of presentation and divided into ALL (unshaded) and NHL (solid). The top histogram shows all cases, including individual cases from a cluster at Cardiff (indicated by a C followed by year of diagnosis). The three lower histograms show the distribution by month of presentation for three centers as indicated.

bimonthly totals starting with February plus March, which gave the lowest combined total for T-cell cases. This combination (Table 3) suggests a reciprocal effect between the types, although, again, the effect depends on particularly high numbers in individual months.

WHITE CELL COUNT AT PRESENTATION

White cell count is known to be a highly significant prognostic factor and so has been analyzed in relation to presentation. Marked variation is seen in each year, but where cases presented at the same time, similar white cell counts have often been observed. With such small numbers, however, the significance of this is unclear.

CLUSTERING OF CASES

Tables 4 and 5 show the data on children from the same locality presenting with ALL of the same phenotype. In the T-cell cases (Table 5), anti-T antisera have shown marked differences in the lymphoblasts.

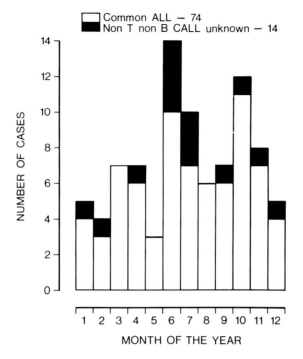

FIG. 5. Common ALL cases (unshaded) and non-T, non-B ALL (cALLA unknown) cases (solid) by month of presentation, January 1976 to December 1981.

TABLE 3. *Bimonthly totals of common and T-cell ALL cases*

Cases	February + March	April + May	June + July	August + September	October + November	December + January
Common ALL and non-T, non-B[a] (88 cases)	11	10	24	13	20	10
T-cell ALL (103 cases)	7	14	13	29	15	25

[a]cALLA status unknown.

CONCLUSIONS

In a mixed racial population in the United Kingdom, the incidence of ALL appears to be low in Afrocaribbean children, whereas the incidence in Asian children is similar to that seen in Caucasian children. The incidence of T-cell cases has varied from year to year, with an unusually high incidence in some years and a lower incidence in others. Seasonal variation appears to be statistically significant in T-cell ALL in the U.K. patients, whereas no statistical significance is seen for common ALL during the year. Clustering of cases of similar phenotype has also been observed. The following questions need to answered: Why is the incidence of ALL

TABLE 4. *Clinical information on a cluster of common ALL patients from the same locality, 1977[a]*

Category	Initials			
	C. S.	S. C.	M. H.	A. B.
Date of presentation	May 26, 1977	May 26, 1977	May 26, 1977	January 7, 1977
Sex	Male	Male	Female	Female
Age	5 years, 9 months	3 years, 2 months	4 years, 1 month	3 years, 8 months
WBC ($\times 10^9$/liter)	57	13.1	8.0	6.2
Hemoglobin (g/dl)	4.3	4.3	6.1	11.5
Platelets ($\times 10^9$/liter)	<10	<10	<10	300
Liver (cm)	7	2	4	4
Spleen (cm)	0	Tip	6	0
Lymphadenopathy	$\pm$[b]	$+++$[c]	$\pm$[b]	$+++$[c]
cALL (%)	85	94	NT[d]	55

[a]No cases from this locality in 1976, 1979, 1980, or 1981. Two cases in 1978.
[b]$\pm$ = small shotty glands.
[c]$+++$ = large lymph nodes and widespread distribution.
[d]NT = Not tested. This patient had non-T, non-B ALL.

TABLE 5. *Clinical and phenotypic data on two patients presenting from the same locality at the same time*

Category	Initials	
	P. B.	M. P.
Date of birth	August 16, 1979	September 18, 1979
Date of presentation	November 5, 1981	November 6, 1981
Sex	Male	Female
Chest X-ray	Thymic shadow	No mediastinal mass
Hemoglobin (g/dl)	6.9	6.8
WBC ($\times 10^9$/liter)	620	1,300
Platelets	23	75
Lymphadenopathy	$+++$	$+++$[a]
Liver (cm)	5	5
Spleen (cm)	7	8
E rosettes	87%	1%
TdT	>90%	Negative
Monoclonal anti-T	T_1 neg, T_3 neg, T_4 56,	T_1 70, T_3 60, T_4 neg,
(% positive cells)	T_6 50, T_8 70, II_A 92	T_6 neg, T_8 5, II_A 70

[a]Large lymph nodes and widespread distribution.

lower in Afrocaribbean children? Why is there seasonal variation in T-cell ALL, and would prospective studies contribute to our understanding of the etiology of this type of leukemia? And do phenotypic, clinical, and hematological data suggest an additional time- and place-related heterogeneity that might explain differences in treatment success?

ACKNOWLEDGMENTS

We wish to thank Drs. J. R. Mann (Birmingham), J. Martin (Liverpool), P. H. Morris Jones (Manchester), and E. N. Thompson (Cardiff) for permission to present data on their patients; Drs. J.2R. Mann and A. Oakhill for permission to present data on their study of Asian children with ALL; Dr. M. F. Greaves (Imperial College Research Fund, London) for providing date of diagnosis on 93 T-cell ALL cases; and Dr. P. Prior (The Cancer Registry, Birmingham) for doing the statistical analysis.

REFERENCES

1. Matthew, P. M., Pragnell, D. R., Cole, A. J. L., Hill, F. G. H., Shah, K. J., Morris Jones, P. H., Martin, J., Palmer, M. K., Thompson, E. N., Eden, O. B., Mott, M. G., and Mann, J. R. (1980): Clinical, haematological and radiological features of children presenting with lymphoblastic mediastinal masses. *Med. Pediatr. Oncol.*, 8:193–204.
2. Oakhill, A., and Mann, J. R. (1983): Poor prognosis of acute lymphoblastic leukaemia in Asian children living in the United Kingdom. *Br. Med. J.*, 286:839–841.

*Pathogenesis of Leukemias and Lymphomas:
Environmental Influences*, edited by
I. T. Magrath, G. T. O'Conor, and B. Ramot.
Raven Press, New York © 1984.

Distribution of Immunological Subtypes of Acute Lymphoblastic Leukemia in White and Mexican Children

*Alice Yu, **Ivor Royston, *Rick Lamb, and *Faith Kung

*Department of Pediatrics, University of California San Diego, Medical Center,
San Diego, California 92103; and **Department of Medicine, University of California
San Diego, School of Medicine and Veterans Administration Medical Center,
La Jolla, California 92161*

The roles of environmental and genetic factors in the genesis of leukemia have long been a focus of interest. The association between the development of leukemia and exposure to radiation and certain chemicals has been well recognized (3,14). The finding that White children have a higher incidence of acute leukemia, especially acute lymphoblastic leukemia (ALL), than Black children has been a matter of discussion (2,4,5). Very little information is available regarding the epidemiology of leukemia in other ethnic groups.

Recently, immunological classification of ALL has revealed that ALL is a heterogeneous disease with many subtypes that differ in clinical features and prognosis (1,12,15). The even more recent advent of the use of monoclonal antibodies and hybridoma technology has added another new dimension to the classification of lymphoid malignancies (8,13,16,17). However, data have been scarce on the epidemiology of the immunological subtypes of lymphoid malignancies.

In this study, we compared the distribution of the subtypes of ALL in White and Mexican children in the San Diego area. Data obtained from patients who were typed at the time of relapse were analyzed separately from data from patients typed at diagnosis to minimize any bias from preselection of patients with poor prognostic characteristics. Our preliminary findings suggested that pre-T ALL constitutes a smaller fraction of ALL in Mexican children.

PATIENTS AND METHODS

Fifty-nine children under 18 years of age with ALL were evaluated at the University of California Medical Center in San Diego, the Naval Regional Medical Center, Children's Hospital and Health Center, and the Kaiser Permanente Medical Center, all in the San Diego area. All patients received a standard therapeutic regimen consisting of induction with vincristine and prednisone, consolidation with

L-asparaginase with or without cyclophosphamide, CNS prophylaxis, and maintenance therapy with 6-mercaptopurine and methotrexate along with vincristine and prednisone pulse reinforcement.

Immunological Classification of ALL

Immunological markers of leukemia lymphoblasts were determined as previously described (16). Briefly, leukemic cells were isolated from heparinized peripheral blood and/or bone marrow by Ficoll-Hypaque density gradient centrifugation. T65 antigens were detected by an indirect immunofluorescence assay using monoclonal antibody T101 (9). This antibody reacts with all cells of thymic origin, i.e., thymus, peripheral blood T cells, and T-cell lines as well as malignant lymphocytes in T-cell lymphomas, T-cell leukemias, and the majority of chronic lymphocytic leukemias. Surface immunoglobulin (sIg) and cytoplasmic immunoglobulin (cIg) were identified by direct immunofluorescent staining procedures. Sheep erythrocyte (E) rosette formation was determined as described (7). The criteria for positivity of each of these evaluations were expressions of the marker by at least 20% of the lymphoblast population. In this study, all 18 patients (four T-ALL, five pre-T, and nine pre-B ALL) who were positive for one or more markers expressed these markers in at least 50% of their lymphoblasts. ALL was classified into four immunological subtypes according to the surface markers as follows: T-ALL—E^+, $T65^+$, sIg^-, cIg^-; pre-T ALL—E^-, $T65^+$, sIg^-, cIg^-; pre-B ALL—E^-, $T65^-$, sIg^-, cIg^+; and null ALL—E^-, $T65^-$, sIg^-, cIg^-.

Statistical Analysis

The age distribution was compared using Student's t-test, and the frequency distribution was compared using Fisher's exact test for independence.

RESULTS

Patient Characteristics

From 1980 to 1982, 59 children with ALL in the San Diego area were analyzed with regard to age, sex, ethnic origin, and immunological subtypes. Of the 59, 31 were White, 22 were Mexican, and the other six included one Black, one Black/White, one Mexican/White, one Japanese/White, one Puerto Rican/Nicaraguan, and one Filipino. Their ages ranged from 1.3 to 16.5 years.

ALL Subtypes and Ethnicity

Table 1 shows the distribution of ALL subtypes among White, Mexican, and other ethnic groups, according to the time of cell marker analysis. Immunological classification of ALL was done at the time of diagnosis in 39 patients, of which 20 were White, 14 were Mexican, and five were other ethnic groups, and at the

TABLE 1. *Distribution of ALL subtypes among ethnic groups*[a]

| | Time of sampling | | | | | | | | | | |
| | Diagnosis | | | | Relapse | | | | Entire population | | | |
ALL subtype	W	M	Other	Total	W	M	Other	Total	W	M	Other	Total
T	1	1	0	2	1	1	0	2	2	2	0	4 (7%)
Pre-T	3	0	1	4	1	0	0	1	4	0	1	5 (8%)
Pre-B	3	3	0	6	3	0	0	3	6	3	0	9 (15%)
Null	13	10	4	27	6	7	1	14	19	17	5	41 (69%)
Total	20	14	5	39	11	8	1	20	31	22	6	59

[a]W = White, M = Mexican. The differences between White and Mexican groups are statistically significant only for pre-T ALL both in the group typed at diagnosis ($p = 0.02$) and in the entire population ($p < 0.01$), and for pre-B ALL typed at relapse ($p = 0.02$).

time of relapse in 20 patients, including 11 White, 8 Mexican, and 1 other. Sixty-nine percent of all 59 patients were of the null cell subtypes, 15% were of pre-B subtype, and 15% were of T-cell lineage (T-ALL and pre-T ALL).

Null cell ALL and T-cell ALL affected Whites and Mexicans equally in both the group typed at diagnosis and the group typed at relapse. However, pre-T ALL was more prevalent in White children than in Mexican children. Of the five cases of pre-T ALL, four were White children, three of them typed at the time of diagnosis and one typed at relapse. The remaining patient was a Black typed at diagnosis. The proportion of pre-T ALL in the group typed at diagnosis was 3/20 in Whites versus 0/14 in Mexicans ($p = 0.02$). For the entire study population, the proportion was 4/31 in White versus 0/22 in Mexican ($p<0.01$). However, the frequency of T-cell ALL of all types in White children (6/31) was not significantly different from that in Mexican children (2/22) ($p = 0.3$). Although the frequency of pre-B ALL was not significantly different in the two ethnic groups typed at diagnosis, pre-B ALL was more common in White (3/11) than in Mexican (0/8) children typed at relapse ($p = 0.02$). In the entire study population, the difference in the proportion of pre-B ALL in White and Mexican children was not statistically significant ($p = 0.6$).

Age Distribution

The mean age of the 59 patients was 7.3 ± 4.5 years, ranging from 1.3 to 16.5 years. There was no significant difference in the mean age of White (7.1 ± 4.3 years) and Mexican (7.8 ± 5.0 years) study populations. As expected from the known association between increasing age and poor prognosis (6,10), the mean age of patients typed at relapse (8.35 ± 5.2 years) was slightly greater than the mean age of patients typed at diagnosis (6.8 ± 4.1 years), although this difference was not statistically significant ($p = 0.2$). This age difference is particularly great for pre-B ALL in White children; the mean age of those typed at diagnosis was 3.7 ± 2.3 years, compared to 13.4 ± 3.3 years for those typed at relapse ($p = 0.01$). The older age of the latter group might have predisposed them to relapse and thereby made their leukemia available for typing and inclusion in the present study. This selection bias might have contributed to the apparently higher frequency of pre-B ALL in White patients than in Mexican patients who were typed at the time of relapse (Table 1). Taken as an entire population, patients with ALL of T-cell lineage had a mean age (10.1 ± 4.8 years) greater than that of patients with null and pre-B subtypes (6.8 ± 4.3 years) ($p = 0.04$). This is in line with recent findings by others (1,12,15). The mean age of 19 White children with null cell ALL was 6.5 ± 3.9 years, compared to 6.9 ± 4.5 years in 17 Mexican patients. For pre-B ALL, the mean ages were 8.6 ± 5.9 years for six White patients and 8.1 ± 6.1 years for three Mexican patients; and for T-ALL, they were 7.3 ± 5.3 years for two White and 14.9 ± 0.6 years for two Mexican patients. Comparison of the mean ages of each ALL subtype for White and Mexican populations revealed no significant differences for these three subtypes of ALL.

Sex Distribution

The population of 59 patients included 32 males and 27 females. Null and pre-B ALL affected males and females equally, with male-female ratios of 20:21 and 4:5, respectively. However, ALL of T-cell lineage had a definite male predominance; the male-female ratios were 4:0 for T-ALL and 4:1 for pre-T ALL. For null cell ALL, the male-female ratios in White and Mexican children were 8:11 and 9:8, respectively, and for pre-B ALL, the sex ratio was 3:3 for the White population and 1:2 for the Mexican population. These differences were not statistically significant.

DISCUSSION

Although the recent advances in the immunological classification of ALL have provided new insights into the heterogeneity of this disease and have added new dimensions to the diagnosis and prognosis of ALL, information on the epidemiology of ALL subtypes is lacking. In this study, we compared for the first time the distribution of various subtypes of ALL in children of two ethnic groups, White and Mexican.

The overall distribution of the 59 patients among the four subtypes of ALL, namely, 69% null ALL, 15% pre-B ALL, and 15% T-ALL and pre-T ALL, was comparable to the results reported in the literature (1,12,15). Our findings of male predominance and the older age of patients with T-ALL and Pre-T ALL were also consistent with recent reports by others (1,12,15). Our data suggested that for null, pre-B, and T-cell ALL, there was no significant difference between White and Mexican patients in the frequency, sex ratio, or mean age of diagnosis. Of special interest was the finding that pre-T ALL seemed to represent a much smaller fraction of ALL in Mexicans than in Whites. This is at variance with the hypothesis recently proposed by Ramot and Magrath (11), based on their preliminary finding of 50% of T-cell ALL in a survey of 29 Black children with ALL and on the observation that ALL of T-cell lineage appears to occur more commonly in less privileged populations. In their study, however, E-rosette formation was the only marker used for the identification of T-ALL. To date, there has been no information regarding the racial distribution of E-rosette-negative T-ALL. Because the sample sizes of both studies are relatively small, definite conclusions must await further studies in larger populations.

ACKNOWLEDGMENTS

We wish to acknowledge Linda Bleeker and Heli Collins for their expert technical assistance; Adele Kayser for her help in the preparation of the manuscript; and Deborah Freeman for assistance in data collection. This work was supported in part by National Cancer Institute grants 5-R01 CA26141-03, 3-R01 CA 28439-03, and N-01-CBH-4250-31 and by the American Cancer Institute grant M-027.

REFERENCES

1. Brouet, J.-C., Valensi, F., Daniel, M.-T., Flandrin, G., Preud'homme, J.-L., and Seligmann, M. (1976): Immunological classification of acute lymphoblastic leukaemias: Evaluation of its clinical significance in a hundred patients. *Br. J. Haematol.*, 33:319–328.
2. Davies, J. N. P. (1965): Leukemia in children in tropical Africa. *Lancet*, 2:65–67.
3. Diamond, E. L., Schmerler, H., and Lilienfeld, A. M. (1973): The relationship of intra-uterine radiation to subsequent mortality and development of leukemia in children: A prospective study. *Am. J. Epidemiol.*, 97:283–313.
4. Ederer, F., Miller, R. W., and Scotto, J. (1965): US childhood cancer mortality patterns, 1950–1959. *JAMA*, 192:593–596.
5. Fraumeni, J. F., Jr., and Miller, R. W. (1967): Epidemiology of human leukemia: Recent observations. *JNCI*, 38:593–605.
6. George, S. L., Fernbach, D. J., Vietti, T. J., Sullivan, M. P., Lane, D. M., Haggard, M. E., Berry, D. H., Lonsdale, D., and Komp, D. (1973): Factors influencing survival in pediatric acute leukemia. *Cancer*, 32:1542–1553.
7. Greaves, M. F., and Brown, G. (1974): Purification of human T and B lymphocytes. *J. Immunol.*, 112:420–423.
8. Lebien, T., McKenna, R., Abramson, D., Gajl-Peczascka, K., Nesbit, M. J., Coccia, P., Bloomfield, C., Brunning, R., and Kersey, J. (1981): The use of monoclonal antibodies, morphology and cytochemistry to probe the cellular heterogeneity of acute leukemia and lymphoma. *Cancer Res.*, 41:4776–4780.
9. Moore, G. E., Wood, L. K., Minowada, J., and Mitchen, J. R. (1973): Establishment of leukemia cell lines with T-cell characteristics. *In Vitro*, 8:434.
10. Pierce, M. I., Borges, W. H., Heyn, R., Wolff, J. A., and Gilbert, E. S. (1969): Epidemiological factors and survival experience in 1770 children with acute leukemia. *Cancer*, 23:1296–1304.
11. Ramot, B., and Magrath, I. (1982): Hypothesis: The environment is a major determinant of the immunological sub-type of lymphoma and acute lymphoblastic leukaemia in children. *Br. J. Haematol.*, 50:183–189.
12. Sen, L., and Borella, L. (1975): Clinical importance of lymphoblasts with T markers in childhood acute leukemia. *N. Engl. J. Med.*, 292:823–833.
13. Sobol, R. E., Dilman, R. D., Beauregard, J. C., Yu, A. L., Lee, J. W., Collins, H., Wormsley, S., Green, M. R., Ellison, R. R., and Royston, I. (1983): Clinical utility of monoclonal antibodies in phenotyping acute and chronic lymphocytic leukemia. In: *Protides of the Biological Fluid. 30th Colloquium*, edited by H. Peters, pp. 413–425. Pergamon Press, Oxford *(in press)*.
14. Thorpe, J. J. (1974): Epidemiologic survey of leukemia in persons potentially exposed to benzene. *J. Occup. Med.*, 16:375–382.
15. Tsukimoto, I., Wong, K. Y., and Lampkin, B. C. (1976): Surface markers and prognostic factors in childhood acute leukemia. *N. Engl. J. Med.*, 294:245–248.

16. Yu, A. L., Royston, I., Leung, K. L., Kung, F. H., Hartman, G. A., Lightsey, A. L., Vangrove, J., and Sobol, R. E. (1982): Utility of monoclonal antibodies in the immunologic phenotyping of acute lymphoblastic leukemia. *Hybridoma*, 1:91–98.
17. Zipf, R. F., Fox, R. I., Dilley, J., and Levy, R. (1981): Definition of the high-risk ALL patients by immunological phenotyping with monoclonal antibodies. *Cancer Res.*, 41:4786–4789.

Pathogenesis of Leukemias and Lymphomas:
Environmental Influences, edited by
I. T. Magrath, G. T. O'Conor, and B. Ramot.
Raven Press, New York © 1984.

Racial Variation in the Frequency of Immunological Subtypes of Childhood Acute Lymphoblastic Leukemia

Gregory H. Reaman and Sanford L. Leikin

Department of Hematology/Oncology, Children's Hospital National Medical Center, and Department of Child Health and Development, George Washington University School of Medicine, Washington, D.C. 20010

The decreased incidence of acute lymphoblastic leukemia (ALL) and its relatively poor prognosis in Black children have been previously documented (18,25,26). The prognostic implications of race for children with this disease appear to relate to differences in the rate of initial remission induction as well as in the duration of continuous complete remission (26).

Organized investigations of large series of children with ALL have resulted in the recognition that certain clinical features at the time of diagnosis demonstrate prognostic significance in childhood ALL (12,17,23). Two such extremely important factors appear to be age at diagnosis and the initial white blood cell (WBC) count (20). Studies from the United States (2,11), Europe (24), Japan (15), and China (16) have confirmed a marked early age peak in the frequency of ALL. This phenomenon, however, had not been observed in Africa (2,11) or, more interestingly, in American Blacks (5,13). Recently, a similar age peak has been described for Black children with ALL (18).

Initial WBC count appears to exert the most significant influence on long-term prognosis in childhood ALL (20). The increased incidence of marked leukocytosis in Black children with ALL has previously been observed (26). This finding has been explained in part by lower socioeconomic status in this population group and its disadvantage in receiving expeditious medical care, resulting in more advanced disease by the time diagnosis is established. However, the mechanism by which peripheral blood leukocytosis occurs is unknown. In addition, the relationship between disease duration and degree of leukocytosis has not been established.

Recent clinical investigations of ALL have resulted in the realization that this disease displays marked biological heterogeneity (17). The intense investigation of normal lymphocyte differentiation antigens, membrane receptors, and other components of the surfaces of neoplastic lymphoid cells has provided further insight into this biological heterogeneity and has resulted in a subclassification of ALL based on surface membrane phenotype (3,4,8,14). This classification scheme has resulted in the recognition of further prognostic variables in childhood ALL (8,21,22). Patients with lymphoblasts of T-cell lineage (T-ALL) have a much poorer prognosis than patients with non-T, non-B ALL. Correlation of clinical features at presentation with leukemic cell phenotypes has resulted in the recognition of nearly distinct clinical syndromes (10). T-ALL is more frequently associated with leukocytosis, male sex, and evidence of a mediastinal mass in children of more advanced age.

To determine if such a biological factor might, in part, explain the worse prognosis for Black children with ALL, we retrospectively reviewed our experience with leukemic cell surface marker characterization in children with this disease.

PATIENTS AND METHODS

The study group consisted of 107 consecutively diagnosed patients with ALL referred to the Department of Hematology/Oncology of the Children's Hospital National Medical Center during the period 1977–1980. This series represents a nearly complete population-based study, because this institution serves as the major pediatric cancer referral center for the metropolitan Washington, D.C. area.

Surface marker phenotyping was performed on the pretreatment bone marrow lymphoblasts of 90 of these patients. Surface marker characterization included ability of leukemic cells to form spontaneous rosettes with neuraminidase-treated sheep erythrocytes, expression of complement receptors with an erythrocyte antibody complement rosette assay, and presence of surface membrane immunoglobulin (sIg) detected by direct fluorescent microscopy using rabbit antihuman immunoglobulin [$F(ab_2)$ specific]. Patients in whom greater than 25% E rosette positive lymphoblasts, confirmed by cytological examination of cytocentrifuge preparations, were observed in the bone marrow were considered to have T-ALL.

Although certain demographic data were available at the time of diagnosis, specific information relating to socioeconomic status was unavailable. However, an estimate of low socioeconomic class was obtained by retrospectively reviewing which families were receiving federally subsidized state aid for medical care, which has as an eligibility requirement that family income be at or near the poverty level.

RESULTS

The study group of 90 patients ranged in age from six months to 17.5 years (Table 1). There were 74 White and 16 Black children. Median age at diagnosis was identical for patients from these two racial groups. WBC at diagnosis ranged from 0.9 to 450×10^9/liter. As has been observed in other studies, the median WBC at diagnosis was significantly higher ($p = 0.01$) in black patients than in white children, namely, 38.2×10^9/liter versus 17.6×10^9/liter.

Eighteen of the 90 patients (20%) had T-ALL, and the remainder had non-T, non-B ALL. This incidence of T-ALL is similar to those reported from much larger series of patients. However, markedly different frequencies of T-ALL were observed in the two racial groups of this study population. Nine of the 16 Black children (56.3%) had T-ALL, whereas this immunological subtype of ALL was observed

TABLE 1. *Characteristics of the study group*

Characteristic	Black	White
Number of patients	16	74
Age (years)		
Range	1–13	0.5–17.5
Median	4	4.2
WBC ($\times 10^9$/liter)		
Range	2.4–415	0.9–450
Median[a]	38.2	17.6
Incidence of T-ALL[b]	9/16 (56.3%)	9/74 (12.2%)

[a]The difference between the two figures is statistically significant ($p = 0.01$).
[b]The difference between the two figures is statistically significant ($p < 0.001$).

TABLE 2. *Clinical characteristics of T-ALL patients*

Characteristic	Black	White
Number of patients	9	9
Age (years)		
Range	1–13	3–16
Median	3	11
WBC ($\times 10^9$/liter)		
Range	6.8–415	42–280
Median	110	94
Male-female ratio	1.3:1	8:1

in only 12.2% of the White patients. The clinical characteristics of the 18 patients with T-ALL are presented in Table 2. The median age at diagnosis of the White children with T-ALL was 11 years, significantly higher than that observed for Black patients (three years). In addition, the marked male predominance was conspicuously absent in the Black children with T-ALL in this series. T-cell phenotypes were observed in the malignant cells of all three Black patients with non-Hodgkin's lymphoma, whereas 80% of the White children had B-cell lymphomas during this same study period.

Nearly one-third of the children in the entire study population were from families of low socioeconomic status (Table 3). No significant racial differences were observed with these small numbers. Furthermore, there was no evidence of a correlation between low socioeconomic status and an increased incidence of T-ALL.

DISCUSSION

Epidemiological evidence indicates that the mortality rate in patients with cancer in the United States is higher in the Black than in the White population (1,6). This observation is documented by the outcome of patients with ALL, the most common childhood neoplastic disease.

TABLE 3. *Low socioeconomic status and ALL*

ALL subtype	Patients of low socioeconomic status		
	Total	Black	White
Total	28/90 (31.1%)	7/16 (43.8%)	21/74 (28.4%)
Non-T, non-B	23/72 (31.9%)	3/7 (42.9%)	20/65 (30.8%)
T-ALL	5/18 (27.8%)	4/9 (44.4%)	1/9 (11.1%)

The recognition of the relationship between certain clinical variables at the time of diagnosis and the outcome for children with this disease has contributed greatly to the understanding of the biological heterogeneity of the disease. Initial WBC count at diagnosis demonstrates profound prognostic significance.

The data in this study confirm previous observations that Black children with ALL present with significantly higher WBC counts than White children (18,25,26). The relationship between race and initial WBC count as prognostic variables in childhood ALL is well demonstrated by a recent multivariate analysis by the Children's Cancer Study Group (20). Race, which previously provided highly significant results when assessed univariately, was no longer found to be a statistically significant predictor of prognosis when the data were adjusted for initial WBC count.

This present study demonstrates a markedly increased incidence of T-ALL in Black children relative to Whites. In addition, intriguing differences in the clinical characteristics of these Black children with T-ALL were observed. The median age at diagnosis and the frequency of T-ALL in females were decidely different from those of the White T-ALL patients. These data suggest a possible biological explanation for the increased incidence of marked leukocytosis in Black children with ALL and, more important, for their worse prognosis. This finding is not supported by a recent report by St. Jude's (19), in which a decrease was observed in the incidence of Black patients presenting with high-risk factors (WBC greater than 100,000, E rosette positive blasts, CNS disease, and mediastinal mass), to the point where the incidence of high-risk factors was the same for Black and White children. This observation represents a change from what this same group had previously reported. The possibility of changes in referral patterns to that institution was not addressed. The data in this present study, however, are derived from a single, relatively homogeneous, geographically based population group.

Furthermore, although a relatively crude assessment of socioeconomic status was used, these data suggest that socioeconomic factors alone are not responsible for the prognostic influence of race in children with ALL. This finding is supported by a previous report demonstrating no significance for race as it relates to socioeconomic status, as a prognostic variable in neuroblastoma, another common childhood malignancy (9).

Recently, six black patients from the West Indies have been reported with adult T-cell lymphoma-leukemia with clinical features similar to those in patients reported from Japan in whom high-titer antibody against the structural core protein of a new human C-type leukemia virus has been observed (7). This suggests that distinctive geographic and racial determinants may be operational in this T-cell proliferative malignancy. It is of interest that none of the Black children in the series reported here were of West Indian descent.

The present study does not suggest that lowered socioeconomic status alone is related to the observed increased incidence of T-ALL in Black children. However, the findings emphasize the need for further prospective epidemiological investigations in large series of patients. These will hopefully provide useful information in delineating the possible association of genetic and/or environmental factors with the incidence of immunological subtypes of childhood ALL.

ACKNOWLEDGMENTS

We wish to gratefully acknowledge the assistance of Ms. Bonnie Dunlop in completing this study and of Ms. Marilyn Adeyemi in the preparation of the manuscript. This study was supported in part by grant CA 03888 from the National Institutes of Health and by a Junior Faculty Clinical Fellowship to G. H. Reaman from the American Cancer Society.

REFERENCES

1. Alderson, M. (1980): The epidemiology of leukemia. *Adv. Cancer Res.*, 31:1–76.
2. Amsel, S., and Nabembezi, J. S. (1974): Two year survey of hematologic malignancies in Uganda. *JNCI*, 52:1397–1401.
3. Bowman, W. P., Melvin, A., and Mauer, A. M. (1980): Cell markers in lymphomas and leukemias. In: *Advances in Internal Medicine*, vol. 25, edited by G. H. Stollerman, pp. 391–425. Year Book Medical Publishers, Chicago.
4. Brouet, J. C., and Seligmann, M. (1978): The immunological classification of acute lymphoblastic leukemias. *Cancer*, 42:817–827.
5. Brown, W. M. C., and Doll, R. (1961): Leukaemia in childhood and young adult life. *Br. Med. J.*, 26:982–992.
6. Burbank, F., and Fraumeni, J. F. (1972): U.S. cancer mortality—Non-white predominance. *JNCI*, 49:649.
7. Catovsky, D., Greaves, M. F., Rose, M., Galton, D. A. G., Goolden, A. W. G., McCluskey, D. R., White, J. M., Lampert, I., Bourikas, G., Ireland, R., Brownell, A. I., Bridges, J. M., Blattner, W. A., and Gallo, R. C. (1982): Adult T-cell lymphoma-leukaemia in Blacks from the West Indies. *Lancet*, 1:639–643.
8. Chessells, J. M., Hardisty, R. M., Rapson, N. T., and Greaves, M. F. (1977): Acute lymphoblastic leukaemia in children: Classification and prognosis. *Lancet*, 2:1307–1309.
9. DiNicola, W., Movassaghi, N., and Leikin, S. (1975): Prognosis in black children with neuroblastoma. *Cancer*, 36:1151–1153.
10. Dow, L. W., Borella, L., Sen, L., Aur, R. J. A., George, S. L., Mauer, A. M., and Simone, J. V., (1977): Initial prognostic factors and lymphoblast-erythrocyte rosette formation in 109 children with acute lymphoblastic leukemia. *Blood*, 50:671–682.
11. Edington, G. M., and Hendrickse, M. (1973): Incidence and frequency of lymphoreticular tumors in Ibadan and the Western State of Nigeria. *JNCI*, 50:1623–1631.
12. George, S. L., Fernbach, D. J., Vietti, T. J., Sullivan, M. P., Lane, D. M., Haggard, M. E., Berry, D. H., Lonsdale, D., and Komp, D. (1973): Factors influencing survival in pediatric acute leukemia. *Cancer*, 32:1542–1553.
13. Gilliam, A. G., and Walter, W. A. (1958): Trends of mortality from leukemia in the United States. *Public Health Rep.*, 73:773.
14. Gupta, S., and Good, R. A. (1980): Markers of human lymphocyte subpopulations in primary immunodeficiency and lymphoproliferative disorders. *Semin. Hematol.*, 17:1–29.

15. Kawashima, K., Suzuki, H., and Yamada, K. (1980): Long-term survival in acute leukemia in Japan, a study of 304 cases. *Cancer* 45:2181–2187.

16. Li, F. P., Chitan, T. D., and Tu, T. G. (1980): Incidence of childhood leukemia in Shanghai. *Int. J. Cancer*, 25:701–703.

17. Miller, D. R., Leikin, S., Albo, V., Vitale, L., Sather, H., Coccia, P., Nesbit, M., Karon, M., and Hammond, D. (1980): Use of prognostic factors in improving the design and efficiency of clinical trials in childhood leukemia. *Cancer Treat. Rep.*, 64:381–392.

18. Pendergrass, T. W., Hoover, R., and Godwin, J. D. (1975): Prognosis of Black children with acute lymphocytic leukemia. *Med. Pediatr. Oncol.*, 1:143–148.

19. Presbury, G., Bowman, P., George, S., Aur, R., Dahl, G., and Simone, J. (1981): Re-examination of race as a prognostic factor in acute lymphocytic leukemia (ALL). *Proc. Am. Soc. Cancer Res. Am. Soc. Clin Oncol.*, 22:480 (abs. C-574).

20. Robison, L. L., Sather, H. N., Coccia, P. F., Nesbit, M. E., and Hammond, D. G. (1980): Assessment of the interrelationship of prognostic factors in childhood acute lymphoblastic leukemia. *Am. J. Pediatr. Hematol. Oncol.*, 2:5–13.

21. Sallen, S. E., Ritz, J., Pesando, J., Gelber, R., O'Brien, C., Hitchcock, S., Coral, F., and Schlossman, S. F. (1980): Cell surface antigens: Prognostic implications in childhood acute lymphoblastic leukemia. *Blood*, 55:395–402.

22. Sen, L., and Borella, L. (1975): Clinical importance of lymphoblasts with T markers in childhood acute leukemias. *N. Engl. J. Med.*, 292:828–832.

23. Simone, J. V., Verzosa, M. S., and Rudy, J. A. (1975): Initial features and prognosis in 363 children with acute lymphocytic leukemia. *Cancer*, 36:2099–2108.

24. Stalsberg, J. (1978): Lymphoreticular tumors in Norway and in other European countries. *JNCI*, 50:1685–1702.

25. Szklo, M., Gordis, L., Tonascia, J., and Kaplan, E. (1978): The changing survivorship of White and Black children with leukemia. *Cancer*, 42:59–66.

26. Walters, T. R., Bushore, M., and Simone, J. (1972): Poor prognosis in Negro children with acute lymphocytic leukemia. *Cancer*, 29:210–214.

27. Young, J. L., Jr., and Miller, R. W. (1975): Incidence of malignant tumors in U.S. children. *J. Pediatr.*, 86:254–258.

Pathogenesis of Leukemias and Lymphomas: Environmental Influences, edited by
I. T. Magrath, G. T. O'Conor, and B. Ramot.
Raven Press, New York © 1984.

A Comparative Analysis of Acute Lymphocytic Leukemia in White and Black Children: Presenting Clinical Features and Immunologic Markers

*W. Paul Bowman, *Gerald Presbury, **Susan L. Melvin,
†Stephen L. George, and *Joseph V. Simone

*Divisions of *Hematology-Oncology, **Pathology, and †Biostatistics,
St. Jude Children's Research Hospital, Memphis, Tennessee 38101*

Acute lymphocytic leukemia (ALL) in North America is more than twice as frequent in White children as in Black children (21). Nevertheless, American Blacks resemble American Whites more than they do African Blacks with respect to childhood lymphoid disease types (20). In Africa, lymphomas predominate, whereas ALL is extremely rare (11). At the moment, the relative contributions of heredity and the environment to the etiology of these diseases are not clear. However, it does appear that the incidence of childhood ALL may be influenced by environmental socioeconomic factors (13). ALL in White children has a striking peak age incidence between two and five years, which has become increasingly apparent in the past 30 to 40 years. This peak age frequency has been reported to be absent or less striking in Black children (2), perhaps accounting for the lower incidence of the disease overall.

With the advent of successful combined modality therapy for ALL in the 1960s, a number of factors associated with poor prognosis were recognized (16). It became evident that Black children tended to have clinical features associated with "more advanced" disease and that they responded less well than white children did to the same therapy (19). In the 1970s, biological correlates of the clinical heterogeneity of childhood ALL were found. Certain unfavorable prognostic factors such as mediastinal mass and high white blood cell (WBC) count were often associated with the presence of T-cell surface markers (6). On the other hand, most patients two to five years old had favorable features such as low white count and a surface marker phenotype now known as common ALL (4).

We review here our 20-year experience with childhood ALL. We compare and contrast the presenting clinical features of White and Black children and present more recent data on cell surface markers in these two populations. We seek to learn if different clinical and biological subsets are overrepresented or underrepresented according to race. We also wish to determine if there is any evidence of change in the epidemiology of childhood ALL during the past two decades. The issue of race and response to therapy will be the subject of a separate report.

MATERIALS AND METHODS

The subjects of this report are the 1,144 children (less than 20 years old) with ALL admitted to St. Jude total therapy protocols I–X from 1962 through December 1981. Of these, 1,035 (90.5%) are White, 109 (9.5%) are Black. The following clinical features at diagnosis were analyzed for differences according to race: age, sex, initial WBC count, presence or absence of mediastinal mass, pretreatment central nervous system (CNS) involvement, hemoglobin and platelet counts, and liver and spleen size. A previous analysis (5) demonstrated that the presence of one or more of the following features is associated with a very poor response to therapy: initial WBC greater than 100×10^9/liter, mediastinal mass, CNS involvement, and E-rosette-forming lymphoblasts. Patients exhibiting any of these features are designated "high risk," the remainder "standard risk." The distribution of patients into these two groups according to their race was also analyzed.

Because of recent observations of a change occurring over a relatively short time in the epidemiology of lymphoid disease in Arabs living in the Gaza Strip (13), we separated our analysis into two consecutive decades. The first decade, 1962–1971, includes the 357 patients entered on studies I–VII; the second decade, 1972–1981, includes 787 patients entered on studies VIII–X. Each of the above features analyzed was examined for the entire 20-year period and for each of the two decades in an effort to learn whether the presenting clinical features of childhood ALL in Whites and Blacks have remained stable or have undergone any change over the period of observation.

The E-rosette test came into routine use in 1975 and has been applied to the blast cells of more than 90% of our newly diagnosed patients with ALL since then. The presence of E-rosette-forming lymphoblasts, defined by heat stability at 37°C, is evidence for T-cell lineage of the malignant cells (10). Patients on studies VIII–X who had E-rosette testing done were analyzed to determine if race is associated with E-positivity.

Additional surface marker studies can be performed to allow a more refined classification of ALL based on immunologic phenotype. Immunofluorescence testing for surface immunoglobulin, T-cell, Ia-like, and "common ALL" antigens reveals patterns of marker expression that may be used to divide patients into four groups (Table 1) (1). T-cell disease is that which is E-rosette-positive and/or anti-T-positive. Cells from E-rosette-positive patients always express T-cell antigens, but the converse is not true, and some cases of ALL with T-cell properties have not formed E rosettes. B-cell ALL is that which is surface-immunoglobulin-positive. Common ALL includes patients whose cells have reactivity with both Ia and common ALL antisera. Finally, only Ia antigen or no marker at all is identified in the undifferentiated group. These groups are not mutually exclusive and areas of overlap

TABLE 1. *Identification of four major ALL groups by membrane markers*

Membrane marker	Groups[a]			
	Common	T-cell	B-cell	Undifferentiated
Erythrocyte receptors	−	±	−	−
T-cell antigens	±	+	−	−
Common ALL antigen	+	±	±	−
Ia-like antigens	+	−	+	±
Immunoglobulin	−	−	+	−
Percentage of patients[b]	72	17	3	8

[a]A minus sign (−) means that marker is absent from all specimens; plus or minus (±) means that marker may be either present or absent; plus (+) means that marker is present on all specimens. Marker patterns enclosed in boxes are those that define the respective groups of patients.
[b]Based on 320 untreated children with ALL.

do exist, as illustrated in Table 1. However, the vast majority of cases are easily classifiable into one of the four groups. From 1977 to 1981, 320 patients (90% of all new ALL cases) were so classified. An analysis has also been done to determine if the subset of 29 Black children differed from the 291 White children with respect to immunologic phenotype.

The statistical analysis used was based on simple contingency table procedures. Significance levels (p values) refer to the chi-square statistic on each table.

RESULTS

A total of 1,144 patients (1,035 white, 109 black) with ALL were entered on protocol studies I–X during the 20-year period. The first decade included 357 entries (315 White, 42 Black), and the second decade included 787 entries (720 White, 67 Black). Because our patient accrual depends on referral, accurate incidence figures cannot be derived from these data. However, the proportion of Black patients (9.5%) is consistent with the lower incidence of ALL in blacks, because the total population from which our patients are derived is at least one-third Black.

Table 2 shows selected clinical features at diagnosis of ALL, with comparison by race. The first pair of columns represent the overall 20-year experience, the second pair studies I–VII, and the third pair studies VIII–X. With respect to age at diagnosis, the following observations are apparent. An overall comparison (I–X) reveals no significant difference by race. The very striking age peak at two to five years is present in both White and Black patients. However, if one examines the two decades separately, a difference is apparent that was masked in the overall analysis: In the first decade, a significantly larger proportion of Black patients were in the 10-year-old or older age group, whereas in the second decade the age distribution of patients is virtually identical in the two races. No change is apparent in the relative age frequencies of White ALL patients during the study period.

TABLE 2. *Clinical features of white and black ALL patients at diagnosis*

Clinical feature	Overall (studies I–X)		1962–1971 (studies I–VII)		1972–1981 (studies VIII–X)	
	White	Black	White	Black	White	Black
Age						
<2	90 (9%)	7 (6%)	31 (10%)	1 (2%)	59 (8%)	6 (9%)
2–5	521 (50%)	45 (41%)	165 (52%)	19 (45%)	356 (49%)	26 (39%)
6–9	186 (18%)	23 (21%)	65 (21%)	7 (17%)	121 (17%)	16 (24%)
≥10	238 (23%)	34 (31%)	54 (17%)	15 (36%)	184 (26%)	19 (28%)
	$p = 0.11$		$p = 0.03$		$p = 0.29$	
WBC (×10⁹/liter)						
<10	498 (48%)	34 (31%)	153 (49%)	9 (21%)	345 (48%)	25 (37%)
10–99.9	420 (41%)	53 (49%)	132 (42%)	19 (45%)	288 (40%)	34 (51%)
≥100.0	117 (11%)	22 (20%)	30 (10%)	14 (33%)	87 (12%)	8 (12%)
	$p < 0.001$		$p < 0.001$		$p = 0.20$	
Mediastinal mass						
No	948 (92%)	89 (82%)	286 (91%)	34 (81%)	662 (92%)	55 (82%)
Yes	87 (8%)	20 (18%)	29 (9%)	8 (19%)	58 (8%)	12 (18%)
	$p = 0.002$		$p = 0.06$		$p = 0.01$	
CNS involved						
No	994 (96%)	100 (92%)	302 (96%)	37 (88%)	692 (96%)	63 (94%)
Yes	41 (4%)	9 (8%)	13 (4%)	5 (12%)	28 (4%)	4 (6%)
	$p = 0.05$		$p = 0.05$		$p = 0.34$	
Total	1,035	109	315	42	720	67

The initial WBC in White children with ALL is below 10×10^9/liter in nearly 50% of cases and above 100×10^9 in only 10 to 12% of cases. This distribution has been constant over the period of study. In contrast, the overall analysis of initial WBC in Blacks reveals a trend toward significantly higher counts, with only 31% below 10×10^9 and 20% above 100×10^9/liter. This racial difference is accounted for entirely by the first decade of observation, in which only 21% of Blacks were under 10×10^9 and 33% were above 100×10^9. In the second decade, initial WBC in Blacks has shifted downward, with 37% below 10×10^9 and only 12% above 100×10^9. This distribution is no longer significantly different from that seen in White patients.

An anterior mediastinal mass is present at diagnosis in 8% of our White ALL patients but 18% of our Black patients. In contrast to the downward shift in presenting age and WBC noted in Black patients during the past two decades, no such change has been noted in the frequency of mediastinal mass, which remains more than twice as common in Black ALL patients as in White. The known association of mediastinal mass with T-cell markers (1,6) is thus strong evidence that Blacks with ALL have a larger proportion of T-cell cases.

Initial CNS involvement is rare in ALL but in our experience has been about twice as frequent in Blacks. Along with the downward shift in age and WBC toward greater similarity between White and Black children has been a parallel decrease in the frequency of CNS leukemia at diagnosis in Blacks, such that there is no longer a significant difference in the second decade.

A high initial WBC count and the presence of a mediastinal mass at diagnosis are strongly correlated (6). Thus, the constancy of mediastinal mass in our Black patients is puzzling in the face of more patients presenting with lower WBC counts in recent years. Table 3 shows, in fact, that this downward shift over time in WBC at diagnosis is restricted to those patients *without* a mediastinal mass. Patients with a mass continue to have higher WBC counts, as is also the case for White patients. In the first decade, initial WBC in Blacks tended to be high regardless of the presence of a mediastinal mass, whereas in the second decade, the Black patients without a mass had significantly lower counts no longer different from those of their White counterparts.

Additional clinical features that are not represented in the table and that were not significantly different in Whites versus Blacks (either overall or by decade) are sex (males 57%, females 43%) and initial hemoglobin and platelet count. Parallel to the observations relative to WBC was the finding that liver and spleen sizes were significantly larger in Black patients in the first decade but not in the second.

Analysis according to "risk status" (Table 4) showed that the proportion of White patients assigned to the high-risk category has been fairly constant at 16 to 20%. In the first decade, 50% of all Black patients fell into this category, whereas in the second decade, the proportion dropped to 31%. This is still significantly greater than the proportion of high-risk White patients and is attributed mainly to the persistently higher frequency of mediastinal mass in Blacks.

E-rosette testing was performed on the lymphoblasts of 72% of White and Black patients admitted to protocols VIII–X (Table 5). The majority of the omissions were in 1973–1975 before the test came into routine use. There is clearly no significant difference in the proportion of E-positive cases according to race. This observation

TABLE 3. *Mediastinal mass (mm) and initial WBC count*

Initial WBC ($\times 10^9$/liter)	White		Black	
	No mm	mm	No mm	mm
Studies I–VII				
<10	146 (51%)	7 (24%)	9 (26%)	0
10–99	120 (42%)	12 (41%)	13 (38%)	6 (75%)
≥100	20 (7%)	10 (34%)	12 (35%)	2 (25%)
	$p < 0.001$		$p = 0.15$	
Subtotals	286	29	34	8
Studies VIII–X				
<10	341 (52%)	4 (7%)	23 (42%)	2 (17%)
10–99	260 (39%)	28 (48%)	28 (51%)	6 (50%)
≥100	61 (9%)	26 (45%)	4 (7%)	4 (33%)
	$p < 0.001$		$p = 0.04$	
Subtotals	662	58	55	12

TABLE 4. Risk status

Risk status	Studies I–X		Studies I–VII		Studies VIII–X	
	White	Black	White	Black	White	Black
Standard	842 (81%)	67 (61%)	264 (84%)	21 (50%)	578 (80%)	46 (69%)
High	193 (19%)	42 (39%)	51 (16%)	21 (50%)	142 (20%)	21 (31%)
	$p < 0.001$		$p < 0.001$		$p = 0.04$	
Total	1,035	109	315	42	720	67

TABLE 5. Heat-stable E-rosette-forming
lymphoblasts (studies VIII–X)

E-rosette-forming lymphoblasts	White	Black
No	461 (64%)	42 (63%)
Yes	58 (8%)	6 (9%)
Unknown	201 (28%)	19 (28%)
	$p = 0.92$	
Total	720	67

TABLE 6. Immunologic surface
phenotype (studies IX and X only)

Phenotype	White	Black
T-cell	45 (15%)	9 (31%)
B-cell	8 (3%)	0
Common ALL	217 (75%)	16 (55%)
Undifferentiated	21 (7%)	4 (14%)
	$p = 0.06$	
Total	291	29

is initially somewhat surprising in view of the increased frequency of mediastinal mass in Black patients.

The issue can be clarified by examining the 320 patients for whom more complete immunologic surface phenotyping is available (Table 6). These data suffer from the small numbers of Black patients so far typed -29- and therefore do not reach conventional statistical significance ($p = 0.06$). However, the results are consistent with earlier findings on mediastinal mass in that T-cell disease (based on definition by anti-T sera) is proportionately twice as frequent in Blacks as in Whites, whereas the common ALL phenotype is relatively underrepresented in Blacks. Only two of the nine T-cell ALL cases in Blacks were E-rosette-positive, and so it appears that the subset of E-negative, anti-T-positive ALL may be specifically increased in Black patients. This is of some interest, because observations by others suggest that E-negative, anti-T-positive ALL may have a uniquely poor response to therapy (7).

DISCUSSION

This survey of 1,144 children with ALL consecutively admitted to St. Jude "total therapy" protocols over a 20-year period reveals that the distribution of initial clinical features in White patients has been quite constant. Males constitute a 57% majority; there is a striking age peak of onset at two to five years; initial WBC count is 10 × 10⁹/liter or less in 50% and over 100 × 10⁹ in about 10%; and mediastinal mass is present in 8% and early CNS involvement in 4%. Immunologic marker studies show that a common ALL phenotype is present in 74% and a T-cell phenotype in 15%; the B-cell and undifferentiated groups are rare. These clinical and immunologic features are quite consistent with observations by others (9,14).

In contrast, the epidemiology of ALL in Blacks appears to be in a dynamic state. Our conclusions must be tentative because our patient population comes to us by referral. However, there is no reason to suspect a selection bias for certain types of Black patients while the clinical features of the White children remain constant. ALL continues to be less frequent in Blacks. However, during the two decades of accrual, we have witnessed a trend for the presenting features of Black ALL patients to become more similar to those of White patients. In summary, the tendency in the 1960s for Black patients to be older and to have a higher initial WBC, larger livers and spleens, and a greater risk for early CNS involvement has disappeared in the 1970s. The only major clinical feature that remains strikingly different between the races is the 18% incidence of mediastinal mass in blacks. This, in turn, is correlated with more Blacks having clinical "high-risk" leukemia and with immunologic marker data that indicate that T-cell disease is about twice as frequent among Black patients with ALL as in Whites.

The reason for the apparent change over time in the clinical features of ALL in Blacks is not obvious. A facile explanation is that improved socioeconomic conditions and better access to medical care imply fewer delays in diagnosis and therefore patients are presenting with less advanced disease. This assumes that the level of WBC, the size of infiltrated organs, and the risk of CNS involvement are functions purely of time. However, clinical experience alone indicates that patients whose disease is most "advanced" often have the shortest clinical histories. The initial WBC count is more likely a function of the growth fraction of the tumor cells, of whether or not the disease had an extramedullary origin such as the thymus, and of little understood factors that lead to the release into the blood or retention of bone marrow-derived blast cells. Preschool children with common ALL characteristically have low initial WBC counts, often in spite of histories of illness of several weeks' duration. Regardless of the above, the greater frequency of documented T-cell disease in the Black patients confirms that previous delays in diagnosis are not the sole explanation for racial differences in childhood ALL.

Changes in the epidemiology of childhood leukemia over relatively short periods of time are not without precedent. A recent report from Baltimore has shown a striking increase there in the occurrence of acute nonlymphocytic leukemia in Blacks (8), and T-cell ALL appears to be on the increase in Arabs living in the Gaza Strip (13).

Our own observations are consistent with the hypothesis of Ramot and Magrath (13) that environmental factors contribute to the subtype of childhood lymphoid disease that occurs in a particular population. Over a 20-year period of observation, clinical T-cell leukemia has remained relatively more frequent in Blacks, but also in Blacks we have begun to see more childhood ALL of "common" type, i.e., preschool-age children with low WBC. It is not yet clear to what degree the lower incidence of ALL in Blacks is the result of genetic protective factors or of lack of exposure to environmental leukemogens. The third decade of observation will be of special interest to see if ALL in Blacks increases in frequency and/or continues to become more similar in clinical behavior to the disease in Whites.

In the meantime, further studies are needed to elucidate the biological basis for our clinical observations, including immunogenetic studies to determine if there are factors that protect against the development of ALL in Blacks (3) and additional cell marker studies such as karyotype and cytoplasmic IgM (18). The variant of ALL known as "pre-B" (about one-third of common ALL) may be associated with higher WBC counts and a poorer response to therapy (12,15). In keeping with the hypothesis of Ramot and Magrath (13), it is possible that the patients seen in the 1960s with more unfavorable prognostic features such as high WBC represented examples of pre-B cell disease. If this is so, studies of present-day Black patients may still yield evidence for a higher frequency of pre-B ALL. Such investigations have been undertaken by the Pediatric Oncology Group.

The response of our Black patients to treatment of ALL will be the subject of a separate report. It is clear that the early reports of poor prognosis were closely associated with a preponderance of high-risk clinical features (19). A Children's Cancer Study Group multivariate analysis of prognostic factors failed to show that race was an independent prognostic variable (14). On the other hand, a survey from the Baltimore area indicated that Blacks had benefited less from recent advances in therapy than had Whites (17). Our own data support the latter conclusion, but the details are beyond the scope of the present chapter.

ACKNOWLEDGMENTS

This work was supported by Cancer Center Support (CORE) Grant CA-21765 and Leukemia Program Project Grant CA-20180 from the National Cancer Institute and by American Lebanese Syrian Associated Charities (ALSAC).

REFERENCES

1. Bowman, W. P., Melvin, S. L., Aur, R. J. A., and Mauer, A. M. (1981): A clinical perspective on cell markers in acute lymphocytic leukemia. *Cancer Res.*, 41:4794–4801.
2. Brown, W. M. C., and Doll, R. (1961): Leukaemia in childhood and young adult life. *Br. Med. J.*, 26:982–992.
3. Budowle, B., Action, R., Barger, B., Blackstock, R., Crist, W., Go, R. C., Humphrey, G. B., Rogab, A., Roper, M. A., Vietti, T., and Dearth, J. (1983): Properdin factor B and acute lymphocytic leukemia. *Cancer (in press)*.
4. Chessells, J. M., Hardisty, R. M., Rapson, N. T., and Greaves, M. F. (1977): Acute lymphoblastic leukaemia in children: Classification and prognosis. *Lancet*, 2:1307–1309.

5. Dahl, G. V., Aur, R. J. A., George, S. L., Rivera, G., and Mauer, A. M. (1978): High risk acute lymphocytic leukemia (ALL): Problem of early relapse. *Blood*, 24:477 (abs.).
6. Dow, L. W., Borella, L., Sen, L., Aur, R. J. A., George, S. L., Mauer, A. M., and Simone, J. V. (1977): Initial prognostic factors and lymphoblast-erythrocyte rosette formation in 109 children with acute lymphoblastic leukemia. *Blood*, 50:671–682.
7. Falletta, J. M., Pincus, J. K., Metzgar, R. S., Pullen, D. J., Humphrey, G. B., Crist, W. M., Boyette, J., and van Eys, J. (1981): Reduced efficacy of vincristine-prednisone in some patients with T cell leukemia. *Clin. Res.*, 29:893a (abs.).
8. Gordis, L., Szklo, M., Thompson, B., Kaplan, E., and Tonascia, J. A. (1981): An apparent increase in the incidence of acute nonlymphocytic leukemia in Black children. *Cancer*, 47:2763–2768.
9. Greaves, M. F., Janossy, G., Peto, J., and Kay, H. (1981): Immunologically defined subclasses of acute lymphoblastic leukaemia in children: Their relationship to presentation features and prognosis. *Br. J. Haematol.*, 48:179–197.
10. Melvin, S. L. (1981): Immunologic definition of leukemic cell surface phenotypes. *Cancer Res.*, 41:4790–4793.
11. Olisa, E. G., Chandra, R., Jackson, M. A., Kennedy, J., and Williams, A. O. (1975): Malignant tumors in American Black and Nigerian children: A comparative study. *JNCI*, 55:281–284.
12. Pullen, D. J., Falletta, J. M., Crist, W. M., Vogler, L. B., Dowell, B., Humphrey, G. B., Blackstock, R., van Eys, J., Cooper, M. D., Metzgar, R. S., and Meydrech, E. F. (1981): Southwest Oncology Group experience with immunological phenotyping in acute lymphocytic leukemia of childhood. *Cancer Res.*, 41:4802–4809.
13. Ramot, B., and Magrath, I. (1982): Hypothesis: The environment is a major determinant of the immunological sub-type of lymphoma and acute lymphoblastic leukaemia in children. *Br. J. Haematol.*, 50:183–189.
14. Robison, L. L., Nesbit, M. E., Sather, H. N., Hammond, G. D., and Coccia, P. F. (1980): Assessment of the interrelationship of prognostic factors in childhood acute lymphoblastic leukemia. *Am. J. Pediatr. Hematol. Oncol.*, 2:5–13.
15. Roper, M., Crist, W., Rogab, A., Pullen, J., Humphrey, G. B., Boyette, J., Metzgar, R. S., van Eys, J., Nix, W., and Cooper, M. (1981): Pre-B cell leukemia differs in its response to therapy. *Blood*, 59:150a.
16. Simone, J. V., Verzosa, M. S., and Rudy, J. A. (1975): Initial features and prognosis in 363 children with acute lymphocytic leukemia. *Cancer*, 36:2099–2108.
17. Szklo, M., Gordis, L., Tonascia, J., and Kaplan, E. (1978): The changing survivorship of white and black children with leukemia. *Cancer*, 42:59–66.
18. Vogler, L. B., Crist, W. M., Bockman, D. E., Pearl, E. R., Lawton, A. R., and Cooper, M. D. (1978): Pre-B-cell leukemia: A new phenotype of childhood lymphoblastic leukemia. *N. Engl. J. Med.*, 298:872–878.
19. Walters, T. R., Bushore, M., and Simone, J. (1972): Poor prognosis in Negro children with acute lymphocytic leukemia. *Cancer*, 29:210–214.
20. Young, J. L., Jr., and Miller, R. W. (1975): Incidence of malignant tumors in U.S. children. *J. Pediatr.*, 86:254–258.
21. Young, J. L., Percy, C. L., and Asire, A. J., editors (1981): *Surveillance, Epidemiology and End Results: Incidence and Mortality Data, 1973–77*. Natl. Cancer Inst. Monogr. 57. National Cancer Institute, Bethesda, MD.

Pathogenesis of Leukemias and Lymphomas:
Environmental Influences, edited by
I. T. Magrath, G. T. O'Conor, and B. Ramot.
Raven Press, New York © 1984.

Differences in the Presentation of Acute Lymphoblastic Leukemia and Non-Hodgkin's Lymphoma in Black Children and White Children: A Report from the Epidemiology Committee of the Childrens Cancer Study Group

Harland Sather, Richard Honour, Richard Sposto, Carolyn Level, and Denman Hammond

Childrens Cancer Study Group, Operations Office, University of Southern California Comprehensive Cancer Center, Los Angeles, California 90031

The Childrens Cancer Study Group (CCSG) is a multi-institution network funded by the National Cancer Institute to conduct clinical trials in pediatric cancer. Most of the 29 primary member institutions (Table 1) have a local or regional network of affiliated hospitals. The total number of affiliated institutions is currently 104.

CCSG has been conducting clinical trials in the treatment of childhood leukemia for more than 25 years. In 1978, the CCSG initiated its first clinical trials in the treatment of non-Hodgkin's lymphoma (NHL). Recent examination of the data from these clinical trials has shown a number of interesting results with regard to the

TABLE 1. *Geographic distribution of the 29 primary member institutions of the Childrens Cancer Study Group*

Ann Arbor, MI	Nova Scotia, CAN
Chicago, IL	Philadelphia, PA
Cincinnati, OH	Pittsburgh, PA
Columbus, OH	Portland, OR
Denver, CO	Rochester, MN
Indianapolis, IN	Rochester, NY
Iowa City, IO	Salt Lake City, UT
Los Angeles, CA	San Antonio, TX
Louisville, KY	San Francisco, CA
Madison, WI	Seattle, WA
Minneapolis, MN	Toronto, CAN
Nashville, TN	Washington, D.C.
New York City, NY	Vancouver, CAN

179

presentation of disease and the eventual treatment outcome for different racial groups with childhood lymphoid cancers.

PATIENT POPULATION

The primary member institutions in the CCSG are required to register all pediatric cancer patients seen within their institutional network with the Operations Office in Los Angeles, even if the patient is not enrolled as part of a CCSG study. These data are regularly entered in the computerized CCSG registration file. For all patients that are part of a CCSG study, additional data are sent to the Operations Office regarding treatment, patient status, and outcome. Key information abstracted from these records is routinely entered in the computer data base for the clinical trials being conducted. In the most recent 12-month period, the U.S. members registered 2,263 children seen for the first time within the CCSG network. These cases represent about one-third of the approximately 6,400 incident cases of pediatric cancer (i.e., patients less than 15 years old at diagnosis) in the United States each year.

The relative distribution of diagnoses for patients registered in CCSG is shown in Fig. 1. As expected, the largest percentage of the children have leukemia (39%), mostly acute lymphoblastic leukemia (ALL). About 11% have lymphomas, with approximately equal percentages of Hodgkin's disease and NHL. Because of the types of oncologic specialties involved in CCSG clinical trials and the associated relationship to referral patterns, these data differ slightly from the relative percentages one would see in a true population-based incidence registry.

The general definition CCSG uses to delineate ALL from NHL is that all patients classified as ALL must have more than 25% lymphoblasts in the marrow at diagnosis. For therapeutic reasons, the small proportion of children with more than 25% blasts and L3 blast morphology in the French-American-British (FAB) classification system (i.e., "Burkitt's leukemia") were treated on the NHL study.

Each patient's race is requested on the CCSG registration form. The categories of classification are White, Black, Latin, American Indian, Asian, and other non-White. About 10% of the patients enrolled in the registry do not have a racial classification because they chose not to provide that information. Table 2 shows the racial classification of all newly diagnosed children with ALL and NHL in a recent one-year period. About 80% of all children registered in these disease categories are White, 7% are Black, and the remaining 13% are other non-White categories. Slightly more Latins than Blacks are enrolled in CCSG (8.6% versus 6.5%). No other racial group constitutes a significant proportion of the children in the registry. In this one-year period, 869 children with ALL and 159 with NHL were registered.

FIG. 1. Distribution by diagnosis of 6,496 patients registered with the Childrens Cancer Study Group.

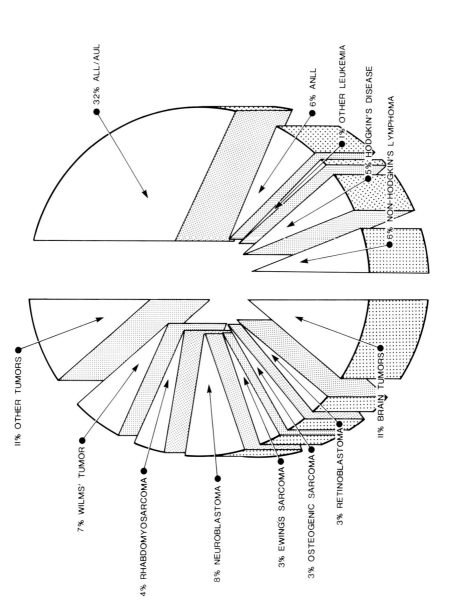

11% OTHER TUMORS

32% ALL/AUL

6% ANLL

1% OTHER LEUKEMIA

HODGKIN'S DISEASE

5%

NON-HODGKIN'S LYMPHOMA

6%

11% BRAIN TUMORS

7% WILMS' TUMOR

4% RHABDOMYOSARCOMA

8% NEUROBLASTOMA

3% EWING'S SARCOMA

3% OSTEOGENIC SARCOMA

3% RETINOBLASTOMA

TABLE 2. *First-time CCSG registrants with
acute lymphoblastic leukemia (ALL)
and non-Hodgkin's lymphoma (NHL)
by racial group, October 1980
through September 1981*

Racial group	ALL	NHL
White	622	118
Black	53	8
Latin	66	14
American Indian	5	2
Asian	16	3
Other non-White	16	2
Unreported	91	12
Total	869	159

RESULTS

Because the CCSG has conducted studies in ALL for many years, the data base for patients with that disease is large. These data are frequently examined for the purpose of identifying prognostic factors and their interrelationships. As other researchers (2,7,13,14) and other studies within CCSG (11) have described, Black children with ALL have a poorer outcome than Whites. Because the proportion of Black children in most large U.S. series is only about 5 to 10%, it is sometimes difficult to obtain accurate statistical estimates of the true difference in treatment outcome between Blacks and Whites. For that reason, we combined our ALL studies from 1972 to the present to better estimate the relative outcomes in these racial groups.

A total of 4,361 newly diagnosed children with ALL were enrolled in these studies. Of this group, 84.6% were White, 5.5% were Black, and 9.9% were other racial categories. All patients in the CCSG studies during this period received prophylactic treatment to the central nervous system and multiagent chemotherapy for induction, consolidation, and maintenance treatment. Figure 2 shows the survival from diagnosis for the racial groups. The estimated survival rate eight years from diagnosis is 61% for Whites, 48% for Blacks, and 59% for others. This result is highly significant ($p<0.0001$), with a life-table-adjusted estimate of the relative mortality rate for Blacks versus Whites of 1.55. Figure 3 shows the disease-free survival (DFS) results for the subset of the original population in which induction therapy was completed and complete remission was achieved. The Black children again had a significantly poorer DFS ($p<0.0001$). At eight years from initial remission, the disease-free survival rates in Whites, Blacks, and others are 56%, 44%, and 46%, respectively. The relative life-table-estimated first adverse event rate for Blacks versus Whites is 1.52.

Because clinical trials by CCSG in NHL were not started until recently, a large data base regarding treatment outcome does not exist. The studies that started in 1978 do not yet have sufficiently long follow-up. A preliminary analysis of these patients has not shown a significantly poorer outcome in Black children compared to White children.

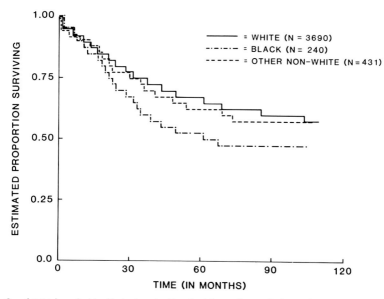

FIG. 2. Acute lymphoblastic leukemia: Survival from diagnosis by racial group, 1972–1982.

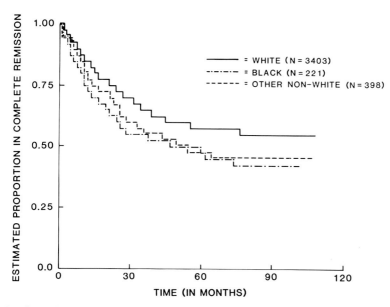

FIG. 3. Acute lymphoblastic leukemia: Disease-free survival from initial remission by racial group, 1972–1982.

In light of the poorer outcome for Black children with ALL, we investigated the characteristics of the disease at diagnosis in Blacks and Whites. A CCSG report covering the period from 1957 to 1964 (8) did not show any important differences between Whites and Blacks in age at diagnosis or type of leukemia [ALL or acute nonlymphoblastic leukemia (ANLL)], but more recent reports suggest that Blacks with ALL are older at diagnosis and that the relative frequency of ALL to ANLL cases may be changing for Blacks as compared to Whites (3,6,13). Other factors that have been mentioned as important to the outcome of treatment and that differ for Blacks and Whites are socioeconomic status, high white blood (WBC) count, central nervous system (CNS) involvement, and presence of a mediastinal mass at diagnosis (3,7,9,13). These reports fail to agree consistently on the presence of such prognostic factors, however.

Prognostic factors have been examined in detail in a number of large CCSG studies of ALL (4,5,11,12). Overall, the studies done by CCSG since 1972 suggest that the following diagnostic characteristics have the most *independent* statistical significance as poor prognostic factors when assessed in a multivariate analysis: high WBC (above 50,000/mm³); age less than one or greater than 10 years; L2 FAB blast cell morphology; marked adenopathy or splenomegaly; high hemoglobin levels (above 10 g/dl); depressed serum immunoglobulin levels; and male sex. Other factors that show significant prognostic effects in a single-variable context, but that are highly associated with certain subsets of the preceding variables, are E-rosette positivity ("T-cell" leukemia), mediastinal mass, CNS involvement, and hepatomegaly.

Because multivariate analysis suggested that the strong univariate prognostic difference between Whites and Blacks was partially explained by other factors, we examined the pattern of disease presentation for Blacks and Whites with respect to most of the preceding factors in our current study of childhood ALL (1978–1982) (Table 3). Four bad prognostic characteristics showed a clear excess in blacks: marked adenopathy, mediastinal mass, high WBC, and E-rosette-positivity. The

TABLE 3. *Prognostic characteristics at diagnosis of ALL in Blacks and Whites, 1978–1982*

Diagnostic characteristic	Blacks[a] (%)	Whites[a] (%)	Odds ratio (for blacks)
E-rosette-positive	13.9	8.6	1.73
Mediastinal mass	14.3	7.4	2.08
Marked adenopathy	15.2	7.1	2.32
WBC above 50,000	33.7	19.9	2.04
Age above 10 years	26.9	21.1	1.38
Hemoglobin above 10 mg/dl	24.3	21.1	1.20
Marked splenomegaly	15.3	16.4	0.92
Male	54.8	56.8	0.92
L2 morphology	5.2	9.0	0.56

[a]At the time of analysis, 103 Black children and 1,692 White children were enrolled in this study. For a few of the characteristics (cell surface immunologic markers, FAB cell morphology), slightly smaller denominators were used because not all patients were evaluated.

relative odds[1] of these factors in Blacks are about twice as high as in Whites. Age ranges and hemoglobin levels characteristic of a poor prognosis were more frequent in Blacks, but this was not statistically significant at a conventional 0.05 level. Splenomegaly and sex ratio show no differences between Blacks and Whites. Blacks had a lower rate of L2 blast morphology, but because of the small number of Black patients with this characteristic, the result was not statistically significant. More children will have to be studied to assess the possible differences in age, hemoglobin level, and FAB morphology between Blacks and Whites.

The poor risk factors mentioned above are frequently associated with one another. In CCSG studies this interrelationship is referred to as "lymphomatous" leukemia because of a hypothesis that presence of these factors may indicate extramedullary origin of disease and secondary spread to the marrow. These patients have a greater risk of disease recurrence in such extramedullary sites as the CNS or testes, as evidenced by a number of CCSG analyses of leukemia subgroups.

A report by Presbury et al. (9) also noted a greater association of poor risk prognostic factors in Black children with ALL treated at St. Jude Children's Hospital. Although this association was highly significant for the period before 1972, it was not statistically significant for the period since 1972. The CCSG data were examined for evidence of a temporal trend in the data, but none was found. However, the patients used in the CCSG analysis were all diagnosed in the period since 1972. It is also important to note that the reported comparative incidence figures of certain poor prognostic features in Blacks are greater than Whites in the St. Jude's data even in the period since 1972 (e.g., mediastinal mass—Blacks 18%, Whites 8%; E-rosette positivity—Blacks 11%, Whites 8%), and that these incidence figures are very similar to the CCSG data in Table 3. Thus, the larger patient population in the CCSG study may have permitted differences of a smaller magnitude to be detected statistically.

An analysis of patient characteristics was performed for the children in the current NHL protocol similar to the analysis for the children with ALL. In this study, the most significant poor prognostic factor at diagnosis was the presence of widely disseminated disease. However, a number of features are of interest for contrasting the presentation of Blacks and Whites; some of these features were examined because of the differences seen in children with ALL. The following additional diagnostic characteristics were examined: E-rosette-positivity, B-cell disease, mediastinal primary, lymphoblastic histology (Rappaport classification), CNS involvement, and sex. To be classified as E-rosette-positive, more than 25% of the malignant cells in the tissue sample had to form rosettes with sheep red blood cells. Similarly, B-cell disease was defined as more than 25% of the malignant cells bearing surface

---

[1]Suppose the number of individuals in group 1 with and without a particular characteristic are n^+ and n^-, respectively, and in group 2 are m^+ and m^-. The odds of having the characteristic in group 1 are defined as n^+/n^- and in group 2 as m^+/m^-. Then the relative odds (or odds ratio) for group 1 compared to group 2 are $(n^+/n^-)/(m^+/m^-)$. An odds ratio of one implies no association between the characteristic and group membership.

immunoglobulin. Table 4 contrasts the distribution of the previously mentioned descriptive characteristics in Blacks and Whites. Note that E-rosette-positivity, mediastinal primary, disseminated disease, and lymphoblastic histology all occur at a higher rate in Blacks, with odds ratios of about 2.0 to 3.5. CNS involvement was slightly higher in blacks but is based on very small numbers. Blacks showed a substantially lower frequency of presentation with B-cell disease and a lower male-female ratio than Whites. It is evident that the diagnostic characteristics that show a higher prevalence in Blacks with NHL correspond closely to the same factors in leukemia that were more fre quent in Blacks.

DISCUSSION

The examination of recent CCSG studies clearly shows a poorer outcome in ALL for Blacks compared to Whites. Multivariate analysis suggested that a substantial proportion of this decrement was caused by a different presentation of disease in the two racial groups. Blacks were diagnosed more frequently with poor prognostic characteristics such as E-rosette-positivity, higher WBC, mediastinal mass, and marked adenopathy. Examination of patients with NHL showed that Blacks more often had E-rosette-positivity, mediastinal presentations, disseminated disease, and lymphoblastic histology. Ramot and Magrath (10) recently suggested the possibility that Blacks differ from Whites in the relative proportion of T-cell disease. The CCSG data support that hypothesis.

Data on socioeconomic status (SES) have not been collected in these studies by the CCSG. Thus, the hypothesis of Ramot and Magrath (10) that the immunologic subtype of childhood lymphoid cancer may be related to environmental factors such as SES could not be examined in these data. Other researchers who have examined the racial and temporal patterns of incidence for children with lymphoid cancer (1,3,7,11) have suggested that SES might be a surrogate measure of a potentially important etiologic factor such as childhood infections that may influence suscep-

TABLE 4. *Prognostic characteristics at diagnosis of NHL in Blacks and Whites, 1977–1982*

Diagnostic characteristic	Blacks[a] (%)	Whites[a] (%)	Odds ratio (for Blacks)
E-rosette-positive	68.4	38.7	3.43
Mediastinal primary	46.0	21.5	3.10
Disseminated disease	83.8	67.0	2.55
Lymphoblastic histology	55.6	35.2	2.30
CNS involvement	5.4	4.3	1.27
B-cell	26.3	37.2	0.60
Male	64.9	78.7	0.50

[a]At the time of analysis, 35 Black children and 419 White children were enrolled in this study. For a few of the characteristics, slightly smaller denominators were used because not all patients were evaluated.

tibility to lymphoid malignancies. Investigation of this issue is a worthwhile objective for future studies of childhood ALL and NHL.

ACKNOWLEDGMENT

Grant support was provided by the Division of Cancer Treatment, National Cancer Institute, National Institutes of Health, Department of Health and Human Services. Contributing CCSG investigators, institutions, and grant numbers are given in Appendix A of this chapter.

REFERENCES

1. Anonymous (1981): Leukaemia in Black and White (editorial). *Lancet*, 2:732–733.
2. George, S. L., Fernbach, D. J., Vietti, T. J., Sullivan, M. P., Lane, D. M., Haggard, M. E., Berry, D. H., Lonsdale, D., and Komp, D. (1973): Factors influencing survival in pediatric acute leukemia. *Cancer*, 32:1542–1553.
3. Gordis, L., Szklo, M., Thompson, B., Kaplan, E., and Tonascia, J. A. (1981): An apparent increase in the incidence of acute nonlymphocytic leukemia in Black children. *Cancer*, 47:2763–2768.
4. Leikin, S., Miller, D., Sather, H., Albo, V., Esber, E., Johnson, A., Rogentine, N., and Hammond, D. (1981): Immunologic evaluation in the prognosis of acute lymphocytic leukemia. *Blood*, 58:501–508.
5. Miller, D. R., Leikin, S., Albo, V., Vitale, L., Sather, H., Coccia, P., Nesbit, M., Karon, M., and Hammond, D. (1980): Use of prognostic factors in improving the design and efficiency of clinical trials in childhood leukemia. *Cancer Treat. Rep.*, 64:381–392.
6. Miller, R. (1977): Ethnic influences in cancer occurrence: Genetic and environmental influences with particular reference to neuroblastoma. In: *Genetics of Human Cancer*, edited by J. Mulvihill, R. Miller, and J. Fraumeni, pp. 1–41. Raven Press, New York.
7. Pendergrass, T. W., Hoover, R., and Godwin, J. D. (1975): Prognosis of black children with acute lymphocytic leukemia. *Med. Pediatr. Oncol.*, 1:143–148.
8. Pierce, M. I., Borges, W. H., Heyn, R., Wolff, J. A., and Gilbert, E. S. (1969): Epidemiological factors and survival experience in 1770 children with acute leukemia. *Cancer*, 23:1296–1304.
9. Presbury, G., Bowman, P., George, S., Aur, R., Dahl, G., and Simone, J. (1981): Re-examination of race as a prognostic factor in acute lymphocytic leukemia (ALL). In: *Proceedings of the 17th Annual Meeting of the American Society of Clinical Oncology; American Ass. Cancer Res.*, 22:480 (abs. C-574).
10. Ramot, B., and Magrath, I. (1982): Hypothesis: The environment is a major determinant of the immunological sub-type of lymphoma and acute lymphoblastic leukaemia in children. *Br. J. Haematol.*, 50:183–189.
11. Robison, L. L., Sather, H. N., Coccia, P. F., Nesbit, M. E., and Hammond, D. G. (1980): Assessment of the interrelationship of prognostic factors in childhood acute lymphoblastic leukemia. *Am. J. Pediatr. Hematol. Oncol.*, 2:5–13.
12. Sather, H., Miller, D., Nesbit, M., Heyn, R., and Hammond, D. (1981): Differences in prognosis for boys and girls with acute lymphoblastic leukemia. *Lancet*, 1:739–743.
13. Szklo, M., Gordis, L., Tonascia, J., and Kaplan, E. (1978): The changing survivorship of White and Black children with leukemia. *Cancer*, 42:59–66.
14. Walters, T. R., Bushore, M., and Simone, J. (1972): Poor prognosis in Negro children with acute lymphocytic leukemia. *Cancer*, 29:210–214.

PRINCIPAL INVESTIGATORS OF THE CHILDRENS
CANCER STUDY GROUP

Institution	Investigator	Grant no.
Group Operations Office University of Southern California Comprehensive Cancer Center Los Angeles, CA	Denman Hammond, M.D. Richard Honour, Ph.D. Harland Sather, Ph.D. Richard Sposto, Ph.D. John Weiner, Dr.P.H.	CA 13539
University of Michigan Medical Center Ann Arbor, MI	Ruth Heyn, M.D.	CA 02971
Children's Hospital National Medical Center George Washington University Washington, DC	Sanford Leikin, M.D.	CA 03888
Memorial Sloan-Kettering Cancer Center Cornell University New York, NY	Denis R. Miller, M.D.	CA 14557
Children's Hospital of Los Angeles University of Southern California Los Angeles, CA	Jorge Ortega, M.D.	CA 02649
Babies Hospital Columbia University New York, NY	Sergio Piomelli, M.D.	CA 03526
Children's Hospital of Pittsburgh University of Pittsburgh Pittsburgh, PA	Vincent Albo, M.D.	CA 07439
Children's Hospital of Columbus Ohio State University Columbus, OH	William Newton, M.D.	CA 03750
Children's Orthopedic Hospital and Medical Center University of Washington Seattle, WA	Ronald Chard, M.D.	CA 10382
University of Wisconsin Hospitals Madison, WI	N. Shahidi, M.D.	CA 05436
University of Minnesota Health Sciences Center Minneapolis, MN	Mark Nesbit, M.D.	CA 07306
Children's Memorial Hospital Northwestern University Chicago, IL	Helen Maurer, M.D.	CA 07431
University of Utah Medical Center Salt Lake City, UT	Richard O'Brien, M.D.	CA 10198
Princess Margaret Hospital University of Toronto Toronto, ONT, Canada	Marilyn Sonley, M.D.	Ontario Cancer Treatment and Research Foundation Grant No. 41-17

Institution	Investigator	Grant no.
Strong Memorial Hospital University of Rochester Rochester, NY	Harvey Cohen, M.D.	CA 11174
University of British Columbia Vancouver, BC, Canada	Mavis Teasdale, M.D.	Vancouver Foundation Grant
Children's Hospital of Philadelphia University of Pennsylvania Philadelphia, PA	Audrey Evans, M.D.	CA 11796
James Whitcomb Riley Hospital for Children Indiana University Indianapolis, IN	Robert Baehner, M.D.	CA 13809
Harbor General Hospital University of California Los Angeles Torrance, CA	Jerry Finklestein, M.D.	CA 14560
University of California Medical Center San Francisco, CA	Arthur Ablin, M.D.	CA 17829
Rainbow Babies and Children's Hospital Case Western Reserve University Cleveland, OH	Peter Coccia, M.D.	CA 20320
Children's Hospital Medical Center University of Cincinnati Cincinnati, OH	Beatrice Lampkin, M.D.	CA 26126
Vanderbilt University School of Medicine Nashville, TN	John Lukens, M.D.	CA 26270
University of Oregon Health Sciences Center Portland, OR	Robert Neerhout, M.D.	CA 26044
University of Texas Health Science Center San Antonio, TX	Paul Zeltzer, M.D.	—
University of California Medical Center Los Angeles, CA	Stephen Feig, M.D.	CA 27678
University of Iowa Hospitals and Clinics Iowa City, IA	C. Thomas Kisker, M.D.	CA 29314
Children's Hospital of Denver Denver, CO	David Tubergen, M.D.	CA 28851
Mayo Clinic Rochester, MN	Gerald Gilchrist, M.D.	CA 28882
Izaak Walton Killam Hospital Halifax, NS, Canada	Allan Pyesmany, M.D.	Province of Nova Scotia

Pathogenesis of Leukemias and Lymphomas:
Environmental Influences, edited by
I. T. Magrath, G. T. O'Conor, and B. Ramot.
Raven Press, New York © 1984.

Clinical and Phenotypic Features of Childhood Acute Lymphocytic Leukemia in Whites, Blacks, and Hispanics: A Pediatric Oncology Group Study

*John M. Falletta, **James Boyett, †D. Jeanette Pullen,
‡William Crist, §Barry Dowell, ‡Maryann Roper,
§§G. Bennett Humphrey, §Richard Metzgar, #Max D. Cooper,
and ##Jan van Eys

*Pediatric Hematology-Oncology, Duke University Medical Center, Durham, North
Carolina 27710; **Pediatric Oncology Group, Veterans Administration Medical Center,
Gainesville, Florida 32602; †Pediatric Hematology-Oncology, University of Mississippi
Medical Center, Jackson, Mississippi 39216; ‡Pediatric Hematology-Oncology,
University of Alabama, Birmingham, Alabama 35294; §Division of Immunology, Duke
University Medical Center, Durham, North Carolina 27710; §§University of Oklahoma
Health Sciences Center, Oklahoma Children's Memorial Hospital, Oklahoma City,
Oklahoma 73126; #Cellular Immunobiology Unit, University of Alabama, Birmingham,
Alabama 35294; and ##Pediatric Oncology, M. D. Anderson Hospital, University of
Texas Cancer Center, Houston, Texas 77030

The Pediatric Oncology Group initiated a study in 1978 (POG 7865) in which all children with untreated acute lymphocytic leukemia (ALL) were evaluated to define the clinical and laboratory characteristics of their disease. In addition to the usual clinical variables quantified at diagnosis, each patient's leukemic cells were characterized morphologically using the French-American-British (FAB) criteria, cytochemically using a battery of special stains, and immunologically (5). Immunologic classification studies included assessment of E-rosette receptors, performed in the patient's home institution; the presence of surface and cytoplasmic immunoglobulin, performed in conjunction with the University of Alabama Reference Laboratory; and identification of membrane antigens Ia, common ALL antigen (cALLA), thymocyte, and other T-lymphocyte-associated antigens, performed by the Duke University Reference Laboratory (5).

Patients were regarded as having pre-B cell leukemia if more than 10% of their leukemic cells contained cytoplasmic mu chains. Patients were regarded as having T-cell leukemia if their leukemic cells possessed T antigen detected by heteroantisera and monoclonal antibodies, whether or not they were E-rosette-positive (5). No patient in this study expressed both T and pre-B markers.

The statistical methods used to analyze the data were as follows. The expected cell frequencies of all contingency tables permitted analysis by the classical chi-square statistic (7), and quantitative variables were analyzed by the Kruskal-Wallis test (2).

RESULTS

During the three years from May 1978, 750 pediatric patients with ALL were registered on the study. Of these, 75% were White, 12% were Black, 11% were of Spanish origin, and 2% were of other origins, including American Indian, Oriental, and Asian Indian. The ratio of male to female patients with ALL was nearly identical for Whites, Blacks, and Hispanics—60 to 62% of each group were male, giving a male predominance of about 1.5:1.

As seen in Table 1, the median peripheral leukocyte count at diagnosis was somewhat higher for Black patients and somewhat lower for Hispanic patients when compared with Whites; the difference is significant ($p<0.05$). These differences also were reflected in the mean leukocyte counts for each group. The median age at diagnosis did not differ substantially among the groups, with the median age being approximately five years.

The distribution of age at diagnosis also did not differ significantly ($p = 0.4$) among the groups (Fig. 1). Each of the patient groups had a peak age at diagnosis in the two- to four-year age range.

When the FAB morphological classification was applied to bone marrow films obtained at diagnosis, 89 to 91% of patients in each racial or ethnic group had L1 morphology ($p = 0.93$). With regard to assessment by cytochemical stains, all patients had leukemic cells that were Sudan black-negative and nonspecific-esterase-negative. Between 59 and 62% of the patients in each group had PAS-positive ALL ($p = 0.90$). Acid-phosphatase-positive leukemic cells predominated in 29% of White patients and in 21% of both Black and Hispanic patients ($p = 0.13$).

About 80% of White and Hispanic children were cALLA-positive, whereas only 58% of Black ALL patients were cALLA-positive, a difference significant at the 0.007 level (Table 2). Ia was expressed on the great majority of patients' leukemic cells, with no significant difference noted among the groups.

When each child's leukemia cell phenotype was classified into one of three mutually exclusive categories (Table 2), it was found that Black children tended

TABLE 1. *Findings at diagnosis of ALL in Whites, Blacks, and Hispanics*[a]

Finding	Whites	Blacks	Hispanics	p
Peripheral leukocyte count ($\times 10^3/\mu L$)				
Median	12.6	15.2	8.4	<0.05
Mean	47.8	72.2	45.1	
Age (years)				
Median	5.14	5.36	4.17	0.30
Mean	6.46	6.57	5.74	

[a]Study population of 727.

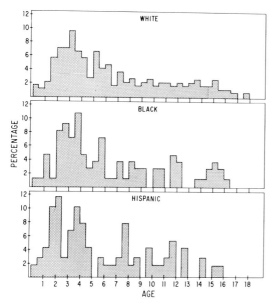

FIG. 1. Age at diagnosis of 727 White, Black, and Hispanic children with ALL, noted at half-year intervals.

TABLE 2. *Antigen expression and leukemia phenotype in Whites, Blacks, and Hispanics with ALL*

Feature	White	Black	Hispanic	p
Antigen expression				
cALLA-positive	241 (78%)	31 (58%)	31 (82%)	0.007
Ia-positive	272 (84%)	41 (76%)	36 (90%)	0.18
Leukemia phenotype				
Non-T, non-B	157 (68%)	17 (52%)	28 (82%)	
Pre-B	42 (18%)	9 (27%)	3 (9%)	0.12
T	32 (14%)	7 (21%)	3 (9%)	

to be more likely to have pre-B or T-cell disease than did White children, and Hispanic children tended to be more likely to have non-T, non-B cell disease than did Whites. The overall p value for the comparison was 0.12.

When all patients who were found to have pre-B cell disease were compared with those who were pre-B-negative (Table 3), Black children were found to have a higher occurrence of pre-B cell disease than White or Hispanic children. The difference between the White and Black children was significant at the 0.02 level, and the difference between Black and Hispanic children was significant at the 0.08 level. The level of significance for the overall comparison was 0.06.

When all patients who had T-cell disease were compared with those who did not (Table 4), Black children were found to have a slightly higher occurrence of T-cell disease than Hispanic children, although the level of significance was at the 0.10 level. Although the percentage of Blacks with T-cell disease was slightly higher than that of Whites, the difference was less apparent and must be regarded as tentative.

TABLE 3. *Occurrence of pre-B cell ALL in Whites, Blacks, and Hispanics*

Group	Pre-B	Non-pre-B	p^a
Whites	55 (16%)	274 (84%)	
Blacks	15 (29%)	36 (71%)	0.02
Hispanics	9 (16%)	49 (84%)	0.08

[a]Overall $p = 0.06$.

TABLE 4. *Occurrence of T-cell ALL in Whites, Blacks, and Hispanics*

Group	T	Non-T	p^a
Whites	56 (17%)	269 (83%)	
Blacks	13 (24%)	42 (76%)	0.25
Hispanics	4 (10%)	35 (90%)	0.10

[a]Overall $p = 0.24$.

DISCUSSION

Many studies have found that Black children with ALL respond less well than do White children to the same program of leukemia therapy (3,6,8). Although this report does not deal with therapy or outcome, the results of the study indicate that Black children are more likely to have cALLA-negative ALL than are White or Hispanic children and that they tend to have pre-B cell leukemia more often than do White or Hispanic children. As a group, children with cALLA-negative, non-T ALL tend to respond less well than do cALLA-positive patients (1), and pre-B cell patients respond less well than do other non-T, non-B cell patients (4). Thus, Black children as a group may respond less well to antileukemic therapy because as a group they have a higher likelihood of having a leukemic cell phenotype that is more resistant to conventional therapy.

These observations suggest the hypothesis that American Black children fare worse than White children or Hispanic children in large part not because of problems of delivery of health care, but because they are more apt to have a type of ALL that is more resistant to available therapy. A corollary to this hypothesis is that, when corrected for phenotype, Black children will be found to have a similar outcome to White children.

These hypotheses are now being tested in a study that has been under way for more than a year. More than 300 patients have now been entered on second-generation Pediatric Oncology Group protocols that link leukemic cell phenotype with therapy. All T-cell patients are treated identically, and pre-B cell patients and cALLA-negative non-T patients are stratified on common treatment arms. As a result of this study, we should soon be able to answer whether race or Spanish origin predict outcome independently of leukemic cell phenotype.

ACKNOWLEDGMENTS

We acknowledge with appreciation the assistance of Martha Timmons in the preparation of the manuscript. This investigation was supported in part by the following grant numbers awarded by the National Cancer Institute: CA-15989, CA-03713, CA-15525, CA-29139, CA-11233, CA-16673, and CA-13148.

REFERENCES

1. Chessells, J. M., Hardisty, R. M., Rapson, N. T., and Greaves, M. F. (1977): Acute lymphoblastic leukaemia in children: Classification and prognosis. *Lancet*, 2:1307–1309.
2. Lehmann, E. L. (1975): *Nonparametrics, Statistical Methods Based on Ranks*. Holden-Day, San Francisco.
3. Pendergrass, T. W., Hoover, R., and Godwin, J. D., II (1975): Prognosis of Black children with actue lymphocytic leukemia. *Med. Pediatr. Oncol.*, 1:143–148.
4. Pullen, D. J., Crist, W. M., Falletta, J. M., Boyett, J. M., Roper, M. A., Dowell, B., van Eys, J., Humphrey, G. B., Head, D., Blackstock, R., Metzgar, R. S., and Cooper, M. D. (1983): Pediatric Oncology Group ALinC 13 Classification Protocol for Acute Lymphocytic Leukemia. Characterization of Immunologic Phenotypes and Correlation with Treatment Results. St. Jude's International Symposium of Leukemia Cell Biology. In: Leukemia Research: Advances in Cell Biology and Treatment, edited by S. Murphy and J. R. Gilbert. Elsevier Scientific Pub. Co., North-Holland.
5. Pullen, D. J., Falletta, J. M., Crist, W. M., Vogler, L. B., Dowell, B., Humphrey, G. B., Blackstock, R., van Eys, J., Cooper, M. D., Metzgar, R. S., and Meydrech, E. F. (1981): Southwest Oncology Group experience with immunological phenotyping in acute lymphocytic leukemia of childhood. *Cancer Res.*, 41:4802–4809.
6. Ramot, B., and Magrath, I. (1982): Hypothesis: The environment is a major determinant of the immunological sub-type of lymphoma and acute lymphoblastic leukaemia in children. *Br. J. Haematol.*, 50:183–189.
7. Snedecor, G. W., and Cochran, W. G. (1980): *Statistical Methods*. 7th edition. The Iowa State University Press, Ames.
8. Walters, T. R., Bushore, M., and Simone, J. (1972): Poor prognosis in Negro children with acute lymphocytic leukemia. *Cancer*, 29:210–214.

Pathogenesis of Leukemias and Lymphomas:
Environmental Influences, edited by
I. T. Magrath, G. T. O'Conor, and B. Ramot.
Raven Press, New York © 1984.

Variations in Acute Lymphoblastic Leukemia and Non-Hodgkin's Lymphoma Phenotypes in Subpopulations: Summary and Comments

Bracha Ramot

Chaim Sheba Medical Center, Tel-Hashomer 52621, Israel

This second section of this volume provides a considerable amount of important information relating to the frequency and characteristics of leukemia and lymphoma in different races in the same country.

Dr. Greaves (Chapter 15) presents surface marker studies in a large series of patients with acute lymphoblastic leukemia (ALL) and elaborates on a number of important points. T-cell leukemia was detected in 11% of 1,269 cases tested between February 1980 and December 1981. Because his center does cell typing for a large number of medical institutions in England, it appears that the frequency of T-cell leukemia in England may be somewhat lower than in previously reported studies indicating that 15 to 25% of patients have T-cell subtype of ALL. This result is very similar, however, to the series reported from the United States in this volume, at least with regard to Whites. Note that the three- to five-year age peak that Dr. Greaves has clearly shown to be caused by common ALL evolved in England in the 1920s and in the United States in the 1940s. Whether there is a continued trend toward an increased incidence of common ALL or a reduction in incidence of T-cell ALL remains to be determined, but the possibility that the relative proportions of ALL subtypes are undergoing continued evolution seems a real one. In evaluating this in the future, the age at diagnosis is a critical factor with regard to the likelihood of any given phenotype and should not be overlooked.

Several different groups of investigators from the United States have extensively reviewed ALL in Blacks. All authors confirmed previous observations that Blacks have a poorer prognosis caused at least in part by the higher preponderance of high-risk patients. In different series, 14 to 50% of Black patients were found to have T-cell markers, but the incidence of leukemia in Blacks is about half that in Whites and, therefore, it is perhaps misleading to refer to a high incidence of T-cell ALL in Blacks. Rather, Blacks appear to have a lower incidence of common ALL. This is quite consistent with the lack of the three- to five-year early age peak in ALL in Blacks that has been previously reported, and was confirmed directly by the POG group (Falletta et al., Chapter 21). The longitudinal studies of the St. Jude's group (W. P. Bowman et al., Chapter 20) are of special interest in this regard. Their analysis of two sequential periods of observation demonstrated no change in the clinical risk factors in Whites, whereas in Blacks in the second observation period the greater frequency of patients with a high white blood cell count disappeared and the age distribution became similar to that observed in Whites. These findings indicate a change in the disease pattern of Blacks in the last decade. No change, however, was observed in the higher frequency of mediastinal tumors in Blacks, and although the percentage of E-rosette-positive blasts was similar in Whites and Blacks in the St. Jude's study, the use of anti-T sera in a smaller group demonstrated that Blacks in fact had twice the frequency of T-cell ALL compared to Whites (31% versus 15%). These results raise the possibility of a high prevalence of E-rosette-negative T-cell leukemia in Blacks. On the other hand, in the CCSE study (Chapter 21) the proportion of Blacks with E-rosette-positive ALL was higher than in Whites. Clearly, the technique of assessing E-rosette formation is critical, and studies with a monoclonal antibody to the E-rosette receptor such as T-11 may shed further light on this phenomenon. Numerous different monoclonal T-cell antibodies and antisera are available and, if only one is to be used, it should react with T-cells at all stages, e.g., the WT-1 antibody proposed by Dr. Greaves. The possibility must also be considered that Blacks, in addition to having an increased frequency of T-cell ALL, also have a greater proportion of other kinds of higher risk leukemia. This possibility is supported by the results of the Pediatric Oncology Group (J. M. Falletta et al., Chapter 22). In this regard, adenosine deaminase levels, which we have found to correlate with a poor prognosis independent of other factors, may be worth measuring and comparing in Blacks and Whites.

In analyzing the relative frequency of T-cell ALL in Blacks and Whites, it should be noted that the separation between T-cell leukemia and T-cell lymphoma in children is quite arbitrary. This is important, because Blacks not only have a higher frequency of T-cell leukemia but also have a higher frequency of T-cell lymphoma, as demonstrated clearly both by the Children's Cancer Study Group data (H. Sather et al., Chapter 21) and Dr. Reaman and Dr. Leikin (Chapter 19). It may be of value to analyze all T-cell malignancies (i.e., both "leukemia" and "lymphoma") in children together. It would also be of interest to evaluate total B-cell malignancies in various childhood populations and the relative proportions of B-cell lymphomas and common ALL, which is a leukemia of the B-cell lineage. At first sight there appears to be a reciprocal relationship between these diseases in children, in whom there is a relatively narrow histological spectrum of B-cell lymphomas.

The possible effect of socioeconomic conditions on leukemia rates and subtype frequencies cannot be determined from the small amount of data presented in this section but is surely worthy of further study and should be pursued with a well-prepared questionnaire, appropriate controls, and well-standardized methods for cell typing. Dr. Greaves is prepared to collaborate on such an undertaking and to provide antibodies to centers that have enough patients and sufficient expertise to carry out efficient phenotyping. It will also be important to study the effect of changing environmental factors in general on the pattern of lymphoid neoplasia, since our observations in the Gaza Strip indicate an increase in the incidence of acute leukemia in Arabs over the past 12 years such that it is now similar to that observed in Jews. This marked change was accompanied by dramatic environmental improvements. In this population—both Arabs and Jews—the incidence of T-cell leukemia is still high compared to that in U.S. Whites, but is similar to that in U.S. Blacks.

Dr. Hill et al. (Chapter 17) present data from England suggesting that climatic factors may in some way influence the incidence of T-cell leukemia. Although apparently statistically significant, this kind of analysis is notoriously difficult, and statistical methodology is of critical importance. Thus, this observation must be confirmed before it can be accepted. Nonetheless, this possibility is intriguing, with its inherent suggestion of a transmissible agent that is etiologically important. Epidemiological information relating the incidence of T-cell ALL to climate and geography as well as to socioeconomic and other environmental factors such as degree of urbanization should be collected. Some of the differences in the data on Blacks presented in these chapters, for example, could relate the differences in the environmental circumstances of the patients included in the various series. As such, information from cooperative groups, in which patients from many different areas are included, may fail to reveal differences that would be apparent in regional, population-based studies.

In conclusion, there are enough suggestive hints from the data that have been presented to justify much more extensive epidemiological studies in ALL in which immunological phenotyping is routinely performed. Extension of the preliminary data to subpopulations other than Blacks and Whites, such as that presented by Dr. Yu et al. (Chapter 18), Dr. Hill et al. (Chapter 17), and the cooperative groups (Chapters 21 and 22), is also likely to be of considerable interest.

Pathogenesis of Leukemias and Lymphomas:
Environmental Influences, edited by
I. T. Magrath, G. T. O'Conor, and B. Ramot.
Raven Press, New York © 1984.

Some Persons at High Risk of Lymphoproliferative Diseases

Robert W. Miller

Clinical Epidemiology Branch, National Cancer Institute, National Institutes of Health,
Bethesda, Maryland 20205

By way of introduction to this section of this volume, I will discuss some highlights of the etiology of lymphoma and of acute lymphocytic leukemia (ALL). Further description is provided in the following chapters.

ENVIRONMENTAL AGENTS

Ionizing Radiation

The first environmental agent known to induce human leukemia was ionizing radiation. The history of this discovery began, as usual, with individual case reports. The second step was to show that the same effect could be obtained in animal experimentation. Then came studies that used the death notices routinely published in the *Journal of the American Medical Association*, an inexpensive form of research, to show an excess of leukemia among radiologists compared with other physicians. After that, prospective studies of Japanese atomic bomb survivors [reviewed by Miller (11)] showed an excess of leukemia among the heavily exposed compared with those less heavily exposed.

It is notable that ionizing radiation did not induce lymphoma (9) or chronic lymphocytic leukemia (CLL), and it induced ALL among atomic bomb survivors primarily or only if they had been exposed when they were under 20 years old (15). These observations indicate that lymphocytes of young people are more susceptible than those of older people to the leukemogenic effect of ionizing radiation.

Drugs

Drugs are rare causes of lymphoma, and none are known to cause lymphocytic leukemia. Case reports strongly suggest that phenytoin induces true lymphoma and causes death, or pseudolymphoma, which regresses when the drug is discontinued (7).

Phenytoin crosses the placenta and may induce a particular constellation of malformations known as the fetal hydantoin syndrome (FHS) (4). Because the drug can induce lymphoma in patients treated for epilepsy, my colleagues and I expected that when pregnant women received it, the child would be affected (too seldom to be detected in clinical practice). Perhaps children with FHS would be especially prone to lymphoma. Much to our surprise, the first case report of FHS and cancer concerned not lymphoma but neuroblastoma and was followed soon after by publication of a second case. Eventually, four cases were reported (1). The tumor and syndrome may be caused by an effect on the neural crest causing maldevelopment of the face and a tumor of the autonomic nervous system. By contrast, phenytoin-induced lymphoma is apparently related to immunosuppression.

Immunosuppressive drugs markedly predispose patients to lymphoma who have received organ transplantation (6). The relative risk is 150 times greater than normal, beginning a few weeks after initiation of immunosuppressive therapy. Transplacental carcinogenesis is possible if pregnant women are heavily immunosuppressed by drugs for medical or surgical reasons, but no such effect has yet been described (17).

HOST SUSCEPTIBILITY

Much more has been learned about the origins of human ALL and lymphoma from genetic studies (and virology, as discussed in the final section of this book) than has been learned from studies of the effects of radiation or drugs.

Hereditary Syndromes

Certain hereditary syndromes carry a high risk of leukemia or lymphoma (2). Among them is ataxia telangiectasia (AT), an autosomal recessive disorder that causes children to stagger when they are old enough to walk and to develop dilation of the conjunctival blood vessels in mid-childhood, among other signs of the disease (10). Persons with AT are predisposed to lymphoma and, to a lesser extent, to ALL (20). Certain other syndromes predispose to leukemia, but not necessarily of the lymphocytic type. The syndromes include Down's, Fanconi's, and Bloom's, each of which involves chromosomal abnormality, although not of the same type (3).

The observations linking genetic syndromes and cancer are first made at the bedside and are elucidated in the laboratory. The relationship between Down's syndrome (DS) and leukemia was established in this way before trisomy 21 was found to be typical of DS. When trisomy was detected, one could appreciate that the associated leukemia was in some way determined prezygotically, when the chromosomal misdivision occurred. In this way, new insight was gained into cancer biology. Leukemia in DS, as in the general pediatric population, is primarily ALL, but the peak is early—at one year rather than at four years of age. This finding provides another clue to the origins of the disease and is in need of an explanation from laboratory research (12). In other syndromes at high risk, leukemia is of the nonlymphocytic type (3). Thus, the genetic disorder affects host susceptibility as it relates to the cell type of leukemia that develops.

According to Dr. Greaves (Chapter 15), the type of ALL that causes the peak in childhood leukemia at four years of age is common ALL, or cALL. When cell surface markers were first recognized, it became possible to subclassify ALL, and epidemiologic studies showed that T-cell leukemia is clinically different from cALL (18).

A Brief History of AT

We have gained new understanding of carcinogenesis from the association of rare diseases with cancer. The astute clinician often plays an important role in linking the diseases, as is well illustrated by the history of AT.

In 1957, Boder and Sedgwick in Los Angeles teased out of a great tangle of neurologic disorders with telangiectasia a separate syndrome that they called "ataxia-telangiectasia." One of their seven cases died of lymphoma. Dr. Boder noticed at autopsy that one of the patients had what seemed to be an absence of the thymus. She called this peculiarity to the attention of Dr. Robert A. Good, and a few years later he and his associates pieced together from their own experience or from reports they had read or heard about, a series of patients with lymphoma and AT (eight cases), Wiskott-Aldrich syndrome (three cases), and X-linked agammaglobulinemia (three cases). From these observations, all of which involved hereditary immuno-deficiency, Good et al. developed the hypothesis that immunodeficiency predisposes to lymphoma. They expected ALL to occur excessively in these syndromes.

In seeking such evidence, I found a family in Oregon in which two children had died of ALL and an unusual form of ataxia. Dr. Fred Hecht examined the only surviving member of the sibship, a 19-year-old male who was neurologically hand-icapped, and found that he had AT. In addition, chromosomes in his lymphocytes were unusually fragile in culture, the first time this had been observed in AT. Photographs of his siblings, who at five and six years of age had not yet developed conjunctival telangiectasia, showed that one of them had this sign of the disease, but it had not been noted in the hospital records [reviewed by Miller (14)]. On repeated examination of lymphocytes from the surviving sibling over four years, clonal evolution of a cell with a D/D chromosomal translocation was observed, increasing in frequency from 1 to 78% of peripheral lymphocytes. The patient did not develop leukemia but died of infection at 23 years of age (5). Before the syndrome had been delineated, physicians on ward rounds, on seeing a patient so handicapped, would be inclined to think, "poor child, let's go on to the next patient." And yet so much has been learned through study of this ailment from this patient and from others.

Shortly thereafter, two case reports were published independently concerning children with AT and lymphoma who overreacted to conventional doses of radio-therapy for the tumor. When another case was observed in Birmingham, England, the clincians called on laboratory scientists for their advice. They offered to expose the patient's skin fibroblasts in culture to various doses of X-ray, and found that cell survival diminished markedly as the radiation dose increased. Soon after, other laboratory scientists found evidence for a defect in the repair of DNA after damage from ionizing radiation [reviewed by Miller (14)]. Although the acute response is caused by an interaction between the genetic disorder and ionizing radiation, lymphoma is not a radiogenic neoplasm and therefore is apparently related to the immunodeficiency characteristic of AT. The relationship between lymphoproliferative neoplasia in this syndrome and the DNA repair defect is unknown.

Ethnic Differences in Lymphocytic Disease Occurrence

CLL is rare among Chinese and Japanese. Less than 2% of adult leukemia is of this type in these ethnic groups, compared with 30% among Caucasians [reviewed by Miller (13)]. Recently, a very low frequency of follicular nodular lymphoma was reported in Japanese—6% of all non-Hodgkin's lymphoma, compared with 35% in the United States. With regard to Hodgkin's disease, Japan, to date, is the only country known not to show the early age peak at 25 to 29 years. Thus, certain lymphoproliferative disorders are much less frequent among the Japanese than among Caucasians.

In the United States, males develop lymphoma about 1.5 times more often than females do, but females develop systemic lupus erythematosus (SLE) five to 10 times more often than males do. This reciprocal relationship between the sex ratio for lymphoma and that for autoimmune disease led researchers to wonder if ethnic groups with low rates for certain lymphomas would have high rates for SLE and perhaps other autoimmune diseases. The question was answered when an epidemiologic study was made in Hawaii to evaluate the clinical impression that SLE was more common in Asians than in Caucasians. SLE proved to be two to three times more common in Asians (8,19). Other autoimmune diseases also appear to be more common in Japanese than in Caucasians. Hashimoto's thyroiditis and Takayasu's aortitis are among them, but Japan has a seeming deficiency of rheumatoid arthritis, Sjögren's syndrome, myasthenia gravis, dermatomyositis, and ankylosing spondylitis. All of these diseases are more common in U.S. females than males, so the failure to find corresponding excesses in Japanese is puzzling. Other little known lymphocytic diseases occur in Japan, however, more commonly than they do in the United States, e.g., subacute necrotizing lymphadenitis, which clusters in women 20 to 35 years old in Hokkaido; plasma cell dyscrasia with polyneuropathy; and subacute mucocutaneous lymph node syndrome (Kawasaki's disease). These ethnic differences suggest dissimilar functions of subsets of lymphocytes that "protect" the Japanese against certain lymphomas but predispose them to some but not all autoimmune diseases (16).

Ethnic host factors are involved here, as contrasted with single-gene disorders that predispose to lymphomas, as described earlier in this chapter. Much remains to be explained about the ethnic differences. Epidemiologists working with laboratory scientists should be able to make rapid progress in these studies.

REFERENCES

1. Allen, R. W., Jr., Ogden, B., Bentley, F. L., and Jung, A. L. (1980): Fetal hydantoin syndrome, neuroblastoma and hemorrhagic disease in a neonate. *JAMA*, 244:1464–1465.
2. Fraumeni, J. F., Jr., and Miller, R. W. (1967): Epidemiology of human leukemia: Recent observations. *JNCI*, 38:593–605.
3. German, J. (1972): Genes which increase chromosomal instability in somatic cells and predispose to cancer. *Prog. Med. Genet.*, 8:61–101.
4. Hanson, J. W., and Smith, D. W. (1975): The fetal hydantoin syndrome. *J. Pediatr.*, 87:285–290.
5. Hecht, F., McCaw, B. K., and Koler, R. D. (1973): Ataxia-telangiectasia—clonal growth of translocation lymphocytes. *N. Engl. J. Med.*, 289:286–291.
6. Hoover, R. (1977): Effects of drugs—immunosuppression. In: *Cold Spring Harbor Conferences on Cell Proliferation, Vol. 4: Origins of Human Cancer, Book A, Incidence of Cancer in Humans*, edited by H. H. Hiatt, J. D. Watson, and J. A. Winsten, pp. 369–379. Cold Spring Harbor Laboratory, Cold Spring Harbor, NY.
7. Hoover, R., and Fraumeni, J. F., Jr. (1975): Drugs. In: *Persons at High Risk of Cancer: An Approach to Cancer Etiology and Control*, edited by J. F. Fraumeni, Jr., pp. 185–198. Academic Press, New York.
8. Kaslow, R. A. (1982): High rate of death caused by systemic lupus erythematosus among U.S. residents of Asian decent. *Arthritis Rheum.*, 25:414–418.
9. Kato, H., and Schull, W. J. (1982): Studies of the mortality of A-bomb survivors. 7. Mortality, 1950–1978: Part 1. Cancer mortality. *Radiat. Res.*, 90:395–432.
10. Kraemer, K. H. (1977): Progressive degenerative diseases associated with defective DNA repair: Xeroderma pigmentosum and ataxia telangiectasia. In: *DNA Repair Processes: Cellular Senescence and Somatic Cell Genetics*, edited by W. W. Nichols and D. G. Murphy, pp. 37–71. Symposia Specialists, Miami, FL.
11. Miller, R. W. (1969): Delayed radiation effects in atomic-bomb survivors. *Science*, 166:569–574.
12. Miller, R. W. (1970): Neoplasia and Down's syndrome. *Ann NY Acad. Sci.*, 171:637–644.
13. Miller, R. W. (1977): Ethnic differences in cancer occurrence: Genetic and environmental influences with particular reference to neuroblastoma. In: *Genetics of Human Cancer*, edited by J. J. Mulvihill, R. W. Miller, and J. F. Fraumeni, Jr., pp. 1–14. Raven Press, New York.
14. Miller, R. W. (1982): Highlights in clinical discoveries relating to ataxia-telangiectasia. In: *Ataxia-Telangiectasia—A Cellular and Molecular Link Between Cancer, Neuropathology, and Immune Deficiency*, edited by B. A. Bridges and D. G. Harnden, pp. 13–21. John Wiley & Sons, New York.
15. Miller, R. W., and Beebe, G. W. (1983): Leukemia, lymphoma and multiple myeloma. In: *Radiation Carcinogenesis*, edited by A. C. Upton. Elsevier/North-Holland, New York *(in press)*.
16. Miller, R. W., Gilman, P. A., and Sugano, H. (1981): Meeting highlights: Differences in lymphocytic diseases in the United States and Japan. *JNCI*, 67:739–740.
17. Scott, J. R. (1977): Fetal growth retardation associated with maternal administration of immunosuppressive drugs. *Am. J. Obstet. Gynecol.*, 128:668–676.
18. Sen, L., and Borella, L. (1975): Clinical importance of lymphoblasts with T markers in childhood acute leukemia. *N. Engl. J. Med.*, 292:828–832.
19. Serdula, M. K., and Rhoads, G. G. (1979): Frequency of systemic lupus erythematosus in different ethnic groups from Hawaii. *Arthritis Rheum.*, 22:328–333.
20. Spector, B. D., Filipovich, A. H., Perry, G. S., III, and Kersey, J. H. (1982): Epidemiology of cancer in ataxia-telangiectasia. In: *Ataxia-Telangiectasia—A Cellular and Molecular Link Between Cancer, Neuropathology, and Immune Deficiency*, edited by B. A. Bridges and D. G. Harnden, pp. 103–138. John Wiley & Sons, New York.

Pathogenesis of Leukemias and Lymphomas:
Environmental Influences, edited by
I. T. Magrath, G. T. O'Conor, and B. Ramot.
Raven Press, New York © 1984.

Ionizing Radiation and Drugs in the Pathogenesis of Lymphoid Neoplasia

Stuart C. Finch

Cooper Medical Center, Rutgers Medical School, Camden, New Jersey 08103

The pathogenic mechanisms of radiation and chemical induction of lymphoma and leukemia show many similarities. Many leukemogenic drugs and chemicals are radiomimetic in their actions. Both radiation and many drugs have the potential for malignant transformation after either chronic low-dose or acute high-dose administration. Almost invariably, a latent period of many months or years passes between the time of exposure to either chemical carcinogens or radiation and the development of any type of hemopoietic neoplasm. Both the duration of the latent period and the incidence of malignant transformation bear some relationship to radiation and drug doses. These are some of the reasons for considering ionizing radiation and drugs together in a discussion of their roles in lymphoid neoplasia induction.

RADIATION-INDUCED LEUKEMIA

The most reliable information concerning radiation-induced leukemia in humans has been derived from study of the atomic bomb survivors of Hiroshima and Nagasaki (61,74) and the ankylosing spondylitis patients treated by radiotherapy in England (33,117). Most low-dose information has been derived by extrapolating the Japanese and ankylosing spondylitis dose-response curves from high-dose levels down through the low-dose range. Extrapolation introduces a great many problems because of uncertainties about the shape of the dose-response curve at low-dose levels, but it is the best information now available (96). Leukemia studies initiated at the former Atomic Bomb Casualty Commission in Japan in the late 1940s have been continued at the Radiation Effects Research Foundation in a fixed population of about 110,000 atomic bomb survivors and their controls. This program is known as the Life Span Study (LSS) (10). The ankylosing spondylitis study group in England consisted of about 14,000 patients who received a single or several closely spaced courses of radiation therapy to the spine during 1935–1954. The average spinal marrow exposure was in the range of 200 to 600 rads, with rather large standard deviations. The average period of follow-up has been about 17 years.

Radiation-induced leukemia first became apparent about three to four years after radiation exposure in Hiroshima and Nagasaki. Peak incidence levels in the heavily exposed survivors were about 40 times normal, six to eight years after exposure. Since then, the excess risk of leukemia in exposed persons in both cities has declined with time (Table 1). In Hiroshima, the downward trend has been slow and the effect has continued through 1978, but in Nagasaki, the excess risk declined sharply with time after exposure and disappeared around 1970 (61). The absolute risk of leukemia in 1950–1954 was about 4 per million person-year-rads (PYR) in both cities, but on the average from 1950 to 1978, it has been about 1.7/10⁶ PYR (Table 1).

Information from the ankylosing spondylitis patients has been only moderately different. The excess risk of leukemia appeared about two years after the initiation of treatment and has persisted for about 20 years (117). Most of the leukemia was acute myeloid in type and showed an incidence increase with age. The absolute risk of leukemia has been estimated at about $0.8/10^6$ PYR over the 20-year observation period (33,117).

Most of the radiation-induced leukemia in the atomic bomb survivors was granulocytic in type. In Hiroshima, a relatively high proportion was chronic granulocytic in comparison to Nagasaki and the radiation spondylitis series. An increase in acute lymphocytic leukemia also was noted in both children and adults. The highest acute lymphocytic leukemia incidence occurred in those who were less than 15 years old at the time of exposure (Table 2). The effect occurred early and disappeared by 1960. Exposed adults, however, tended to develop their acute lymphocytic leukemia later in life (Table 3). One of the striking features of significant exposure in young persons has been the relatively high incidence of chronic granulocytic leukemia (Table 3). The overall incidence of leukemia in the atomic bomb survivors was relatively high during the early years of life and increased again with age after early adulthood (72) (Table 4). These findings were the net result of increased risks of acute granulocytic leukemia with increasing age at the time of the bomb and decreased risk of chronic granulocytic leukemia with increasing age at the time of the bomb (Table 3). No evidence has been found of increased chronic lymphocytic

TABLE 1. *Absolute risk of leukemia among Hiroshima and Nagasaki atomic-bomb survivors, at intervals from 1950 to 1978*[a]

Years	Excess deaths/ 10⁶ PYR[b]	90% Confidence intervals
1950–54	4.15	3.72–4.57
1954–58	2.28	1.87–2.68
1958–62	1.80	1.43–2.16
1962–66	0.91	0.58–1.24
1966–70	1.14	0.75–1.52
1970–74	0.42	0.03–0.81
1975–78	0.47	0.00–0.95
Total period	1.74	1.59–1.89

[a]Life Span Study sample, ages and sexes combined.
[b]Person-year-rads.
From Kato and Schull (74).

TABLE 2. Incidence[a] of acute lymphocytic leukemia in persons in Hiroshima and Nagasaki exposed to 100 rads or more, by age,[b] at intervals from 1950 to 1978

Period	Age[b] (years)			
	Under 15	15–29	30–44	45 and above
Oct. 1950–Sept. 1955	53.0	29.8	0.0	0.0
Oct. 1955–Sept. 1960	13.5	10.1	0.0	0.0
Oct. 1960–Sept. 1970	0.0	5.2	8.7	15.5
Oct. 1970–Dec. 1978	0.0	0.0	12.5	0.0
Total period	12.1	9.2	6.2	5.3

[a]Annual incidence rate per 100,000. Life Span Study.
[b]Age at the time of the atomic bomb.
From Ichimaru et al. (61).

TABLE 3. Incidence[a] of leukemia in persons in Hiroshima and Nagasaki exposed to 100 rads or more, by age[b] and type of leukemia, 1950–1978

Type of Leukemia	Age[b] (years)			
	Under 15	15–29	30–44	45 and above
Acute lymphocytic	12.1	9.2	6.2	5.3
Chronic granulocytic	14.5	7.3	15.5	5.3
Acute granulocytic	2.4	12.8	27.9	36.8
Other acute	12.1	9.2	6.2	5.3

[a]Annual incidence rate per 100,000. Life Span Study.
[b]Age at the time of the atomic bomb.
From Ichimaru et al. (61).

leukemia or any of its variants in the exposed populations. There is little or no evidence of significant bone marrow aplasia or preleukemia developing before the onset of leukemia (43).

The best available data on therapeutic radiation leukemogenesis in patients with tumors come from a number of large centers where patients with Hodgkin's disease are being aggressively treated with local or total nodal radiation with or without combination chemotherapy (7,8,19,24,30,37,38,47,107,128). The relative risk of developing leukemia after radiation received as the sole form of therapy for Hodgkin's disease has been reported to be approximately three to four times normal (7,37,107). In several other larger lymphoma series, however, radiation therapy as the sole form of therapy has not resulted in increased occurrence of leukemia (19,30,47,128). Radiation induction of acute leukemia in patients with non-Hodgkin's lymphoma or chronic lymphocyte leukemia is uncommon, but a few instances of each have been reported (99,138). In most treated lymphoma patients, the latent period for the development of leukemia varies from three to five years or longer.

TABLE 4. *Absolute risk of leukemia in atomic-bomb survivors by age[a], Hiroshima and Nagasaki, 1950–1978*

Age[a] (years)	Excess deaths/10[6] PYR[b]	90% Confidence interval
0–9	2.83	2.48–3.18
10–19	0.78	0.55–1.01
20–34	1.64	1.35–1.93
35–49	1.93	1.53–2.33
50+	3.31	2.61–4.01
All ages	1.74	1.59–1.89

[a]Age at the time of the atomic bomb.
[b]Person-year-rads.
From Kato and Schull (74). Life Span Study.

It usually is preceded for periods of two to 18 months by a preleukemic or mye-loproliferative syndrome picture (24). Once leukemia develops, it usually is acute myeloid in type or one of its variants (i.e., erythroleukemia, myelomonocytic leukemia, monocytic leukemia, etc.). Rarely does it respond to any form of therapy.

Thirteen patients with Hodgkin's disease have been reported to have developed acute lymphocytic leukemia following radiation therapy, with or without chemotherapy (21,38,107). Only two of the 13 were lymphocyte-subtyped; both of these had T-cell disorders and both had received radiation therapy followed by combination chemotherapy (21,38). A possible corollary to these observations is a recent report of radiation as a possible etiologic factor in hairy cell leukemia (leukemic reticuloendotheliosis) (123). In a group of 23 patients with the disorder, eight had had a significant history of prior radiation exposure, and five had thyroid nodules.

Increased risks of leukemia have been reported following external radiation therapy for benign gynecologic disorders (116) and breast cancer (27,106), but not for cancer of the cervix (17). There are few reliable estimates of the risk of developing leukemia after radiotherapy for most other disorders. Nonsignificant increases in leukemia incidence have been reported in children who received either thymic radiation (54,113) for presumed thymic hyperplasia or cranial radiation (91,115) for the treatment of tinea capitis. Most of the leukemia has been acute nonlymphocytic, but some has been of unspecified types.

Increased leukemia risks have been associated with the use of Thorotrast® (thorium dioxide) for diagnostic purposes (42,57,68,71,92,93), radium dial painting (102), and treatment of polycythemia vera with radioactive phosphorus (11). Most of the leukemia has been acute nonlymphocytic, but the relative risk of acute lymphocytic leukemia in the best controlled thorotrast series was 0.9 (71).

Most reports of increased leukemia following low-dose radiation exposure have involved preconception or intrauterine radiation (15,35,88,121), occupational exposure (34,75,81,85,95,136), adult diagnostic X-ray (122), increased background radiation (49,55,56), fallout from nuclear testing (83), or direct exposure from atomic bomb testing (25). Many of the low dose radiation reports have been seriously criticized on the basis of bias, improper epidemiologic design, the application of unproven assumptions, improper interpretation of data, inaccurate dosimetry, or results that are implausible in terms of current knowledge of dose-related effects in man (9,20, 41,58,64,79,84,105,132,133). In any consideration of low-dose leukemogenesis, it should be noted that patients with acute and chronic granulocytic leukemia tend to have greater exposure to medical radiation than the average population (52,114). It also has been demonstrated that less than 3% of cancer deaths in the United States can be attributed to radiation effects (63). All of these factors must be considered in the evaluation of any low-dose radiation effects.

Several epidemiologic studies have suggested a relationship between either pre-conception parental irradiation or fetal irradiation at low levels and the subsequent development of increased childhood leukemias (15,35,88,121). Leukemia risks as high as 50 times normal have been claimed for 1% of the children exposed to low-dose radiation in a three-city study (22). An absolute leukemia risk of $572/10^6$ PYR and a relative risk of 1.47 during the first 10 years of life have been estimated following *in utero* and prenatal diagnostic X-ray exposures, respectively (15,121). These estimates are believed to be much too high because a number of unlikely assumptions were made (64,84,133). Furthermore, the largest single study of leu-kemia occurrence in children following exposure to prenatal diagnostic X-ray has not demonstrated an increased risk during the first postnatal years of life (35). Studies of the atomic bomb survivors exposed *in utero* also have been negative for leukemia, but the population at risk is small (62,84).

The report of increased leukemia among military personnel who may have been exposed to average radiation doses of about 0.5 rem during atomic bomb testing in the late 1950s (25) has been criticized, because the population of about 3,000 at risk is too small to reliably demonstrate a low-dose effect (20). Nine cases of leukemia were reported, of which seven were myeloid, one was lymphocytic, and one was hairy cell in type. The Lyon et al. report (83) of increased leukemia in children from the fallout of atomic bomb testing in the western United States during the 1950s also has been questioned because of several peculiarities (9,41,79,133). Reanalysis of the data (75) that showed an association between occupational ra-diation exposure and the development of leukemia in Hanford workers has failed to confirm an increased risk of leukemia caused by radiation exposure (58). The reported incidence in leukemia among Portsmouth Naval Shipyard workers (95) has not been confirmed. Cancer mortality comparisons with the U.S. white male population and nonradiation workers showed no increased risk among naval nuclear shipyard workers for either leukemia or any form of lymphoma (105). Despite background radiation in Denver, Colorado, that is at least two to four times that of cities along the eastern seaboard, the leukemia rate in Denver is no higher and is possibly even lower than it is in several of the larger cities on the East Coast (55). Leukemia rates have shown no statistically significant increase in areas of the world, such as portions of India, China, Madagascar, and Brazil, where the levels of background terrestrial radiation may be as much as 10 times the usual (49,55,56,132).

Some of the more persuasive studies in support of a chronic low-dose leukemic effect are those involving the causes of death among U.S. radiologists between 1948 and 1961 (81,85). In that group, there was a statistically significant increased incidence of leukemia, but radiation doses are not well established and may have been rather substantial. A similar study of British radiologists has demonstrated no increased risk of leukemia for the period 1920–1957, although there may have been an increased risk before 1920 (34). Some of the more important negative low-dose leukemia studies include analyses of U.S. and British radiologist information during recent years (34,85), World-War-II-trained X-ray technologists (65), the *in utero* exposed in England (35) and Japan (62,84), uranium mill workers (6), and women exposed to repeated fluoroscopic examinations of the chest (18).

It has been stated recently that more than 40 studies have found an association between low-dose radiation exposure and leukemia, but it also was noted that as many or more studies have failed to demonstrate a leukemogenic effect for humans at low exposure levels (5). Probably the safest assumptions at this time for the risk of developing leukemia from low-dose radiation are those derived from the linear extrapolation of the atomic bomb and ankylosing spondylitis dose-response curves for leukemia down through the low-dose range. The likelihood of any epidemiologic study showing a clear relationship between low-dose irradiation and the occurrence of leukemia is quite small.

RADIATION-INDUCED LYMPHOMA

Information is scanty concerning the radiation induction of lymphomas. Studies of atomic bomb survivors exposed to less than 100 rads show no evidence of radiation-induced lymphomas in either city (74; M. Ichimaru and T. Ishimaru, *personal communication*). Increased prevalence rates are noted in the Hiroshima LSS sample for individuals who received 100 or more rads in Hiroshima and 200 or more rads in Nagasaki. These data are based on nine lymphomas in Hiroshima and five in Nagasaki in persons exposed to more than 100 rads. The trend statistics, however, for all malignant lymphomas for increased incidence with dose for the period 1950–1978, based on LSS death certificates, is not significant ($p = 0.29$) (74). Hodgkin's disease constitutes 25% of the lymphomas in the control population but only 14% of the lymphomas that have occurred in the 100+ rads exposure group. Most of the non-Hodgkin's lymphomas in the control and exposed groups are reticulum cell or diffuse histiocytic in type. The onset of lymphoma in exposed individuals has been much later than it was for radiation-related leukemia. An early lymphoma peak in exposed young persons, similar to that observed with leukemia, has not occurred. The absolute risk of lymphoma during 1950–1978 in the LSS population was 0.04 excess deaths per 10^6 PYR (confidence interval of -0.07 to 0.15) (74). The relative risk during that 28-year interval for persons exposed to 200+ rads was about 1.6, with wide 90% confidence intervals.

Increased risks of lymphoma development have been noted for American radiologists since 1939 (85) and uranium industrial workers who were exposed in the early 1950s (6). Relative risks for these groups have been in the range of 4 to 5. The lymphoma risk in persons who received radiation therapy for ankylosing spondylitis for a period of six or more years was about 2, with a ratio of leukemia to lymphoma risk of about 3 (117). In all of these studies, the onset of radiation-related lymphomas appears to be considerably later than it was for leukemia. Repeated fluoroscopic examinations of a group of women have not resulted in increased lymphoma (18), and the lymphoma-induction effects of thymus gland irradiation during childhood are equivocal (54,113).

The occurrence of mulitple myeloma has been associated with radiation exposure in the atomic bomb survivors of both Hiroshima and Nagasaki (60,74). A cumulative increase in multiple myeloma in individuals whose bone marrows were exposed to more than 50 rads appeared in the early 1960s and has become progressively larger. Significant increases are noted only for persons exposed during the middle years of life. The elderly probably died of other causes before multiple myeloma became apparent, and it is also likely that the exposed youths will develop increased radiation-related myeloma at a later date. This information is consistent with the long natural latent period of 20 to 35 years or more for multiple myeloma. The excess risk of multiple myeloma, based on incidence studies in the LSS population for persons aged 20 to 59 at the time of the atomic bomb is estimated to be approximately $0.48/10^6$ PYR of bone marrow exposure (60). The standardized relative risk for persons in the LSS population with bone marrow exposure to $50+$ rads for the period 1950–1977 is about 3. The absolute risk based on mortality data for the period 1950–1978 is 0.11 excess cases per 10^6 PYR (74). There is a significant trend statistic with dose ($p = 0.0006$).

Hanford employees who were exposed chronically to low-dose radiation and American radiologists for the period of 1948–1961 have been reported to show an increased incidence of multiple myeloma (75,81). Myeloma mortality among American radiologists has been increasing since 1939, even though radiation doses have been decreasing (85). The German thorotrast data suggest a possible myeloma and lymphoma effect, but the results are not definite (71).

DRUG INDUCTION OF LEUKEMIA

Before the late 1960s, only a handful of reports concerning the leukemogenic effects of chemotherapeutic agents had appeared in the medical literature. Subsequently, there have been many reports of the late occurrence of leukemia in patients with Hodgkin's disease, non-Hodgkin's lymphoma, multiple myeloma, and several other disorders. These reports began to appear in the early 1960s, following the widespread use of multiple chemotherapeutic agents and total nodal radiation for the treatment of these disorders (29).

In recent years, it has become clear that the incidence of leukemia is increased in long-surviving patients who have been treated with cytotoxic drugs, either with or without radiation therapy (1,3,29,45,90). The leukemogenic effects of the alkylating agents, particularly cyclophosphamide, procarbazine, melphalan, and chlorambucil, have been derived from studies of their use in patients with Hodgkin's disease (7,8,19,21,24,30,37,38,47,72,107,109,127,128), non-Hodgkin's lymphomas (16,26,31,39,72,99,108,120,134,139), multiple myeloma (8,16,26,73,107–109), chronic lymphocytic leukemia (8,26,28,72,89,99,107,138), various carcinomas (8,27,40,50,72,80,87,98,103,104,109,124), autoimmune and other benign disorders (1,8,11,12,51,66,70,72,76,94,109,111,112,131,135), and renal allografts (15,66,67,100,112,126). Azathioprine not infrequently has been included as one of the drugs in the treatment of patients with nonmalignant autoimmune disorders who have developed leukemia.

The incidence of acute leukemia in patients with Hodgkin's disease treated with intensive combination chemotherapy or with various combinations of chemotherapy and radiation therapy usually is reported to be somewhere between 2 and 5% seven to 10 years after the initiation of therapy (19,30,47,128). Relative risks of leukemia development for these patients may be as high as 100 to 300 or more over a 10-year period. The occurrence of leukemia in long-term Hodgkin's disease survivors has been reported to be much lower (2 to 3%) in patients treated with either radiation therapy or chemotherapy alone than in patients treated with both of these modalities of therapy (7,37). Leukemia induction has been reported to be the highest (18.4%) if radiation therapy is given before rather than after combination chemotherapy (37). The incidence of leukemia also varies with the aggressiveness of therapy, length of time after therapy, and type of chemotherapeutic drugs used.

Most of the leukemias that have developed in long-term Hodgkin's disease survivors treated with chemotherapy have been acute nonlymphocytic. Relatively few acute lymphocytic types have been reported (21,38,107). An almost invariable prerequisite for the ultimate development of leukemia is the late occurrence of moderate to severe bone marrow depression before the actual development of rapidly fatal acute leukemia (8,107,109). The preleukemic phase, which is characterized by pancytopenia, a megaloblastic marrow, and nucleated red blood cells in the peripheral blood, appears to be clearly related to previous cytotoxic drug therapy (4,24). Latent periods between the cessation of chemotherapy and the onset of leukemia have varied from months to 15 or more years, with an average of about six to seven years. A relatively large number of variant forms of myelocytic leukemia have been reported, including erythroleukemia, aleukemic myeloid leukemia, and myelomonocytic leukemia (48,109). The leukemia conversion results of single or multiple alkylating agents in the therapy of non-Hodgkin's lymphoma have been similar to that experienced with Hodgkin's disease, but reliable incidence figures are more difficult to obtain (16,26,31,39,72,99,107,109,120,134,139). Latent periods have averaged about six years, with a range of 1.5 to more than 12 years. Chronic lymphocytic leukemia with low-dose administration of a single alkylating agent has 1 to 2% predicted leukemia conversion in five to seven years after the onset of therapy (107,138). Most patients with multiple myeloma who have developed acute leukemia have had long-term therapy with either melphalan or cyclophosphamide (8,16,78,107,108). The relative risk of developing acute nonlymphocytic leukemia in myeloma patients treated for five or 10 years with alkylating agents probably is in the range of 20 to 25 (73). In a recent large polycythemia vera cooperative study, treatment with chlorambucil was associated with a risk of acute nonlymphocytic leukemia 2.3 times greater than in the group treated with radioactive phosphorus and 13 times greater than in those treated only with phlebotomy (11).

Acute leukemia has developed in a number of patients who have received cytotoxic drugs for the treatment of cancer of the ovary (40,104), breast (27,80,98, 103,109), and lung (107,124). In a large series of more than 5,000 women treated with alkylating agents for ovarian carcinoma, the risk of acute nonlymphocytic leukemia was said to have been increased by a factor of 36 over a period of five years (104). A sevenfold increase in acute leukemia has been reported in patients with breast cancer, most of whom were treated with alkylating agents, sometimes in combination with radiotherapy (109).

An impressive number of patients with nonneoplastic diseases has developed acute leukemia following the use of chemotherapeutic agents (1,8,17,18,51,66,70, 72,76,94,109,111,112,131,135). Most of the leukemias are myeloid in type, but a few have been lymphocytic (51). A few renal transplant patients, who have been treated with various immunosuppressive agents and corticosteroids with or without antilymphocyte or antithymocyte serum, also have developed leukemia (12,66,112).

In summary, the characteristics of the leukemia transformation process and the clinical manifestations of leukemia that follows the administration of cancer chemotherapeutic agents bear a considerable resemblance to radiation therapy-induced leukemia. Acute nonlymphocytic leukemia induction rates in long-term survivors are high. The characteristics of the underlying diseases being treated, however, appear to have some influence on the type of leukemia expressed. Leukemia developing in patients with multiple myeloma is about equally divided between myelocytic and monocytic or myelomonocytic types. Patients with chronic lymphocytic leukemia develop acute lymphocytic and acute myelocytic leukemias with about equal frequencies. Patients with Hodgkin's disease usually develop acute granulocytic leukemia and occasionally acute T-cell leukemia (21,38).

Strong evidence for the direct leukemogenic effect of the alkylating agents is provided by the data from patients treated for nonlymphomatous neoplasms and nonneoplastic disorders. Leukemia rarely develops in these patients unless they receive one or more alkylating agents for a prolonged period of time. The most likely cause of the leukemogenicity of these agents is their ability to produce mutations in hemopoietic stem cells. They may act synergistically with radiation. Recently, an increased risk for certain types of cancer based on genetic susceptibility concerning the Ah locus has been suggested (97). This may account for the fact that most of the leukemias are myeloid rather than lymphoid in type and would mitigate against a pure immunologic mechanism.

Leukemogenic effects have been claimed for both chloramphenicol and phenylbutazone, but the relationships are weak (1,3,16,45). Those patients reported to have developed leukemia following administration of these drugs have had similar clinical courses. The few patients reported have experienced a prolonged period of aplasia or reduced bone marrow function before the development of acute nonlymphocytic leukemia.

Recently, some attention has been focused on lithium as a possible leukemogenic agent. Six patients now have been reported to have developed various forms of myeloid leukemia following or during many months to several years of drug administration (44). Lithium appears to be a potent myelopoietic stimulant, but it would be premature to conclude that it is leukemogenic on the basis of current information.

The leukemogenic effect of benzene and its derivatives seems well established (1,2,3,45), but the extent of low-dose exposure risk is uncertain. Exposure to either a single large amount of benzene or multiple small doses may result in the development of acute or chronic progressive pancytopenia. A small proportion of these individuals eventually will develop acute nonlymphocytic leukemia, many months or years after the initial exposure. Several epidemiologic surveys suggest that chronic low-dose occupational exposure to benzene derivatives increased the risk of developing acute myeloid leukemia (110,130). Duration of exposure has varied from one to 15 years, with a relative risk for developing leukemia ranging from two to 20 times normal. The results of some of the studies are difficult to assess, because the largest epidemiologic study conducted in a high-benzene-exposure population demonstrated no increased risk for myeloid leukemia but a weak association with lymphocytic leukemia (137). Furthermore, persons exposed to benzene usually are exposed to a number of other substances, and the leukemogenicity of benzene in experimental animals has been rather inconsistent. Controversy regarding the leukemogenicity of low-dose benzene exposure surrounds a recent report of the International Agency for Research on Cancer of the World Health Organization in which it was calculated that exposure over a lifetime to 10 ppm of benzene might result in 17 excess leukemia deaths per 1,000 persons exposed (125). Despite these weaknesses, the association between benzene and leukemia is stronger than it is for either chloramphenicol or phenylbutazone.

A number of other chemical agents have been reported to be leukemogenic for humans, but very little substantial evidence supports these claims. Some of the drugs and chemicals suggested have been griseofulvin, ethylene oxide, chloroquine, lysergic acid diethylamide, methoxypsoralen, streptozotocin, razoxane, and several antimetabolic chemotherapeutic agents (e.g., 6-mercaptopurine, methotrexate, and aminopterin) (1,3,45,50,69,109).

DRUG INDUCTION OF LYMPHOMA

The drug induction of lymphoma is more difficult to document than is the drug induction of leukemia. Combination chemotherapy involving the use of an alkylating agent and radiotherapy has been associated with subsequent development of non-Hodgkin's lymphoma in a small number of patients treated for Hodgkin's disease (32,36,77,82,128). The risk of developing non-Hodgkin's lymphoma at 10 years after all modalities of therapy for Hodgkin's disease is said to involve about 4.4%

of all patients treated (77). The use of combination chemotherapy and radiotherapy increased this figure to 15.2%. One of three patients who developed non-Hodgkin's lymphoma and was lymphocyte-subtyped had T-cell disease (82). It is of further interest that eight of nine patients described in the literature with Hodgkin's disease who have developed non-Hodgkin's lymphoma have had lymphoma involvement of the gastrointestinal tract (32,36,77,82). In only three instances have alkylating agents been associated with subsequent development of a malignant plasma cell dyscrasia in patients with Hodgkin's disease (46). The latent periods before the development of leukemia have ranged from 14 months to five years.

Immunosuppression for the management of renal and cardiac transplants has been associated with a significant number of cases of non-Hodgkin's lymphoma (12,66, 100,109,112,127). The agents most commonly used in various combinations are methotrexate, azathioprine, cyclophosphamide, melphalan, actinomycin D, adreno-corticosteroids, antilymphocyte globulin, and antithymocyte globulin. The Denver Transplant Tumor Registry has reported that 29% of the neoplasms encountered in renal transplant patients have been lymphomas, in contrast to a lymphoma incidence of 3 to 4% of all tumors in the general population (127). Most of the tumors were large-cell lymphomas with cells resembling activated lymphocytes or the B-cell type. Only 2% of the lymphomas were Hodgkin's disease, in comparison to about 34% of all lymphomas that occur naturally in the general population. The mortality from non-Hodgkin's lymphoma in transplant recipients is more than 40 times greater than that observed in the general population (101). Most of the lymphomas have occurred in fairly young individuals and have appeared only a few months following transplantation. Another unusual feature of these tumors is their predilection for central nervous system and renal homograft involvement (90,101). In one large series, 19% had involvement of the renal homograft (101). Of the patients with localized lymphoma, 60% had lesions in the central nervous system. There is good evidence that these tumors are a consequence of immunosuppression, as judged by their histologic appearance and biological behavior.

In a series of 124 patients at risk at three months after heart transplantation, 10 lymphomas have been observed, of which two have occurred at the injection sites of antithymocyte globulin (12). Human heart transplant recipients managed by conventional immunosuppressive agents have shown conversion rates to histiocytic lymphomas that are greatly increased with retransplantation and are inversely proportional to age. These observations suggest that the characteristics of the underlying disorder may have considerable influence on the ultimate expression of the type of neoplasia. The role of immunosuppression per se in the etiology of these disorders also is strengthened. Recently, cyclosporin A has been introduced as a potent immunosuppressive agent in the field of cardiac transplantation. About 5% of a small number of postrenal transplant patients treated with cyclosporin A have developed a lymphoma within four to 11 months (126). Some direct experimental evidence suggests that this may represent Epstein-Barr virus activation (81). The possible lymphoma induction role of cyclosporin A is strengthened in another report on cardiac transplants in primates, with about 10% developing histiocytic lymphoma (13).

The capacity of other drugs and chemicals to induce lymphomas is much less well documented. Hydantoin derivatives will induce psuedolymphomas that usually regress with cessation of drug therapy (23,45,59,86). There are, however, at least 10 instances in the older literature of either direct development of a malignant lymphoma following the long-term administration of a hydantoin compound or the ultimate conversion of a pseudolymphoma into a lymphoma. The risk of developing a true lymphoma from a hydantoin compound is uncertain but must be low. None of the studies has been well controlled. Phenytoin probably suppresses both humoral and cell-mediated immunity (86,119).

Two of 158 exposed workers in the manufacture of pentachlorophenol have been reported to have developed non-Hodgkin's lymphoma of the scalp (14). It has been suggested that the "dioxins" that are contaminants in the intermediate stages of manufacturing pentachlorophenol are responsible. Workers in this field also are exposed to benzene and various aromatic hydrocarbons. In a case control study, it was noted that 36.1% of 169 patients with lymphomas had been exposed to organic solvents, phenoxy acids, or chlorophenols (53), compared to only 9.6% of 333 controls. The relative risk of lymphoma in the exposed group was estimated to be 5.3. Combined exposure to the various chemicals appeared to increase the risk. Benzene has also been incriminated in the etiology of both Hodgkin's disease and non-Hodgkin's lymphoma (129). At least one large study has been unable to confirm this observation, which has been rather poorly documented (118).

REFERENCES

1. Adamson, R. H., and Sieber, S. M. (1981): Chemically induced leukemia in humans. *Environ. Health Perspect.*, 39:93–103.
2. Aksoy, M. (1980): Malignancies due to occupational exposure to benzene. *Haematologica (Pavia)*, 65:370–373.
3. Alderson, M. (1980): The epidemiology of leukemia. *Adv. Cancer Res.*, 31:1–77.
4. Anderson, R. L., Bagby, G. C., Jr., Richert-Boe, K., Magenis, R. E., and Koler, R. D. (1981): Therapy-related preleukemic syndrome. *Cancer*, 47:1867–1871.
5. Archer, V. E. (1981): Epidemiological studies of low-level radiation effects (letter). *Health Phys.*, 40:129.
6. Archer, V. E., Wagoner, J. K., and Lundin, F. (1973): Cancer mortality among uranium mill workers. *JOM*, 15:11–14.
7. Arseneau, J. C., Canellos, G. P., Johnson, R., and DeVita, V. T., Jr. (1977): Risk of new cancers in patients with Hodgkin's disease. *Cancer*, 40:1912–1916.
8. Auclerc, G., Jacquillat, C., Auclerc, M. F., Weil, M., and Bernard, J. (1979): Post therapeutic acute leukemia. *Cancer*, 44:2017–2025.
9. Bader, M. (1979): Leukemia from atomic fallout (letter). *N. Engl. J. Med.*, 300:1491.
10. Beebe, G. W., Ishida, M., and Jablon, S. (1962): Studies of the mortality of A-bomb survivors. 1. Plan of study and mortality in the medical subsample (selection 1), 1950–1958. *Radiat. Res.*, 16:253–280.
11. Berk, P. D., Goldberg, J. D., Silverstein, M. N., Weinfeld, A., Donovan, P. B., Ellis, J. T., Landaw, S. A., Laszlo, J., Najean, Y., Pisciotta, A. V., and Wasserman, L. R. (1981): Increased incidence of acute leukemia in polycythemia vera associated with chlorambucil therapy. *N. Engl. J. Med.*, 304:441–447.
12. Bieber, C. P., Hunt, S. A., Schwinn, D. A., Jamieson, S. A., Reitz, B. A., Oyer, P. E., Shum-

way, N. E., and Stinson, E. B. (1981): Complications in long-term survivors of cardiac transplantation. *Transplant. Proc.*, 13:207–211.

13. Bieber, C. P., Reitz, B. A., Jamieson, S. W., Oyer, P. E., and Stinson, E. B. (1980): Malignant lymphoma in Cyclosporin A treated allograft recipients. *Lancet*, 1:43.

14. Bishop, C. M., and Jones, A. H. (1981): Non-Hodgkin's lymphoma of the scalp in workers exposed to dioxins (letter). *Lancet*, 2:369.

15. Bithell, J. F., and Stewart, A. M. (1975): Pre-natal irradiation and childhood malignancy: a review of British data from the Oxford survey. *Br. J. Cancer*, 31:271–287.

16. Bloomfield, C. D., and Brunning, R. D. (1976): Acute leukemia as a terminal event in nonleukemic hematopoietic disorders. *Semin. Oncol.*, 3:297–317.

17. Boice, J. D., and Hutchinson, G. B. (1980): Leukemia in women following radiotherapy for cervical cancer: ten-year follow-up of an international study. *JNCI*, 65:115–129.

18. Boice, J. D. Monson, R. R., and Rosenstein, M. (1981): Cancer mortality in women after repeated fluoroscopic examinations of the chest. *JNCI*, 66:863–867.

19. Boivin, J. F., and Hutchison, G. B. (1981): Leukemia and other cancers after radiotherapy and chemotherapy for Hodgkin's disease. *JNCI*, 67:751–760.

20. Bond, V. P., and Hamilton, L. D. (1980): Leukemia in the Nevada "Smoky" bomb test (editorial). *JAMA*, 244:1610.

21. Boucheix, C., Zittoun, R., Reynes, M., Diebold, J., Bernadou, A., and Bilski-Pasquier, G. (1979): Atypical T-cell leukemia terminating Hodgkin's Disease. *Cancer*, 44:1403–1407.

22. Bross, I. D. J., and Natarajan, N. (1980): Cumulative genetic damage in children exposed to preconception and intrauterine radiation. *Invest. Radiol.*, 15:52–64.

23. Cacatian, A. A., and Rando, J. (1981): Diphenylhydantoin-induced pseudolymphoma syndrome with severe thrombocytopenia. *NY State J. Med.*, 81:1085–1087.

24. Cadman, E. C., Capizzi, R. L., and Bertino, J. R. (1977): Acute non-lymphocytic leukemia. A delayed complication of Hodgkin's Disease therapy: analysis of 109 cases. *Cancer*, 40:1280–1296.

25. Caldwell, G. G., Kelley, D. B., and Heath, C. W., Jr. (1980): Leukemia among participants in military maneuvers at a nuclear bomb test. A preliminary report. *JAMA*, 244:1575–1578.

26. Cardamone, J. M., Kimmerle, R. I., and Marshall, E. Y. (1974): Development of acute erythroleukemia in B-cell immunoproliferative disorders after prolonged therapy with alkylating drugs. *Am. J. Med.*, 57:836–842.

27. Carey, R. W., Holland, J. F., Sheehe, P. R., and Saxon, G. (1967): Association of cancer of the breast and acute myelocytic leukemia. *Cancer*, 20:1080–1088.

28. Catovsky, D., and Galton, D. A. G. (1971): Myelomonocytic leukemia supervening on chronic lymphocytic leukaemia. *Lancet*, 1:478–479.

29. Chabner, B. A. (1977): Second neoplasm—A complication of cancer chemotherapy. *N. Engl. J. Med.*, 297:213–214.

30. Coleman, C. N., Williams, C. J., Flint, A., Glatstein, E. J., Rosenberg, S. A., and Kaplan, H. S. (1977): Hematologic neoplasia in patients treated for Hodgkin's disease. *N. Engl. J. Med.*, 297:1249–1252.

31. Collins, A. J., Bloomfield, C. D., Peterson, B. A., and McKenna, R. W. (1977): Acute nonlymphocytic leukemia in patients with nodular lymphoma. *Cancer*, 40:1748–1754.

32. Come, S. E., and Long, J. C. (1980): A 24-year-old man with previous Hodgkin's disease and an abdominal mass (case records of the Massachusetts General Hospital). *N. Engl. J. Med.*, 302:389–395.

33. Court Brown, W. M., and Doll, R. (1957): Leukemia and aplastic anemia in patients irradiated for ankylosing spondylitis. Medical Research Council Report 295. Her Majesty's Stationery Office, London.

34. Court Brown, W. M., and Doll R. (1958): Expectation of life and mortality from cancer among British radiologists. *Br. Med. J.*, 2:181–187.

35. Court Brown, W. M., Doll, R., and Hill, A. B. (1960): Incidence of leukaemia after exposure to diagnostic radiation *in utero*. *Br. Med. J.*, 2:1539–1545.

36. D'Agostino, R. S. (1979): Non-Hodgkin's lymphoma after radiotherapy for Hodgkin's disease. *N. Engl. J. Med.*, 301:1289.

37. DeVita, V. T., Jr. (1981): The consequences of the chemotherapy of Hodgkin's disease: The 10th David A. Karnofsky Memorial Lecture. *Cancer*, 47:1–13.

38. Dick, F. R., Maca, R. D., and Hankenson, R. (1978): Hodgkin's disease terminating in a T-cell immunoblastic leukemia. *Cancer*, 42:1325–1329.
39. Dumont, J., Thiery, J. P., Mazabraud, A., Natali, J. C., Trapet, P., and Vilcoq, J. R. (1980): Acute myeloid leukemia following non-Hodgkin's lymphoma: danger of prolonged use of chlorambucil as maintenance therapy. *Nouv. Rev. Fr. Hematol.*, 22:391–404.
40. Einhorn, N., (1978): Acute leukemia after chemotherapy (melphalan). *Cancer*, 41:444–447.
41. Enstrom, J. E. (1979): Leukemia from atomic fallout (letter). *N. Engl. J. Med.*, 300:1491.
42. Faber, M. (1978): Malignancies in Danish thorotrast patients. *Health Phys.*, 35:153.
43. Finch, S. C., Hoshino, T., Lamphere, J. P., and Ishimaru, T. (1977): Peripheral blood changes preceding the development of leukemia in atomic bomb survivors of Hiroshima and Nagasaki. In: *Topics in Hematology, Proceedings of the 16th International Congress of Hematology*, edited by S. Seno, S. Takaku, and S. Irino, pp. 97–98. Excerpta Medica, Amsterdam.
44. Gauwerky, C. E., and Golde, D. W. (1982): Lithium enhances growth of human leukaemia cells in vitro. *Br. J. Haematol.*, 51:431–438.
45. Geary, C. G. (1980): Lymphoma and leukemia due to drugs. *Br. J. Hosp. Med.*, 24:538–547.
46. Gelmann, E. P., and Dennis, L. H. (1981): Plasma-cell dyscrasia after alkylating-agent therapy for Hodgkin's disease (letter). *N. Engl. J. Med.*, 305:1350.
47. Glicksman, A. S. (1981): Side effects of various Hodgkin's therapies (medical news). *JAMA*, 246:1877 1878.
48. Goldhirsch, A., Pirovino, M., Coninx, S., Tschopp, L., and Sonntag, R. W. (1980): Case report. Acute erythroleukemia following chemotherapy for Hodgkin's disease. *Am. J. Med. Sci.*, 280:53–56.
49. Gopal-Ayengar, A. R., Sundaram, K., Mistry, K. B., Sunta, C. M., Nambi, K. S. V., Kathuria, S. P., Basu, A. S., and David, M. (1972): Evaluation of long-term effects of high background radiation on selected population groups on the Kerala coast. In: *Peaceful Uses of Atomic Energy*, Vol. II, pp. 31–51. United Nations and IAEA, New York and Vienna.
50. Green, M. R., and Anderson, R. E. (1981): Acute myelocytic leukemia following prolonged streptozotocin therapy. *Cancer*, 47:1963–1965.
51. Grunwald, H., and Rosner, F. (1979): Acute leukemia and immunosuppressive drug use. A review of patients undergoing immunosuppressive therapy for nonneoplastic diseases. *Arch. Intern. Med.*, 139:461–466.
52. Gunz, F. W., and Atkinson, H. R. (1964): Medical radiation and leukaemia: a retrospective survey. *Br. Med. J.*, 1:389–393.
53. Hardell, L., Eriksson, M., Lenner, P., and Lundgren, E. (1981): Malignant lymphoma and exposure to chemicals, especially organic solvents, chlorophenols and phenoxy acids: a case-control study. *Br. J. Cancer*, 43:169–176.
54. Hempelmann, L. H., Hall, W. J., Phillips, M., Cooper R. A., and Ames, W. R. (1975): Neoplasms in persons treated with X-rays in infancy: fourth survey in 20 years. *JNCI*, 55:519–530.
55. Hickey, R. J., Bowers, E. J., Spence, D. E., Zemel, B. S., Clelland, A. B., and Clelland, R. C. (1981): Low level ionizing radiation and human mortality: multi-regional epidemiological studies. A preliminary report. *Health Phys.*, 40:625–641.
56. High Background Radiation Research Group (1980): Health survey in high background radiation areas in China. *Science*, 209:877–880.
57. Horta, J. D., DaMotta, C. L., and Tavares, M. H. (1974): Thorium dioxide effects in man: epidemiological, clinical and pathological studies. *Environ. Res.*, 8:131–159.
58. Hutchinson, G. B., MacMahon, B., Jablon, S., and Land, C. E. (1979): Review of report by Mancuso, Stewart and Kneale of radiation exposure of Hanford workers. *Health Phys.*, 37:207–220.
59. Hyman, G. A., Sommers, S. C. (1966): The development of Hodgkin's disease and lymphoma during anticonvulsant therapy. *Blood*, 28:416–427.
60. Ichimaru, M., Ishimaru, T., Mikami, M., and Matsunaga, M. (1982): Multiple myeloma among atomic bomb survivors Hiroshima and Nagasaki, 1950–76: Relationship to radiation dose absorbed by marrow. *JCNI*, 69:323–328.
61. Ichimaru, M., Ishimaru, T., Mikami, M., Yamada, Y., and Ohkita, T. (1981): Incidence of leukemia in atomic bomb survivors and controls in a fixed cohort, Hiroshima and Nagasaki, October 1950–December 1978. Radiation Effects Research Foundation Technical Report 13–81.
62. Ishimaru, T., Ichimaru, M., and Mikami, M. (1981): Leukemia incidence among individuals

exposed *in utero*, children of atomic bomb survivors, and their controls: Hiroshima and Nagasaki, 1945–79. Radiation Effects Research Foundation Technical Report 11-81.

63. Jablon, S., and Bailar, J. C., III (1980): The contribution of ionizing radiation to cancer mortality in the United States. *Prev. Med.*, 9:219–226.

64. Jablon, S., and Kato, H. (1970): Childhood cancer in relation to prenatal exposure to atomic-bomb radiation. *Lancet*, 2:1000–1003.

65. Jablon, S., and Miller, R. W. (1978): Army technologists: 29-year follow up for cause of death. *Radiology*, 126:677–679.

66. Jacobs, C., Brunner, F. P., Brynger, H., Chantler, C., Donckerwolcke, R. A., Hathway, R. A., Kramer, P., Selwood, N. H., and Wing, A. J. (1981): Malignant diseases in patients treated by dialysis and transplantation in Europe. *Transplant. Proc.*, 13:729–732.

67. Jacobs, P., and Gordon-Smith, E. C. (1980): Cyclosporin-A, transplantation, and lymphoma. *Lancet*, 2:1296.

68. Johnson, S. A. N., Bateman, C. J. T., Beard, M. E. J., Whitehouse, J. M. A., and Waters, A. H. (1977): Long-term haematological complications of thorotrast. *Q. J. Med.*, 46:259–271.

69. Joshi, R., Smith, B., Phillips, R. H., and Barrett, A. J. (1981): Acute myelomonocytic leukaemia after razoxone therapy (letter). *Lancet*, 2:1343.

70. Kahn, M. F., Arlet, J., Bloch-Michel, H., Caroit, M., Chaouat, Y., and Renler, J. C. (1979): Leucemies aigues apres traitement par agents cytoxiques en rheumatologie. 19 observations chez 2006 patients. *Nouve. Presse Med.*, 8:1393.

71. Kaick, G. van, and Scheer, K. E. (1973): Actual status of the German Thorotrast Study. *Proceedings of the Third International Meeting on the Toxicity of Thorotrast*, p. 157. Riso Report No. 294:157–162. Danish Atomic Energy Commission, Roskilde.

72. Kapadia, S. B., Krause, J. R., Ellis, L. D., Pan, S. F., and Wald, N. (1980): Induced acute non-lymphocytic leukemia following long-term chemotherapy: A study of 20 cases. *Cancer*, 45:1315–1321.

73. Karchmer, R. K., Amare, M., Larsen, W. E., Mallouk, A. G., and Caldwell, G. G. (1974): Alkylating agents as leukemogens in multiple myeloma. *Cancer*, 33:1103–1107.

74. Kato, H., and Schull, W. J. (1982): Studies on the mortality of A-bomb survivors. 7. Mortality, 1950–1978: Part 1. Cancer mortality. *Radiat. Res.*, 90:395–432.

75. Kneale, G. W., Stewart, A. M., and Mancuso, T. F. (1978): Re-analysis of data relating to the Hanford study of the cancer risks of radiation workers. In: *Late Biological Effects of Ionizing Radiation*, Vol. 1, pp. 386–412. International Atomic Energy Agency, Vienna.

76. Krause, J. R. (1981): Acute nonlymphocytic leukemia after cyclophosphamide therapy for refractory idiopathic thrombocytopenic purpura. *South. Med. J.*, 74:891–892.

77. Krikorian, J. G., Burke, J. S., Rosenberg, S. A., and Kaplan, H. S. (1979): Occurrence of non-Hodgkin's lymphoma after therapy for Hodgkin's disease. *N. Engl. J. Med.*, 300:452–458.

78. Kyle, R. A., Pierre, R. V., and Bayrd, E. D. (1975): Multiple myeloma and acute leukemia associated with alkylating agents. *Arch. Intern. Med.*, 135:185–192.

79. Land, C. E. (1979): The hazards of fallout or of epidemiologic research? (editorial). *N. Engl. J. Med.*, 300:431–432.

80. Lerner, H. J. (1978): Acute myelogenous leukemia in patients receiving chlorambucil as long-term adjuvant chemotherapy for stage II breast cancer. *Cancer Treat. Rep.*, 62:1135–1138.

81. Lewis, E. B. (1963): Leukemia, multiple myeloma, and aplastic anemia in American radiologists. *Science*, 142:1492–1494.

82. Lowenthal, R. M., Harlow, R. W. H., Mead, A. E., Tuck, D., and Challis, D. R. (1981): T-cell non-Hodgkin's lymphoma after radiotherapy and chemotherapy for Hodgkin's disease. *Cancer*, 48:1586–1589.

83. Lyon, J. L., Klauber, M. R., Gardner, J. W., and Udall, K. S. (1979): Childhood leukemias associated with fallout from nuclear testing. *N. Engl. J. Med.*, 300:397–402.

84. MacMahon, B. (1972): Susceptibility to radiation-induced leukemia? *N. Engl. J. Med.*, 287:144–145.

85. Matanoski, G. M., Seltser, R., Sartwell, P. E., Diamond, E. L., and Elliott, E. A. (1975): The current mortality rates of radiologists and other physican specialists: specific causes of death. *Am. J. Epidemiol.*, 101:199–210.

86. Matzner, Y., and Polliack, A. (1978): Lymphoproliferative disorders in four patients receiving chronic diphenylhydantoin therapy: etiologic correlation or chance association? *Isr. J. Med. Sci.*, 14:865–869.

87. May, J. T., Hsu, S. D., and Costanzi, J. J. (1981): Acute leukemia following combination chemotherapy for cancer of the lung. *Oncology*, 38:134–137.
88. MacMahon, B., and Hutchinson, G. B. (1964): Prenatal X-ray and childhood cancer. A Review. *Acta Union Int. Contre Cancer*, 20:1172–1174.
89. McPhedran, P., and Heath, C. W., Jr. (1970): Acute leukemia occurring during chronic lymphocytic leukemia. *Blood*, 35:7–11.
90. Miller, R. W. (1978): Environmental causes of cancer in childhood. *Adv. Pediatr.*, 25:97.
91. Modan, B., Baidatz, D., Mart, H., Steinitz, R., and Levin, S. (1974): Radiation-induced head and neck tumors. *Lancet*, 1:277–279.
92. Mole, R. H. (1978): The radiobiological significance of the studies with ^{224}Ra and Thorotrast. *Health Phys.*, 35:167–174.
93. Mori, T., Nozue, Y., Miyazi, T., and Takahashi, S., (1973): Thorotrast injury in Japan. *Proceedings of the Third International Meeting on the Toxicity of Thorotrast*, pp. 175–192. Riso Report No. 294. Danish Atomic Energy Commission, Roskilde.
94. Muller, W., and Brandis, M. (1981): Acute leukemia after cytotoxic treatment for nonmalignant disease in childhood. A case report and review of the literature. *Eur. J. Pediatr.*, 136:105–108.
95. Najarian, T., and Colton, T. (1978): Mortality from leukaemia and cancer in shipyard nuclear workers. *Lancet*, 1:1018–1020.
96. National Research Council, Committee on the Biological Effects of Ionizing Radiations (1980): The effects on populations of exposure to low levels of ionizing radiation. National Academy Press, Washington, D.C.
97. Nebert, D. W. (1981): Genetic differences in susceptibility to chemically induced myelotoxicity and leukemia. *Environ. Health Perspect.*, 39:11.
98. Nowell, P., Glick, J. H., Bucolo, A., Finan, J., and Creech, R. (1981): Cytogenetic studies of bone marrow in breast cancer patients after adjuvant chemotherapy. *Cancer*, 48:667–673.
99. O'Donnell, J. F., Brereton, H. D., Greco, F. A., Gralnick, H. R., and Johnson, R. E. (1979): Acute nonlymphocytic leukemia and acute myeloproliferative syndrome following radiation therapy for non-Hodgkin's lymphoma and chronic lymphocytic leukemia: clinical studies. *Cancer*, 44:1930.
100. Penn, I. (1978): Development of cancer in transplantation patients. *Adv. Surg.*, 12:155.
101. Penn, I. (1981): Malignant lymphomas in organ transplant recipients. *Transplant. Proc.*, 13:736–738.
102. Polednak, A. P., Stehney, A. F., and Rowland, R. E. (1978): Mortality among women first employed before 1930 in the U.S. radium dial painting industry. *Am. J. Epidemiol.*, 107:179–193.
103. Portugal, M. A., Falkson, H. C., Stevens, K., and Falkson, G. (1979): Acute leukemia as a complication of long-term treatment of advanced breast cancer. *Cancer Treat. Rep.*, 63:177–181.
104. Reimer, R. R., Hoover, R., Fraumeni, J. F., Jr., and Young, R. C. (1977): Acute leukemia after alkylating-agent therapy of ovarian cancer. *N. Engl. J. Med.*, 297:177–181.
105. Rinsky, R. A., Zumwalde, R. D., Waxweiler, R. J., Murray, W. E., Jr., Bierbaum, P. J., Landrigan, P. J., Terpilak, M., and Cox, C. (1981): Cancer mortality at a naval nuclear shipyard. *Lancet*, 1:231–235.
106. Robins, H. I., Ershler, W. B., Hafez, G. R., Dohlberg, S., and Arndt, C. (1980): Acute nonlymphocytic leukaemia in breast cancer: therapy related or *do novo*? (letter). *Lancet*, 1:91–92.
107. Rosner, F. (1976): Acute leukemia as a delayed consequence of cancer chemotherapy. *Cancer*, 37:1033–1036.
108. Rosner, F., and Grunwald, H. (1974): Multiple myeloma terminating in acute leukemia: report of 12 cases and review of the literature. *Am. J. Med.*, 57:927–939.
109. Rosner, F., and Grunwald, H. W. (1980): Cytotoxic drugs and leukemogenesis. *Clin. Haematol.*, 9:663–681.
110. Rushton, L., and Alderson, M. R. (1981): A case-control study to investigate the association between exposure to benzene and deaths from leukaemia in oil refinery workers. *Br. J. Cancer*, 43:77–84.
111. Sheibani, K., Bukowski, R. M., Tubbs, R. R., Savage, R. A., Sebek, B. A., and Hoffman, G. C. (1980): Acute nonlymphocytic leukemia in patients receiving chemotherapy for nonmalignant diseases. *Hum. Pathol.*, 11:175–178.
112. Sheil, A. G. R., Mahony, J. F., Horvath, J. J., Johnson, J. R., Tiller, D. J., Stewart, J. H., and May, J. (1981): Cancer following successful cadaveric donor renal transplantation. *Transplant. Proc.*, 13:733–735.

113. Shimaoka, K., and Sokal, J. E. (1977): Thymic irradiation and chronic myelogenous leukemia. *NY State J. Med.*, 77:2226.
114. Shimaoka, K., and Sokal, J. E. (1978): Radiation-associated chronic myelogenous leukaemia in younger people. In: *Late Biological Effects of Ionizing Radiation*. Vol. 1, pp. 197–203. International Atomic Energy Agency, Vienna.
115. Shore, R. E., Albert, R. E., and Pasternack, B. S. (1976): Follow-up study of patients treated by X-ray epilation for tinea capitis: Resurvey of post-treatment illness and mortality experience. *Arch. Environ. Health*, 31:21–28.
116. Smith, P. G. (1977): Leukemia and other cancers following radiation treatment of pelvic disease. *Cancer*, 39:1901–1905.
117. Smith, P. G., and Doll, R. (1978): Age- and time-dependent changes in the rates of radiation-induced cancers in patients with ankylosing spondylitis following a single course of X-ray treatment. In: *Late Biological Effects of Ionizing Radiation*. Vol. 1, pp. 205–214. International Atomic Energy Agency, Vienna.
118. Smith, P. R., and Lickiss, J. N. (1980): Benzene and lymphomas (letter). *Lancet*, 1:719.
119. Sorrell, T. C., Forbes, I. J., Burness, F. R., and Rischbieth, R. C. (1971): Depression of immunological function in patients treated with phenytoin sodium (sodium diphenylhydantoin). *Lancet*, 2:1233–1235.
120. Steigbigel, R. T., Kim, H., Potolsky, A., and Schrier, S. L. (1974): Acute myeloproliferative disorder following long term chlorambucil therapy. *Arch. Intern. Med.*, 134:728–731.
121. Stewart, A., and Kneale, G. W. (1970): Radiation dose effects in relation to obstetric X-rays and childhood cancers. *Lancet*, 1:1185–1188.
122. Stewart, A., Pennybacker, W., and Barber, R. (1962): Adult leukaemias and diagnostic X-rays. *Br. Med. J.*, 2:882–890.
123. Stewart, D. J., and Keating, M. J. (1980): Radiation exposure as a possible etiologic factor in hairy cell leukemia (leukemic reticuloendotheliosis). *Cancer*, 46:1577–1580.
124. Stott, H., Fox, W., Girling, D. J., Stephens, R. J., and Gralton, D. A. G. (1977): Acute leukaemia after busulfan. *Br. Med. J.*, 2:1513–1517.
125. Sun, M. (1982): Risk estimate vanishes from benzene report. *Science*, 217:914–915.
126. Thiru, S., Calne, R. Y., and Nagington, J. (1981): Lymphoma in renal allograft patients treated with Cyclosporin-A as one of the immunosuppressive agents. *Transplant. Proc.*, 13:359–364.
127. Trump, D. L., and Cowall, D. E. (1977): Acute myelogenous leukemia as a late complication of the multimodality therapy for Hodgkin's disease. *Johns Hopkins Med. J.*, 14:249–251.
128. Valagussa, P., Santoro, A., Kenda, R., Fossati Bellani, F., Franchi, F., Banfi, A., Rilke, F., and Bonadonna, G. (1980): Second malignancies in Hodgkin's disease: A complication of certain forms of treatment. *Br. Med. J.*, 280:216–219.
129. Vianna, N. J., and Polan, A. (1979): Lymphomas and occupational benzene exposure. *Lancet*, 1:1394–1395.
130. Vigliani, E. C., and Forni, A. (1976): Benzene and leukaemia. *Environ. Res.*, 11:122.
131. Wanders, J., Wattendorff, A. R., Endtz, L. J., denNijs, J. J., and Leeksma, C. H. W. (1981): Chronic myeloid leukemia in myasthenia gravis after long-term treatment with 6-mercaptopurine. *Acta Med. Scand.*, 210:235–238.
132. Warren, S. (1980): Risk of cancer subsequent to low-dose radiation. *J. Forensic. Sci.*, 25:721–726.
133. Webster, E. W. (1981): On the question of cancer induction by small X-ray doses. *AJR*, 137:647–666.
134. Weiss, R. B., Brunning, R. D., and Kennedy, B. J. (1972): Lymphosarcoma terminating in acute myelogenous leukemia. *Cancer*, 30:1275–1278.
135. Wheeler, G. E. (1981): Cyclophosphamide-associated leukemia in Wegener's granulomatosis. *Ann. Intern. Med.*, 94:361–363.
136. White, S. C., and Frey, N. W. (1977): An estimation of somatic hazards to the United States population from dental radiography. *Oral Surg.*, 43:152–159.
137. Wolf, P. H., Andjelkovich, D., Smith, A., and Tyroler, H. (1981): A case-control study of leukemia in the U.S. rubber industry. *JOM*, 23:103–108.
138. Zarrabi, M. H., Grunwald, H. W., and Rosner, F. (1977): Chronic lymphocytic leukemia terminating in acute leukemia. *Arch. Intern. Med.*, 137:1059–1064.
139. Zarrabi, M. H., Rosner, F., and Bennett, J. M. (1978): Acute leukemia and non-Hodgkin's lymphoma. *N. Engl. J. Med.*, 298:280.

Pathogenesis of Leukemias and Lymphomas:
Environmental Influences, edited by
I. T. Magrath, G. T. O'Conor, and B. Ramot.
Raven Press, New York © 1984.

Lymphomas in Persons with Naturally Occurring Immunodeficiency Disorders

A. H. Filipovich, D. Zerbe, B. D. Spector, and J. H. Kersey

Immunodeficiency Cancer Registry, University of Minnesota Hospitals,
Minneapolis, Minnesota 55455

The increased incidence of tumors in association with naturally occurring immunodeficiency disorders (NOID), also referred to as primary or genetically determined immunodeficiencies, has been documented in numerous published reports in the past decade (1,6,9,11,22). Lymphoproliferative disorders are the predominant tumor type in patients with underlying disorders classified as primary immunodeficiencies by the World Health Organization (WHO) (25). Similarly, among solid organ transplant recipients treated with postoperative immunosuppression, lymphoproliferative disorders represent the major proportion of *de novo* tumors, excluding nonmelanomatous skin cancer and *in situ* carcinoma of the cervix (14).

Historically, lymphoproliferative disorders in NOID patients as well as allograft recipients have been viewed as lymphomas on the basis of histologic resemblance to malignant lymphoid tumors in nonimmunodeficient individuals and the often rapidly fatal clinical outcome. More recently, results of two different approaches to the diagnosis of lymphoproliferative disorders in immunodeficient persons at the University of Minnesota have led to recognition of the heterogeneity and atypia of these "lymphomas." The first approach has been systematic histopathologic review of tumor material from cases previously reported to our Immunodeficiency Cancer Registry (ICR) (8). Secondly, newly diagnosed "lymphomas" from immunodeficient patients, primarily renal transplant recipients, have been studied with a battery of lymphocyte surface markers (including monoclonal antibodies), cytogenetic techniques, and virologic probes (7). It appears from these studies that the predominant morphologic categories of lymphoproliferative tumors among immunodeficient patients share features compatible with large-cell lymphomas classified as reticulum cell sarcomas, histiocytic lymphomas, and B immunoblastic sarcomas. However, many such tumors show cytologic polymorphism (7) and polyclonal cellular characteristics by surface marker analysis (10,12). Multiple case reports in the past few years have emphasized the role of infection with Epstein-Barr virus (EBV) in the pathogenesis of lymphoproliferative disorders in patients with NOID as well as transplant recipients (10,16).

In this report we have updated descriptive data regarding host and tumor characteristics for the cases of "lymphomas" recorded by the ICR during the past 10 years. This body of retrospective information continues to serve as a background for more definitive prospective investigation of the association between immuno-deficiency and life-threatening lymphoproliferative disorders.

MATERIALS AND METHODS

The ICR was established at the University of Minnesota in 1973 for the purpose of collecting data about malignancies that had developed in individuals with one of the 14 categories of NOID [classified as primary specific immunodeficiencies by the WHO Committee on Immunodeficiency (25)]. The ICR has used physician reporting of case material through literature review, voluntary communication, and ICR-generated in-quiries and surveys. Case holdings are approximately evenly divided between previously published cases and those reported directly to the ICR. Currently, 404 patients and 420 tumors have been registered. Excluding nonmalignant tumors (by reported histology) and cases for which the diagnosis of immunodeficiency has not been verified before the diagnosis of cancer, 385 cases remain.

The distribution of ICR cases according to general histologic type of all malig-nancies is shown in Table 1. (Tumor histologies contributed by the reporting phy-sician have been used for all tabulations in this chapter, unless otherwise stated.) The four immunodeficiency categories with the most lymphomas are ataxia-telan-giectasia (AT) (3); 130 total cancer cases; Wiskott-Aldrich syndrome (WAS) (15), 62 total cancer cases; common variable immunodeficiency disease (CVID) (2), 88 total cancer cases; and severe combined immunodeficiency disease (SCID) (2), 24 total cancer cases. The remaining 81 cancer cases in the ICR were associated with other WHO immunodeficiency categories, including DiGeorge syndrome (two cases), transient hypogammaglobulinemia of infancy (two cases), "other" selective antibody deficiencies (one case), hyper-IgE syndrome (one case), immunodeficiency with thymoma (eight cases), purine nucleoside phosporylase deficiency (one case), se-lective IgA deficiency (30 cases), immunodeficiency with increased IgM (10 cases), X-linked hypogammaglobulinemia (15 cases), and selective IgM deficiency (11 cases).

The Denver Tumor Transplant Registry (DTTR) (14), operated by Dr. Israel Penn at the Veterans Administration Hospital in Denver, Colorado, since 1968, is

TABLE 1. *Summary of cases on file, immunodeficiency cancer registry, March 1982*

General histologic type of first malignancy	Immunodeficiency diagnosis					Totals
	AT	WAS	CVID	SCID	Others	
Non-Hodgkin's lymphoma	58 (42%)	41 (70%)	37 (42%)	12 (50%)	20 (25%)	168 (44%)
Carcinomas	23 (17%)	2 (3%)	39 (44%)	1 (4%)	25 (31%)	90 (23%)
Leukemias	29 (22%)	6 (10%)	6 (7%)	6 (25%)	10 (12%)	57 (15%)
Hodgkin's disease	13 (10%)	3 (5%)	5 (6%)	1 (4%)	7 (9%)	29 (7%)
Others (includes NOS)	10 (7%)	7 (12%)	1 (1%)	4 (17%)	19 (23%)	41 (11%)
Totals	133	59	88	24	81	385

an informal data bank of malignancies arising in patients who have received immunosuppressive therapy following organ transplantation. As of September 1981, data on 1,275 patients who developed 1,354 types of cancers *de novo* post-transplant have been recorded. Of these, 1,252 patients received renal transplants, 21 received cardiac allografts, and two each received bone marrow or liver allografts.

TUMOR HISTOLOGIES IN THE ICR

The cancer cases in the ICR represent a young population at risk. The mean age at diagnosis of non-Hodgkin's lymphoma for the entire ICR was 15.2 years. The immunodeficiency categories represented in the ICR differ according to their underlying genetic defects, symptom complexes, and prognoses for survival as well as the frequency of development of various types of neoplasm. They all show, however, a predisposition to recurrent and chronic infections. Several categories of immunodeficiency disorders demonstrate increased risk of developing tumors of the immune system ("lymphomas"). In some immunodeficiency categories, selected carcinomas (20) occur in proportional excess compared to similar tumors in the general population. Tumors among cases within certain immunodeficiency categories frequently bear similarities to one another (e.g., histiocytic lymphomas in WAS) and occasionally to tumors in other immunodeficiency categories with like immunoregulatory defects (e.g., some cases of histiocytic lymphomas in SCID and CVID). Conversely, tumors in some immunodeficient individuals appear to represent incidental events or malignant outcomes in persons genetically predisposed to cancer on some basis other than the underlying or concurrent immunodeficiency (e.g., multiple tumor types in AT).

Table 1 presents a summary of malignancies in the ICR. Non-Hodgkin's lymphomas account for 44% (168/385) of tumors among all 14 WHO immunodeficiency categories. Non-Hodgkin's lymphomas are the predominant tumor described in WAS (71%), SCID (50%), and AT (42%), and they rival carcinomas (primarily of the stomach) (20) in CVID (42%). The overall incidence of Hodgkin's disease (8%) is not greater than that expected in the general population. Host and tumor characteristics for lymphoma cases in the four major ICR categories (AT, WAS, CVID, and SCID) are shown in Table 2.

Non-Hodgkin's Lymphomas in Ataxia Telangiectasia

Comparison of lymphoid tumors (including leukemias) among AT cases from the United States with expected age and sex-adjusted tumor proportions from the Third National Cancer Survey (24) reflects an excess risk of 15.4 for males and 7.3 for females with AT (21). The array of histologic types contributing to the non-Hodgkin's lymphomas in AT is the most heterogeneous for any ICR NOID category: Burkitt's lymphoma (three cases); lymphosarcoma, not otherwise specified (NOS) (13 cases); lymphoblastic lymphoma (five cases); histiocytic lymphoma (16 cases); and malignant lymphoma, NOS (21 cases). The overall male predominance (1.39)

TABLE 2. *Host and tumor characteristics of lymphomas in immunodeficient persons*

Tumor	NOID category			
	AT	WAS	CVID	SCID
Histiocytic lymphoma[a]				
Number of cases	16	24	15	7
Mean age and range (years)	11 (3–22)	7.9 (1.6–22.3)	29.5 (8–75)	2.2 (0.6–5)
Male-female ratio	1.14:1	—	0.88:1	5.0:1
Proportion with known tumor site	10/16	22/24	7/15	6/7
Primary sites[b]	1. Multiple LN 2. Brain	1. Brain 2. Multiple sites	1. Multiple sites 2. LN	1. Multiple sites 2. Brain
Other lymphomas[c]				
Number of cases	42	17	22	5
Mean and range (years)	9.7 (3–21.2)	7.1 (0.75–20.2)	38.8 (3.7–69.6)	1.9 (1.8–2.0)
Male-female ratio	1.6:1	—	1.44:1	4.0:1
Proportion with known tumor site	27/42	14/17	11/22	3/5
Primary sites[b]	1. LN 2. GI tract	1. Brain 2. Multiple sites	1. LN 2. Multiple sites	1. Multiple sites 2. Brain
Hodgkin's disease				
Number of cases	13	3	5	1
Mean age and range (years)	10 (4–18)	19.1 (7–33)	41.2 (10–63)	.5
Male-female ratio	1.17:1	—	4.0:1	Male

[a]Reticulum cell sarcoma, B immunoblastic lymphoma.
[b]LN = lymph node; GI tract = gastrointestinal tract.
[c]Malignant lymphoma (not otherwise specified), Burkitt's lymphoma (three cases in AT), lymphosarcoma, lymphoblastic lymphoma.

in the incidence of non-Hodgkin's lymphomas is seen in cases of histiocytic as well as all other lymphomas (Table 2).

Three cases or Burkitt's lymphoma occurring at a mean age of 6.5 years have been reported (2/3 abdominal primaries). Mean age at diagnosis for other lymphomas including histiocytic lymphoma is 10 to 11 years, in contrast to the mean age at diagnosis of carcinomas in AT of 25 years.

Six ICR cases in AT have undergone independent histologic review (8). Five were found to represent malignancies involving B lymphocytes representing large cleaved follicular center cells (FCC) (one case), small FCC (one case), and large noncleaved FCC (three cases), the counterparts of activated lymphocytes within a normal lymph node. These tumors are similar to those encountered in nonimmunodeficient children. Whether such lymphomas occur with increased incidence in AT has not yet been determined.

Primary sites for histiocytic lymphomas in AT were the concurrent presentation in multiple lymph nodes or brain. The gastrointestinal tract was frequently involved at diagnosis of the other non-Hodgkin's lymphomas.

In earlier reports (5,21), we examined the role of immunodeficiency in the development of lymphoid tumors in AT. We first established that immunologic abnormalities present in AT cancer patients did not differ significantly from those in other series of AT patients who were tumor-free (21). To our surprise, the proportional distribution of tumors (non-Hodgkin's lymphomas, leukemias, carcinomas, and Hodgkin's disease) did not vary with the degree of documented immunodeficiency and was similar in AT cancer patients with dysgammaglobulinemia alone (IgA deficiency), with defective cell-mediated immunity with normal immunoglobulins, or with a combined defect of humoral cell-mediated immunity (5). These data suggest that aberrations of immune function in AT cannot be used alone to predict which individuals will develop cancer or which histologic types of tumors are more likely to be found.

Non-Hodgkin's Lymphomas in Wiskott-Aldrich Syndrome

An estimated 12% of WAS patients develop tumors (15). An age-adjusted cancer incidence rate of 128 × that expected on the basis of the nonimmunodeficient U.S. population has been calculated (15). The great majority of these tumors—70% by reported histology—are non-Hodgkin's lymphomas (41/24). Fifty-nine percent (24/41) of these have been categorized as histiocytic lymphomas. The remaining 17 cases were reported as lymphosarcoma and malignant lymphoma, NOS.

Thirty-two tumor specimens from WAS patients are in the process of independent histopathologic review by the ICR. Twenty-seven of these represent tumor material from cases reported as non-Hodgkin's lymphomas, and 26 of these have been found to be generally compatible with the categories of histiocytic or large-cell lymphoma. More careful perusal suggests that many of these WAS "lymphomas" resemble B immunoblastic sarcomas (8), and others are reminiscent of the polymorphic B-cell hyperplasias and lymphomas observed in renal allograft recipients (7). Eleven of

32 cases in the current review at Minnesota were discovered at autopsy. Review of the clinical histories has revealed that some of these patients showed symptoms of tumors pre-mortem but that the symptoms were attributed to ongoing infections that contributed to death.

The retrospective ascertainment of these tumors does not permit investigation of associated viral infections in most cases. Study of the polyclonal or monoclonal characteristics of these B-cell lymphoproliferative processes using the few suitably preserved tissue specimens demonstrates that both monoclonal and polyclonal patterns are seen.

The mean age at diagnosis of histiocytic lymphomas and other lymphomas in WAS was 7.9 and 7.1 years, respectively (Table 2). The similarity in mean age probably reflects the similarity of tumors reported in both categories. Indeed, the most frequent primary tumor site for both reported histologies was the brain (Table 2), occurring in 31% of all non-Hodgkin's lymphomas.

Non-Hodgkin's Lymphomas in CVID and SCID

Non-Hodgkin's lymphomas in CVID can also be divided into the histiocytic lymphomas (15 cases), presenting at a mean age of 29.5 years with a slight female predominance (male-female ratio of 0.88:1) (Table 2), and other lymphomas, including lymphoblastic lymphoma (two cases), lymphosarcoma (four cases), and malignant lymphoma, undifferentiated (three cases), poorly differentiated, or NOS (13 cases), presenting at a mean age of 38.8 years with a male predominance (male-female ratio of 1.44:1) (Table 2). Disseminated disease with multiple involved sites at tumor presentation was the rule in patients with histiocytic lymphoma; patients with "other" lymphomas most often initially presented with tumor in a single nodal area (Table 2).

Twelve cases of non-Hodgkin's lymphoma in SCID are listed in the ICR. Of these, six have received immunotherapy in the form of cultured thymic epithelium, thymic factor, fetal thymus, thymosin, or some combination thereof (4,13). The remaining six SCID patients who developed fatal lymphoproliferative disorders were not treated with exogenous thymic replacement (13). Sex and age distribution as well as reported tumor histology are similar in the two groups (13), suggesting that immunotherapy is not prerequisite for the development of "lymphomas" in individuals with the most severe of inborn immunologic impairments.

Most often, the lymphoproliferative disorders in SCID are widely disseminated anatomically at the time of clinical recognition; the brain has been identified as the most prevalent single primary site (Table 2). The mean age at diagnosis for lymphoma in SCID patients is two years. Tumors have been documented as early as three months of age. The distinct male predominance in SCID lymphomas reflects in part the male excess in SCID disorders (2).

Association Between Acute Lymphocytic Leukemia and Non-Hodgkin's Lymphomas in NOID

Although the overall incidence of multiple primary tumors reported to the ICR (4.1%) is not markedly greater than that reported for the general nonimmunodeficient population (24), the sequential occurrence of acute lymphocytic leukemia (ALL) before or after the diagnosis of non-Hodgkin's lymphoma in a significant number of NOID patients requires further investigation. Chromosomal instability may pre-dispose such patients to tumors of proliferating cell populations in AT, including lymphocytes. Ten AT patients with non-Hodgkin's lymphomas also experienced ALL and in some cases additional skin and genital tumors. Two cases of ALL are known to have preceded the diagnosis of lymphoma in AT by three and five years, respectively. However, most cases of ALL, believed to be distinct tumors, were diagnosed 0.7 to 21 years after the lymphoma. Unfortunately, lymphocytic surface marker data is not available for any of these tumors.

Three patients (of 11) with SCID were diagnosed with non-Hodgkin's lymphoma and ALL on separate occasions. Two cases of ALL are known to have preceded the lymphoma by four and 12 months. ALL was reported in only one of 20 CVID patients, five years after the diagnosis of lymphoma. No WAS patients (0/44) with lymphoma known to the ICR have developed ALL. Although six cases of acute myelogenous leukemia have been reported in WAS, independent histologic review of four cases has shown two of the four to be a benign form of myeloid metaplasia and a third case to represent histiocytic lymphoma in the bone marrow.

Hodgkin's Disease in the ICR

Hodgkin's disease, the most frequently occurring tumor of lymphoid tissue in the general population, may represent a primary neoplasm of monocyte-macro-phages. Thirteen cases of Hodgkin's disease in AT have been reported (Table 2). The young mean age at tumor diagnosis, 10 years, and preliminary findings of a major proportion of tumors consistent with the rare lymphocyte-depletion subtype of Hodgkin's disease (8) suggest an unusual predisposition to this tumor in AT. Other cases of Hodgkin's disease in the ICR are similar in their characteristics to Hodgkin's tumors reported in the general population. The mean age for the three cases in WAS was 19.5 years, and for the five cases in CVID, 41.2 years. Reported histologies included nodular sclerosis, mixed cellularity, and NOS subtypes. The single case of Hodgkin's disease in a six-month-old male with SCID has not yet been verified by independent histologic review.

TUMOR HISTOLOGIES IN THE DENVER TUMOR TRANSPLANT REGISTRY

The overall cancer incidence among renal transplant recipients has been estimated at between 2 and 16%. In one center, 26% of patients surviving to one year had developed cancer. Among cardiac allograft recipients, the crude incidence is 8%, with an actuarial risk of $25.6 \pm 11.0\%$ after one year (14). Of 1,354 tumors in the DTTR, 521 were nonmelanomatous cancers of the skin and lips. Solid lymphomas accounted for 252 of the remaining 833 tumors (30%). Of the 252 solid lymphomas, 131 were histiocytic lymphomas (also classified as reticulum cell sarcomas, B immunoblastic lymphomas, and microgliomas). In 39% of lymphoma patients (excluding individuals with Kaposi's sarcoma), the brain and spinal cord were involved, compared to an incidence of less than 2% in the general population (14). Indeed, 32% of all solid lymphomas were confined to the brain (14). Virtually all lymphomas arising in transplant recipients are believed to be of host origin.

The 2:1 male predominance in lymphomatous as well as nonlymphomatous *de novo* tumors among allograft recipients is similar to the male-female ratio of patients receiving transplants. The mean age of patients developing lymphoma is slightly younger (38.2 years) than that of patients with other primary tumors (40.2 years). Lymphomas show a shorter latency period post-transplant, 30 months, than other tumors (50 months).

The proportional incidence of Hodgkin's disease in the DTTR, 3%, is lower than that in the general population (14).

TRANSITIONAL, "PREMALIGNANT," AND POLYCLONAL LYMPHOPROLIFERATIVE PROCESSES

Intermittent lymphadenopathy, intestinal nodular lymphoid hyperplasia, and hepatosplenomegaly are frequent clinical findings in several NOID disorders, including WAS, CVID, and some cases of AT. Although histologically benign reactive hyperplasia is most often documented, atypical infiltrates of transformed B lymphocytes, such as foci of B immunoblasts (19) or small cleaved FCC (18), are occasionally identified. Chronic atypical lymphocyte infiltrates of hepatic portal areas have been observed in patients with a variety of underlying immunodeficiencies following exposure to EBV or hepatitis A (17). Although such lesions can resemble malignancies histologically, our experience has shown that many of these focal or multifocal lymphoproliferative processes are polyclonal (e.g., consist of $\kappa + \lambda$ bearing cells) and can resolve spontaneously or following immunotherapy.

Other polyclonal "lymphomas" associated with EBV infection and/or antecedent immunotherapy (13) or arising spontaneously behave in a malignant manner by virtue of massive proliferation that interferes with normal function. This is particularly true if uncontrolled lymphoproliferation proceeds intracranially in NOID patients as well as renal allograft recipients.

Sequential analyses of lymphoid tumors in renal allograft recipients by histology and cell markers have demonstrated that monoclonal populations of lymphocytes fitting the strict definition of malignancy can emerge amid polyclonal proliferation (8,10). An analogous evolution from benign to malignant lymphoid tumor has also been demonstrated in a patient with congenital immunodeficiency who was monitored prospectively (23).

SUMMARY AND DISCUSSION

Patients with NOID and immunosuppressed individuals, specifically allograft recipients, experience an increased risk of developing lymphoproliferative disorders. "Lymphomas" in these two immunodeficient populations share a number of characteristics. Non-Hodgkin's lymphomas of the histiocytic or large-cell morphologies predominate. The central nervous system is a major primary site. "Lymphomas" occur in younger patients than nonlymphoid tumors and show a shorter latency period after onset of immunosuppression (14). Transitional or hyperplastic "pre-malignant" lesions are observed in both populations as well as polyclonal tumors that are clinically aggressive. A frequent association with EBV and possibly other viruses is now being recognized for lymphoproliferative disorders in NOID and renal transplant recipients.

Many authors, including ourselves, have postulated that ineffective immunoreg-ulation predisposes to the increased incidence and early occurrence of tumors of activated B lymphocytes observed in partial immunodeficiencies. Immunoregulation is a term used to describe internal modulation of constituent populations of the immune system during periods of homeostasis and activation. Cellular subtypes involved in immunoregulation have been previously described (6). Many patients with NOID disorders have demonstrated defects in T suppressor function, T cytolytic function, natural killer function, or a combination of defects. Furthermore, func-tional capacities of the various immune subsets can vary over time in WAS, CVID, and allograft recipients *(unpublished observations)* such that the immunodeficient host may be more susceptible to developing a lymphoproliferative disorder at certain times. We postulate that in most cases, polyclonal proliferation is the early event. Continued activation of B and T lymphocytes, if improperly regulated, can progress to a polyclonal tumor mass(es). Alternatively, a monoclonal malignancy may arise if a new cytogenetic defect occurs in one or more of the proliferating lymphocytes.

ACKNOWLEDGMENTS

This study is a report of the Immunodeficiency Cancer Registry, University of Minnesota, 1982, and was supported by USPHS Contract NO1-CP-43384. The authors wish to thank M. Munro for assistance in preparing the manuscript.

REFERENCES

1. Aiuti, F., Guinchi, G., Bardare, M., Baroni, C., Bonomo, L., Dammacco, F., Tursi, A., Borrone, C., Burgio, G. R., Ugazio, R., Businco, L., Rezza, E., Calvani, M., Bricarelli, F. D., Mosuatelli, P., Fontana, L., Franchesci, C., Masi, P., Paducci, G., Casagni, G., Imperato, C., Carapella, E., Massimo, L., Nicola, P., Pamizon, G., Agasti, F., Ricci, G., Segni, P., Vaccaro, G., Vierucci, A., and Zanussi, C. (1978): Le immunodeficienze primitive in Italia. *Folia Allergol. Immunol. Clin.*, 25:7–15.
2. Ammann, A. J. (1977): T cell and T-B cell immunodeficiency disorders. *Pediatr. Clin. North Am.*, 24:293–311.
3. Boder, E., and Sedgwick, R. P. (1958): Ataxia-telangiectasia. A familial syndrome of progressive cerebellar ataxia, oculocutaneous telangiectasia and frequent pulmonary infection. *Pediatrics*, 21:526–554.
4. Borzy, M. S., Hong, R., Horowitz, S. D., Gilbert, E., Kaufman, D., De Mendonca, W., Oxelius, V. A., Dictor, M., and Pachman, L. (1979): Fatal lymphoma after transplantation of cultured thymus in children with combined immunodeficiency disease. *N. Engl. J. Med.*, 301:565–568.
5. Filipovich, A. H., and Spector, B. D. (1981): Immunodeficiency (ID) as a susceptibility factor for malignancy in ataxia-telangiectasia (A-T): Report from the Immunodeficiency Cancer Registry (ICR). *Pediatr. Res.*, 15:A806.
6. Filipovich, A. H., Spector, B. D., and Kersey, J. H. (1980): Malignancies in the immunocom-

promised human. In: *The Role of Viruses in Human Cancer*, Vol. 1, edited by G. Giraldo and E. Beth, pp. 237–253. Elsevier/North-Holland, New York.

7. Frizzera, G., Hanto, D. W., Gajl-Peczalska, K. J., Rosai, J., McKenna, R. W., Sibley, R. K., Holahan, K. P., and Lindquist, L. L. (1981): Polymorphic diffuse B-cell hyperplasias and lymphomas in renal transplant recipients. *Cancer Res.*, 41:4262–4279.

8. Frizzera, G., Rosai, J., Dehner, L., Spector, B. D., and Kersey, J. H. (1980): Lymphoreticular disorders in primary immunodeficiencies: new findings based on an up-to-date histologic classification of 35 cases. *Cancer*, 46:692–698.

9. Gatti, R. H., and Good, R. A. (1971): Occurrence of malignancy in immunodeficiency diseases. A literature review. *Cancer*, 28:89–98.

10. Hanto, D. W., Frizzera, G., Gajl-Peczalska, K. J., Sakamoto, K., Purtilo, D. T., Balfour, H. H., Jr., Simmons, R. L., and Najarian, J. S. (1982): Epstein-Barr virus-induced B-cell lymphoma after renal transplantation: Acyclovir therapy and transition from polyclonal to monoclonal B-cell proliferation. *N. Engl. J. Med.*, 306:913–918.

11. Hayakawa, H., Iizuka, N., Yata, J., Yamada, K., and Kobayashi, N. (1978): Analysis of registered cases of immunodeficiency in Japan. In: *Immunodeficiency in Human Diseases*, edited by Japan Medical Research Foundation, pp. 271–281. University of Tokyo Press, Tokyo.

12. Hertel, B. F., Rosai, J., Dehner, L. P., and Simmons, R. L. (1977): Lymphoproliferative disorders in organ transplant recipients. *Lab. Invest.*, 36:340.

13. Kersey, J. H., Filipovich, A. H., Spector, B. D., and Frizzera, G. (1980): Lymphoma after thymus transplantation (letter). *N. Engl. J. Med.*, 302:301–302.

14. Penn, I. (1981): The price of immunotherapy. *Curr. Probl. Surg.*, 18:713–728.

15. Perry, G., Spector, B., Schuman, L., Mandel, J., Anderson, V. E., McHugh, R., Hanson, M., Fahlstrom, S., Krivit, W., and Kersey, J. H. (1980): The Wiskott-Aldrich syndrome in the United States and Canada (1892–1979). *J. Pediatr.*, 97:72–78.

16. Reece, E. R., Gartner, J. G., Seemayer, T. A., Joncas, J. H., and Pagano, J. S. (1981): Epstein-Barr virus in a malignant lymphoproliferative disorder of B cells occurring after thymic epithelial transplantation for combined immunodeficiency. *Cancer Res.*, 41:4243–4247.

17. Snover, D., Filipovich, A. H., and Dehner, L. P. (1983): Immunodeficiency-disease associated with atypical chronic hepatitis: A clinicopathological study. *Pediatr. Pathol.*, 1:229–241.

18. Snover, D., Filipovich, A. H., Dehner, L. P., and Krivit, W. (1981): "Pseudolymphoma," a case associated with primary immunodeficiency disease and polyglandular failure syndrome. *Arch. Pathol. Lab. Med.*, 105:46–49.

19. Snover, D., Frizzera, G., Spector, B. D., Perry, G., and Kersey, J. (1981): Wiskott-Aldrich syndrome: histopathologic findings in the lymph node and spleens of 15 patients. *Hum. Pathol.*, 12:821–831.

20. Spector, B. D., and Filipovich, A. H. (1980): Nonlymphoid cancers as a complication of naturally-occurring immunodeficiency (NOID): Report of 58 cases. *Am. Assoc. Cancer Res. Am. Soc. Clin. Oncol. Proc.*, 21:A603.

21. Spector, B. D., Filipovich, A. H., Perry, G., and Kersey, J. H. (1982): Epidemiology of cancer in ataxia-telangiectasia. In: *Ataxia-Telangiectasia: A Cellular and Molecular Link Between Cancer, Neuropathology and Immune Deficiency*, edited by B. A. Bridges and D. G. Harnden, pp. 103–138. John Wiley & Sons, New York.

22. Spector, B. D., Perry, G., and Kersey, J. H. (1978): Genetically determined immunodeficiency diseases (GDID) and malignancy: Report from the Immunodeficiency Cancer Registry. *Clin. Immunol. Immunopathol.*, 11:12–29.

23. Thestrup-Pedersen, K., Esmann, V., Jensen, J. R., Hastrup, J., Thorling, K., Saemundson, A. K., Bisballe, S., Oallesen, G., Madsen, M., Grazia-Masucci, M., and Emberg, I. (1980): Epstein-Barr virus-induced lymphoproliferative disorder converting to fatal Burkitt-like lymphoma in a boy with interferon-inducible chromosomal defect. *Lancet*, 2:997–1001.

24. Third National Cancer Survey (1975): Incidence data. Natl. Cancer Inst. Monogr. 41, DHEW (NIH) 75-787. National Cancer Institute, Bethesda, MD.

25. WHO (1979): Immunodeficiency report of a WHO scientific group. *Clin. Immunol. Immunopathol.*, 13:296–359.

Pathogenesis of Leukemias and Lymphomas:
Environmental Influences, edited by
I. T. Magrath, G. T. O'Conor, and B. Ramot.
Raven Press, New York © 1984.

Immunoregulatory Defects and Epstein-Barr Virus-Associated Lymphoid Disorders

David Purtilo, Shinji Harada, Thomas Bechtold, Joanne Yetz,
Geraldine Rogers, and Beerelli Seshi

Department of Pathology and Laboratory Medicine, Pediatrics and Eppley Institute for Research in Cancer and Allied Diseases, University of Nebraska Medical Center, Omaha, Nebraska 68105

Immunity or immunoregulation is probably a critical factor in lymphomagenesis. Two related groups of inherited disorders predispose to lymphoreticular malignancies: immune deficiency and chromosomal breakage (5). The second major component of the ecogenetic equation, environmental factors, can accentuate or directly bring about immunoregulatory disturbances and/or chromosomal instability in lymphoid cells (45). The Leukemia/Lymphoma Task Force of Nebraska has begun to investigate some of these factors that might be responsible for the inordinately high incidence of these malignancies in our region. The etiological factors we are studying are germane to understanding the etiology and pathogenesis of lymphoma and leukemia worldwide.

Beyond genetic factors, socioeconomic class seems to be a very important factor in determining the various subtypes of lymphomas found in specific locales (4,14). Similarly, the clinical expressions of Epstein-Barr virus (EBV) infections are determined by socioeconomic factors (22,65). Socioeconomic conditions often determine the size of families, location and type of domicile, sanitation, and nutrition. Moreover, socioeconomic conditions often determine who is exposed to various environmental agents that may influence immunoregulation and chromosomal integrity. For example, exposure to infectious agents naturally or by vaccination may be important events in lymphomagenesis. Interrelated matters of nutrition and parasitism may also render an individual immune-deficient or disturbed with regard to immunoregulation (57,64). In agricultural areas, exposure to organic dusts that may be mitogenic to lymphocytes (49) and contamination of water and soil by pesticides, herbicides, fertilizers, and radiochemicals potentially could be deleterious to the immune system and the genetic apparatus. Finally, socioeconomic factors determine the extent of medical care. For example, exposure to ionizing radiation and cytotoxic drugs is more likely in societies with extensive health care programs. Any or all of these factors may alter immunoregulatory responses to EBV.

Here we describe and discuss the impact of immunoregulatory defects in rendering individuals vulnerable to diverse EBV-induced diseases. Inherited immunodeficiency, including the X-linked lymphoproliferative syndrome (XLP) (50,59,71) and other primary immune deficiencies, will be described in this context. Acquired immunodeficiencies and EBV-induced diseases in individuals undergoing allograft of kidney, heart, or bone marrow or treatment for leukemia or lymphoma will be discussed. A group of unusual disorders that have a high frequency in tropical Africa where Burkitt's lymphoma is endemic and their association with immunodeficiency to EBV will also be briefly considered. Evidence for immune deficiency as a factor responsible for lymphadenomegaly and Kaposi's sarcoma in male homosexuals will be examined, and a relevant animal model for EBV-induced lymphoproliferative diseases, namely, the cotton-topped marmoset, will be described. Finally, our testable hypothesis as to how EBV, together with cytogenetic aberrations, may permit lymphomagenesis in immune-deficient individuals is summarized.

IMMUNOREGULATORY DEFECTS TO EBV IN X-LINKED LYMPHOPROLIFERATIVE SYNDROME

The finding of X-linked vulnerability to EBV-associated diseases, including infectious mononucleosis (IM), agammaglobulinemia following IM, and malignant B-cell lymphoma following IM, and the observation of marked depletion of T cells in thymus gland and T-cell regions in lymph nodes and spleen in a family prompted us to adopt the name "X-linked recessive progressive combined variable immunodeficiency disease" for this complex of presumptively related pathological features (70). A large unrelated family was also described in which there were variable phenotypic expressions of XLP (59). Thus, a hypothesis was developed, based on the findings in these two kindreds, that might account for the progression of the immune defects and the various phenotypes of XLP (50) (Fig. 1). In 1976, subsets of suppressor and helper T-cells had not yet been described in man. However, Gershon et al. in 1972 (11) had presented convincing evidence that immunoregulatory subsets of T cells governed B-cell responses in the mouse. Thus we reasoned that immunoregulatory T-cell subpopulations were present in human beings and that disorders of such populations were responsible for XLP. We designated the locus on the X chromosome responsible for XLP the lymphoproliferative control locus (X_{LC}).

In 1978, a registry of XLP was established to define diagnostic criteria, describe phenotypes (Fig. 2), test the above hypothesis (50) prospectively and retrospectively, and provide consultation for clinicians and pathologists encountering families thought to have the syndrome. The registry has proven to be a successful vehicle for studying this rare disorder. To date, approximately 28 kindreds, including 115 affected males with 20 survivors, have been enrolled in the registry for study (16). Before we describe the immunoregulatory defects in males with XLP and the EBV-specific immune deficiencies, we will briefly review the normal immune responses to EBV.

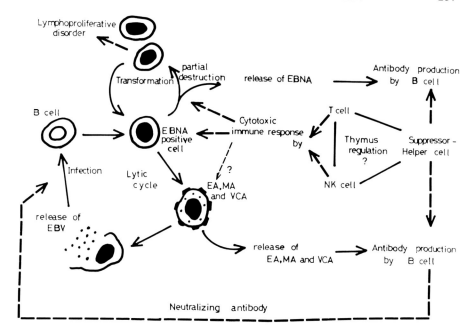

FIG. 1. Hypothesis regarding pathogenesis of EBV-induced lymphoproliferative diseases in X-linked lymphoproliferative syndrome. Inherited thymus regulatory defects lead to failure of natural killer cell (NK) and cytotoxic T cell responses to control Epstein-Barr virus (EBV) induced lymphoproliferative diseases. Abbreviations: EA, early antigen; MA, membrane antigen; VCA, viral capsid antigen; EBNA, EB nuclear-associated antigen.

EBV is a ubiquitous virus that infects nearly 85% of individuals by adulthood (22). During early childhood, the infection occurs silently, whereas approximately two-thirds of adolescent individuals will manifest IM at the time of primary infection. Multiple immune defenses have evolved to protect against this potentially life-threatening virus. EBV infects B-cells that possess receptors for it (Fig. 3). Following B-cell infection and activation, normal immunoregulatory cells are activated and control the infection (53–55). Perhaps the first line of defense against primary EBV infection is the natural killer cell (NK) (54,85–87,91). The activity of NK cells is boosted *in vitro* when interferon is added (54). Also activated rapidly during acute IM are suppressor T cells (74,93). During acute IM, an estimated 1 to 2% of circulating B cells are EBV-genome-positive, whereas during convalescence, approximately one in 1 million circulating B cells harbor EBV (Fig. 3) (54). Shortly after infection, an array of EBV-specific antibodies including IgM anti-viral capsid antigen (VCA) antibody, anti-early antigen (EA) antibody, and anti-membrane antigen develop. Anti-EB nuclear-associated antigen (EBNA) appears later. These antibodies neutralize virus, and some may opsonize infected B cells for phagocytosis and destruction. The virus infection remains latent after the initial clinical episode, apparently because of the presence of NK cells and memory T cells, which appear during convalescence (54).

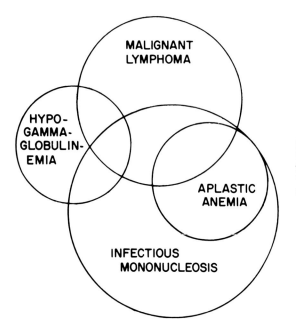

FIG. 2. Venn diagram illustrating the relative frequency of the four major phenotypes of the initial 100 cases of XLP. (From Purtilo, ref. 66.)

The surviving males with XLP exhibit a variety of immunoregulatory defects. Our first effort to test the hypothesis developed in 1976 (50) involved the measurement of EBV-specific antibodies in surviving males with XLP. We found that affected males fell into several categories according to the measured deficiencies in EBV-specific antibodies (79). Some failed to form antibodies to the virus despite infection; others showed persistent anti-VCA and anti-EA activity; and all of the patients lacked significant anti-EBNA titers. Anti-EBNA antibodies require an adequate T-cell competency for their production. Males with XLP lack this capacity. Conversely, males with anti-EBNA titers of greater than 1:10 in XLP families have not manifested the syndrome. Another useful way to detect males with XLP has been to measure the EBV antibodies of mothers of male children with phenotypes of XLP. Paradoxically elevated antibodies against VCA and EA have been found in the majority of obligate female carriers of XLP (82). We have reasoned that the elevated titers in the carrier females reflect humoral compensation for partial T-cell defects. Their hemizygosity probably produces partial immune defects.

Also requiring an explanation is the apparent increased frequency of birth defects, especially involving the heart, in both male and female children born to obligate carriers of XLP (63). Purtilo et al. (60) have demonstrated depressed cellular immunity in normal pregnant women. Based on this and the observation that female carriers have high titers of anti-EBV antibodies, we postulated that the partial immune defect of carriers of XLP would be potentiated when the mothers became pregnant. A study of normal pregnant women has revealed reactivation of the virus

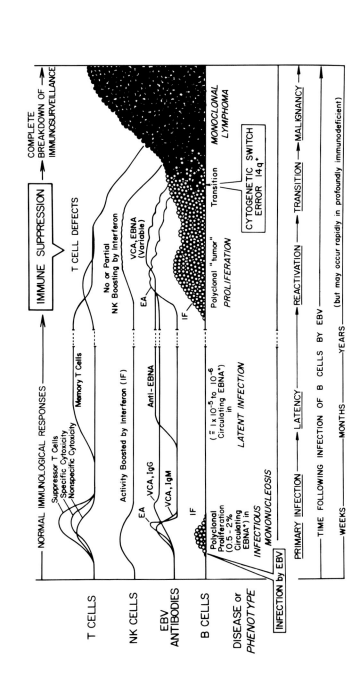

FIG. 3. Hypothesis summarizing cellular and humoral EBV immune responses. Normal immune responses to primary infection are shown at the left. Reactivation of EBV and resumption of B-cell proliferation in the immune-suppressed renal transplant recipient is shown at right. EA = early antigen; VCA = viral capsid antigen; EBNA = nuclear-associated antigen; NK = natural killer cells. (From Purtilo, ref. 54, with permission.)

in most individuals (65,81). Prospective studies are being made to determine if *in utero* infection is responsible for the cardiac defects in families with XLP.

NK cells have been regarded by some as a major deterrent against viral infections and malignancies (23). Thus we measured NK activity in 15 surviving males with XLP who had previously been exposed to EBV and manifested various phenotypes (90). Using the erythroleukemia line K-562 as a target, we found that approximately 80% of the boys with the syndrome showed extensive defects. However, a dying male with IM showed markedly increased NK activity (91). Lipinski et al. (39) have discovered NK defects in children with primary immune defects involving T cells. We have reasoned that the NK defect found in survivors of XLP might be an acquired phenomenon. Thus a study of males at risk for XLP was instituted to determine the immunoregulatory function before EBV infection. We found that males before or shortly after EBV infection showed normal NK activity (85,88). Our finding of additional immunoregulatory defects following EBV infections in XLP also supports this view.

Subsets of T cells are abnormal in number in most patients with XLP (38,84–86). Using OKT monoclonal antibodies (Ortho Diagnostics, Raritan, NJ), we have enumerated subpopulations of T cells (Fig. 4). The variability in the expression of the syndrome in members of families with XLP was noted in the first family study, i.e., fatal IM, aplastic anemia, agammaglobulinemia, and B-cell lymphoma (70). However, the marked variability of immune responses to EBV and the clinical problems we have observed in patients over periods of years were not envisaged at the outset of our studies (Fig. 5). For example, an eleven-year-old male with partial IgA deficiency has been studied for eight years (1974–1982) (61,71). After his primary infection by EBV in 1974, his serum IgM became elevated (71). Surprisingly, he has developed acute IM approximately seven and a half years after documentation of primary EBV infection. Preceding the acute IM, pure red cell aplasia had developed. The patient had an abnormal T4 (helper/inducer) to T8 (suppressor/lytic) ratio of 2.7:1, and five weeks later when acute IM occurred, the ratio became 0.2:1. This T-cell suppressor/lytic ratio was appropriate for a normal immune-competent individual developing acute IM. However, he developed hypogammaglobulinemia and lacks circulating B cells.

Enumeration of subsets of T cells using monoclonal antibodies is not an adequate measure of immunoregulation. Therefore, we have performed functional studies, i.e., measurement of proliferative responses to mitogens such as phytohemagglutinin (PHA), pokeweed (PWM), and EBV (87). In XLP patients we have found slightly reduced lymphoproliferative responses and markedly reduced secretion of immunoglobulin *in vitro* by lymphocytes stimulated by these mitogens. Especially defective has been the production of Ig in response to PWM. This mitogen requires helper T-cell activity (38,88). The helper T-cell defect has been further elaborated by studies using φX174 as an antigen. Males with XLP show a relatively normal primary response to challenge with φX174, whereas defective secondary responses arise, with failure to switch from IgM to IgG production. The various immune defects found in XLP are summarized in Table 1.

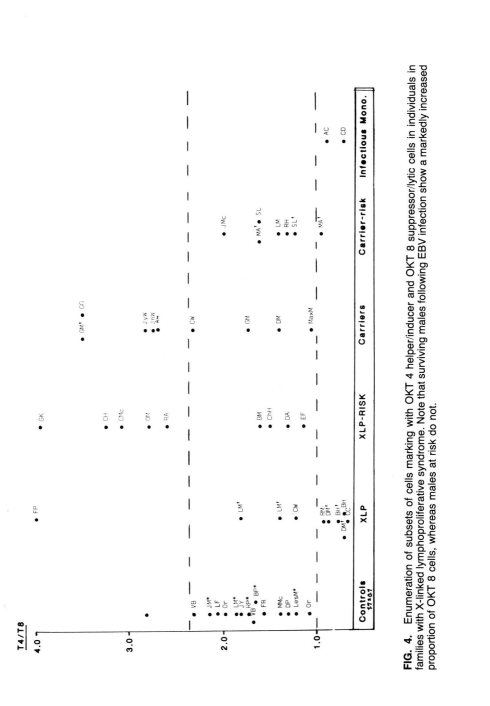

FIG. 4. Enumeration of subsets of cells marking with OKT 4 helper/inducer and OKT 8 suppressor/lytic cells in individuals in families with X-linked lymphoproliferative syndrome. Note that surviving males following EBV infection show a markedly increased proportion of OKT 8 cells, whereas males at risk do not.

AGE AT WHICH EVENTS OCCURRED (YEARS)

PEDIGREE #	1	2	3	4	5	6	7	8	9	10	11	12	13	14	15	16	17	18	19	20	21	22	23
K1-IV-28										EBV								IM-A					
K2-IV-32										IM-H											A		
K2-V-19			ML														IM-D						
K3-IV-46							IM			HC	PL	A											
K4-II-8							ML				ML				IM-HC					A			
K4-III-1			ML-HC									ML	A										

TABLE 1. *Defective immune functions in X-linked lymphoproliferative syndrome*

Defects
  Immunoregulatory function
    Suppression of mitogen-induced Ig production by B cells
    Deficient secondary response to ΦX174, i.e., poor switching from IgM to IgG
    Poor development of memory T cells to EBV
  Abnormal levels and ratios of OKT 4 cells and OKT 8 cells
  Thymic epithelial destruction and T-cell depletion after EBV infection
  Low natural killer cell activity, acquired after EBV infection
  EBV-specific antibody production, especially anti-EBNA, is lacking
Normal
  Normal white blood differential count when not acutely infected
  Normal levels of OKT 3-positive, Ia-positive, and surface-Ig-positive cells
  Normal proliferative responses to mitogens (PHA, PWM, EBV)

A commonly asked question is "Why are males with XLP so vulnerable to EBV?" Perhaps the reason is that males with XLP have an immunoregulatory defect that antedates infection by the virus. This virus uniquely infects the immune system and normally, immunoregulatory responses control the infection and induce a state of clinical latency. The progression of the immune defect and the variability of the phenotypic expression are possibly the result of destruction of thymic epithelium and loss of this important source of immune regulation (66). The immunopathogenic mechanisms of thymic destruction are unknown; however, uncontrolled cytotoxic T cells or NK cells are implicated.

To a lesser extent, individuals with other primary immune deficiency or acquired immune defects may develop immunoregulatory disturbances comparable to those found in XLP. The patients probably can thereby manifest some of the phenotypes found in XLP, especially B-cell lymphomatous proliferations following infection by the virus.

PRIMARY IMMUNOREGULATORY DISTURBANCES AND EBV INFECTIONS

Evidence is mounting that EBV may be a major etiological agent responsible for a variety of lymphoproliferative diseases including B-cell lymphoma in patients with acquired immune deficiency. The overall frequency of malignancy in individuals with primary immunodeficiency disorders has been estimated at 4% (10). Table 2 summarizes various immune deficiency disorders and the documentation of EBV-induced lymphoproliferative diseases. Severe combined immune deficiency (SCID), Wiskott-Aldrich syndrome (WAS), ataxia telangiectasia (AT), XLP, and X-linked agammaglobulinemia (XAg) are discussed and compared with regard to immune deficiency to EBV.

FIG. 5. Representative display of chronological evolution of various phenotypes of X-linked lymphoproliferative syndrome in patients studied over several years. K = Kindred, HG = hypogammaglobulinemia, ML = malignant lymphoma, AA = aplastic anemia, PL = pseudo-lymphoma, D = death, and A = alive. (From Purtilo, ref. 66.)

TABLE 2. *Immune deficiency and EBV-induced lymphoproliferative disorders*[a]

Factor	SCID	AT	XLP	WAS	XAg	RTR	CTM
Genetics	AR,XR	AR	XR	XR	XR	—	Chimera ±
Lymphoma	1%	5%	35%	14%	0.5%	1%	30%
Fatal IM	?	?	65%	?	0	Rare + ML	?35%
Other	1%	5% ALL+HD	36% −HD	1% −HD	0 −HD	Carcinoma, Kaposi	
NK defect	+	+	+ acquired	+, −	−	+, −	−
T defect	++	+	++	++	−	+	+
B defect	+, −	+IgA	+	+	Pre-B	−, ?	−
Secretion	?	?	+	?	?	+ ATG	+
EBV							
Anti-EA	?	++	−, +	−, +	?	+	+
Anti-VCA	?	++	−, +	−, +	?	+ ATG delay	+
Anti-EBNA	?	−	−	+	?	+, −	+
EBV DNA	+	+	+	+	?	+	+
Monoclonal	−	?	++	?	?	+	−
Polyclonal	+	?	+	?	?	+	+
Karyotype	?	14q+	?	+	?	−, +	Diploid
Comments	Post-thymic transplant lymphoma	Breakage and immune defect	Immunoregulatory defect	Immunoregulatory defect	B-cell target defect	ATG-EBV severe	Unnatural host

[a]SCID = severe combined immunodeficiency, AT = ataxia telangiectasia, XLP = X-linked lymphoproliferative syndrome, WAS = Wiskott-Aldrich syndrome, XAg = X-linked agammaglobulinemia, RTR = renal transplant recipient, CTM = cotton-topped marmoset, AR = autosomal recessive, XR = X-linked recessive, IM = infectious mononucleosis, NK = natural killer cell, + = present, − = absent, ATG = antithymocyte globulin, ALL = acute lymphocytic leukemia, HD = Hodgkin's Disease, EA = early antigen, VCA = viral capsid antigen, ML = malignant lymphoma.

Borzy et al. (3) reported polyclonal B-cell lymphoma occurring in three of 30 patients with combined immune deficiency disorders following transplantation of cultured thymus. They proposed that the thymic epithelium influenced the B-cell proliferation and that EBV may have been the etiological agent. Subsequently, Reece et al. (72) demonstrated by molecular hybridization techniques that a tumor in a patient with SCID was polyclonal and contained EBV genome. The role of the transplanted thymic epithelium in the pathogenesis of lymphoproliferative diseases in patients with SCID is unclear, especially in light of a report of nine cases of lymphoma in patients with combined immunodeficiency, five of whom had not received thymic epithelial transplants (31).

Patients with AT have propensities for chromosomal breakage and progressive immunodeficiency and develop malignant lymphoproliferative malignancy in approximately 11% of cases (10). Curiously, patients with AT develop Hodgkin's disease more commonly than patients with any of the other immunodeficiency disorders. Perhaps this is related to their also having a propensity to develop chromosomal breakage and transpositions. An abnormal antibody response to EBV is found in patients with AT. For example, Joncas et al. (30) have found antibodies to VCA in eight patients, and four of them also had antibodies to EA. Antibodies to EBNA, however, were deficient. We have found similar abnormal antibody profiles in patients with AT (67). Patients with AT show T-cell defects that may be partly or wholly responsible for these abnormalities (37). The anti-VCA titers in various immunodeficiency/lymphoproliferative disorders are shown in Fig. 6.

Saemundsen and associates (77) have demonstrated 50 to 70 EBV genome equivalents per cell in a malignant lymphoma in a child with AT. We speculate that the progressive immune deficiency of AT may be related to defective immunoregulatory responses to EBV, as abnormal immune responses to EBV are comparable to those in XLP.

WAS is complicated by malignant lymphoreticular disorders in approximately 15% of cases (10). These malignancies occur at a frequency approximately 100-fold above age-matched individuals (48).

Recently we have been provided with the opportunity to study aspects of immunoregulation in a family affected by WAS (57). The 15-year-old proband had suffered from recurrent lymphadenomegaly, fever, and thrombocytopenia since infancy. His younger brother had also developed similar symptoms, but to a lesser extent. Enumeration of T cells (i.e., OKT3-pan-T-positive cells) showed severe reduction in the proband, lesser reduction in the younger brother, and partial reduction in the mother. A similar gradient of abnormally elevated antibody titers to VCA, EA, and EBNA was found in the three individuals; i.e., proband> brother>mother. The mother, being an obligate hemizygote for the WAS gene, possibly showed partial immune defects; however, she has remained asymptomatic. The findings of abnormal antibody responses to EBV were analogous to those in carrier females of XLP (82).

Schwaber and associates (84) have demonstrated a deficiency of EBV receptor on B cells from certain patients with agammaglobulinemia. Patients with XAg

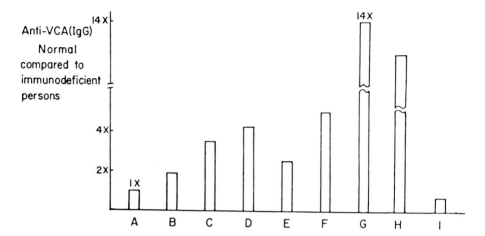

FIG. 6. Anti-VCA titers in patients with various immunodeficiencies/lymphoproliferative disorders: normal **(A)**; Hodgkin's disease (From Henle, ref. 21a) **(B)**; XLP carrier females (From Sakamoto, ref. 79) **(C)**; ataxia telangiectasia (From Berkel, ref. 2a) **(D)**; renal transplant recipients without (From Cheesman, ref. 5a) **(E)**; and with **(F)**; antithymocyte globulin; hairy cell leukemia **(G)**; Burkitt's lymphoma (From Henle, ref. 21b) **(H)**; and XLP males (From Sakamoto, ref. 79) **(I)**.

rarely develop malignant lymphoproliferative disorders (10). Perhaps their B cells are incapable of being transformed by EBV because of a lack of viral receptors. Alternatively, they may lack the capacity for B-cell proliferation to be induced by other agents. An analogous situation prevails in the CBA/N mouse having an X-linked immune deficiency. Lee and Ihle (36) have demonstrated that male CBA/N mice have a much lower frequency of Moloney virus-induced lymphomas. The viremic CBA/N mice lack subpopulations of T lymphocytes capable of proliferating in response to the Moloney viral proteins, and hence lymphomagenesis does not occur.

We have documented (2,68) families with common variable immunodeficiency (CVID) with chronic IM. Growing evidence suggests that some cases of CVID could arise from aberrant immunoregulatory responses to EBV (74). In addition, fatal IM has occurred in siblings (68). The type of immune deficiency in many of these families is poorly characterized (55). Finally, we have observed diverse malignancies and immunodeficiencies in a family, including partial IgM deficiency complicated by an EBV-carrying immunoblastic sarcoma of B cells (62).

A comparison of EBV-related disorders is summarized in Table 2. As noted above, in patients with primary immunodeficiency disorders, some protection from EBV infection may be afforded by altered susceptibility or numbers of target cells (e.g., patients with XAg lack mature B cells). Conversely, vulnerability may depend on the extent of immunoregulatory defects. For example, patients with XLP show the most marked immunoregulatory defects and in WAS less severe immunoregulatory defects occur; WAS patients manifest lymphoma approximately half as often as XLP patients. Another contrast is the lack of fatal IM in the immunodeficiency disorders other than XLP.

The cotton-topped marmoset (CTM) is a New-World monkey that serves as an animal model (Table 2) for EBV-associated lymphomas such as those in XLP and transplant recipients (44). This monkey has apparently been shielded by geographical events. EBV probably arose from a common herpes virus progenitor in Africa after the continents of South America and Africa separated some 50 million years ago (Donald Johnson, *personal communication*). Owing to lack of exposure to EBV, CTM probably failed to develop the genetic apparatus necessary for mounting a vigorous immune response to the virus. A study by Miller et al. (44) of 20 animals inoculated with EBV revealed large tumors in 30%, marked to moderate hyperplasia in 35%, and no abnormalities in the remaining animals. The anti-VCA and anti-EA titers were in a range comparable to those found in seropositive immune-competent human beings with IM. In contrast, the CTM failed to produce significant anti-EBNA titers. With respect to variability of pathological expression and the lack of anti-EBNA, CTMs resemble males with XLP. Johnson et al. (27) have demonstrated that the lymphoproliferative diseases provoked by EBV inoculation in CTM are polyclonal and normal diploid. Thus CTM appears to be a good model for the profound immune deficiency seen in most individuals with XLP or comparable to renal transplant recipients who are seronegative and then acquire immune deficiency followed by primary infection (17,20).

DIVERSE GENETIC DISORDERS WITH POSSIBLE IMMUNOREGULATORY DEFECTS TO EBV

Joncas et al. (28) have described a Canadian family with diverse EBV-associated diseases apparently occurring on a familial basis. Two of the individuals have experienced nasopharyngeal carcinoma, two Burkitt's lymphoma, one multiple myeloma, and one acute lymphocytic leukemia, and several family members have partial IgA deficiency. This family offers an opportunity to evaluate the role of EBV and immunoregulatory disturbances in the pathogenesis of these disorders (29). Many of the family members have shown abnormally elevated EBV-specific antibody titers, and various T-cell aberrations were found.

Familial Hodgkin's disease requires investigation for the role of EBV as a possible etiological agent (43). We have investigated several families with familial Hodgkin's disease. These individuals frequently have demonstrated elevated EBV-specific antibody profiles and immunoregulatory defects. We have actively sought collaborative studies on a family reported by McBride and Fennelly from Ireland (43). Previous immunological studies had revealed CVID in the affected family members and siblings as well as the mother. T-cell function was diminished as was cutaneous skin reactivity to antigen stimuli. The mother had increased immunoglobulin levels. During 1980, we obtained serum samples on the family members and found markedly elevated antibody profiles to EBV, indicating chronic active infection by this agent (D. Purtilo, *unpublished*).

Green et al. (12) have reported a family with Hodgkin's disease affecting two of three young siblings, following IM. The events began in the family in mid-1972, when a 15-year-old developed IM with persistent Paul-Bunnell reactivity for seven months and subsequent good health. In 1974, her 25-year-old brother developed IM followed by Hodgkin's disease in 1978. His 18-year-old sister developed IM the year following his bout with the disease and developed Hodgkin's disease. These findings could have occurred by chance; however, high-risk families for Hodgkin's disease should be studied for immune defects to EBV. The immunological studies to define immune deficiency and serological studies for EBV have not been completed in the family. Many additional families could be summarized. Such families at high risk for Hodgkin's disease should be entered into prospective studies to evaluate the role of EBV and immunoregulatory disturbances in the pathogenesis.

Chédiak-Higashi disease (CHD) often terminates in a fatal lymphoproliferative disease (35). Haliotis et al. (15) have described defective NK cell function in individuals with CHD. They proposed this defect as a major reason for the development of fatal lymphoproliferative disorders. However, Krueger et al. (35) have noted, at autopsy, defective thymic epithelium in patients with CHD, suggesting immunoregulatory defects. Moreover, collaborative studies have shown elevated EBV-specific antibody titers and increased suppressor T-cell numbers in individuals with CHD (F. Merino and D. Purtilo, *unpublished*).

Patients with Bloom's syndrome show both chromosomal breakage and immune deficiency (5,25). Lymphomas are overrepresented in children with this autosomal recessive disease. Such patients should be examined for immunoregulatory defects to EBV.

Louie and Schwartz (41) have noted increased B-cell lymphoproliferative malignancies in individuals with rheumatoid arthritis and autoimmune disturbances. Patients with rheumatoid arthritis show defective EBV-specific suppressor T-cell function (94). A case can also be made for investigating the role of EBV in the B-cell lymphomas of patients with Sjögren's syndrome (95).

DISORDERS CLUSTERED WHERE BURKITT'S LYMPHOMA IS PREVALENT

Several rare disorders are seen in high frequency in tropical Africa where Burkitt's lymphoma is prevalent. These disorders could arise in part from immunodeficiency to EBV. For example, histiocytic medullary reticulosis (HMR) (24,89) is seen in tropical Africa and in patients with various immunodeficiencies, including children with acute lymphocytic leukemia in remission (46). Moreover, XLP is misdiagnosed as HMR (63).

Another unusual disorder, big spleen disease, is found commonly in tropical Africa in areas of holoendemic malaria. Such patients show lymphocytic infiltration in the liver (6) that mimics IM hepatitis.

Kaposi's sarcoma is also common in tropical Africa (92). This disease is known to complicate individuals with immune deficiency, such as renal transplant recipients

(47). Moreover, an alarming number of Kaposi's sarcomas have appeared in homosexual men (26). These men have shown immunoregulatory disturbances associated with lymphadenomegaly and EBV-genome-positive Burkitt's lymphoma (D. Abrams and D. Purtilo, *unpublished*). Kaposi's sarcoma is probably caused by immune deficiency to cytomegalovirus (9). The lack of Kaposi's sarcoma in female prostitutes who have multiple sexual partners is noteworthy. Perhaps this is because of immunological superiority of females (69). Females show lower morbidity and mortality for infectious agents and malignant lymphomas (52), which can be explained in part by X-linked immunoregulatory genes.

ALLOGRAFT RECIPIENTS AND EBV INFECTIONS

Renal transplant recipients (RTR) (47), cardiac transplant patients (1), and thymus epithelial transplant recipients (83) are at increased risk for developing lymphoproliferative neoplasia. Our collaborative studies of lymphoproliferative diseases in RTR with investigators in Minneapolis and Stockholm have revealed that these neoplasms carry EBV (17–20,77). The young individuals immunosuppressed before primary infection by EBV tend to develop the fatal IM phenotype of XLP. They show low-titer anti-VCA and EA and often lack anti-EBNA responses (Table 3). In contrast, elderly individuals who experienced primary infection before immune suppression show a reactivation profile with elevated titers to VCA, EA, and EBNA. The youths tend to develop lymphoproliferation after a short incubation period, and it is rapidly lethal and widely disseminated. The elderly patients show longer incubation periods from time of immune suppression to emergence of tumors. The lymphomas tend to be localized, but nevertheless, most of these are polyclonal (19).

Cardiac transplant patients showing idiopathic cardiomyopathy are at high risk for developing malignant lymphomas. The patients generally are young males, and they show suppressor cell dysfunction (1). Three of the lymphomas recently studied by EBV cRNA/DNA molecular hybridization contained EBV genome (G. Klein, *personal communication*).

Bone marrow transplant recipients are remarkably free of malignant B-cell lymphomas complicating their transplantation. Recently, however, an EBV-carrying immunoblastic sarcoma of donor origin has been documented (83). Perhaps the reason lymphomas are uncommon in this population is that recipients of bone-marrow transplants show activation of T-suppressor cells and hypogammaglobulinemia (33).

Depending on the age of the individual, the underlying disease, and the type and degree of immune suppression resulting from cytotoxic drugs or irradiation, an increased risk of malignant lymphoproliferative diseases induced by EBV can be anticipated. Our experience has been that approximately one in 100 renal transplant recipients develops a lethal post-transplant lymphoproliferative disorder (20).

TABLE 3. *EBV-induced lymphoproliferative diseases in renal transplant recipients*

Age (years)	Time after transplant	Cytotoxic agents	EBV antibody titers[a]			Lymphoproliferative disease location/clonality	EBV genome[b]	Comments
			Anti-VCA	Anti-EA	Anti-EBNA			
Young (14–16)	3–9 months	Multiple	60	<10	8	Oropharynx/poly (2), disseminated/mono (1)	9	Primary infection
Elderly (50–63)	4–6 years	Multiple	1,500	80	160	Oropharynx/poly (3), localized/mono (1)	8	Reactivation; trisomy 14
Control			100	<10	50			

[a]Absolute numbers are reciprocal mean values of the dilution.
[b]Mean numbers of EBV genome equivalents per cell.

TABLE 4. *Expressions of Epstein-Barr virus infection are determined by age and immunocompetence*

Age	In-utero	6–60 mos	6–10 yrs	11–17 yrs	18–35 yrs	36–85 yrs
% Sero-positive in immunocompetents	60–85	0–60	30–70	50–75	60–80	89–90
	Rare birth defects	Silent infection	Silent infection	IM 66%	IM 50%	Lifelong latency
Immunodeficients	Rare birth defects	Fatal IM, agamma, ML	Fatal IM, agamma, aplastic anemia, ML	Chiefly ML?	Transplant recipients chiefly fatal IM	Transplant recipients chiefly ML

Abbreviations: IM = infectious mononucleosis, ML = malignant lymphoma, agamma = agammaglobulinemia.

ACQUIRED IMMUNODEFICIENCY TO EBV IN PATIENTS WITH LEUKEMIA OR LYMPHOMA

Malignant B-cell lymphomas can emerge in patients in remission from Hodgkin's disease or leukemia. For example, Look et al. (40) have described a fatal EBV-induced lymphoproliferative disease in a child with acute lymphocytic leukemia in remission. Similarly, we have documented immunodeficiency to EBV and marked hyperplasia of gut-associated lymphoid tissues that bordered on malignant lymphoma in a patient in remission with acute lymphocytic leukemia. He had developed hypogammaglobulinemia and had cellular and humoral defects in anti-EBV responses. (C. Hardy and D. T. Purtilo, *unpublished*). Patients in remission for acute lymphocytic leukemia may show hypogammaglobulinemia (73) and a variety of cellular immune defects. Approximately 4.4% of patients treated for Hodgkin's disease develop non-Hodgkin's lymphoma (34). Patients who have received both chemotherapy and radiotherapy are at greatest risk. Because these patients are probably immune-compromised, they should be evaluated for EBV as an etiological agent in the B-cell lymphomas.

EBV infects virtually all adults and is held in lifelong latency by immunoregulatory defenses. In immunosuppressed patients with leukemias or lymphomas these defenses prevent life-threatening reactivation of EBV. For example, patients with hairy cell leukemia cope with latent EBV by elevating antibodies to EBV (78). Figure 6 summarizes anti-VCA titers in patients with various immunodeficiency states.

AGE, SEX, IMMUNOCOMPETENCE, AND SOCIOECONOMIC FACTORS DETERMINE OUTCOME OF EBV INFECTION AND POSSIBLY MALIGNANT LYMPHOMAS

Evaluation of the possible outcomes of EBV infection suggests that the clinical and pathological expressions of EBV infections are governed by socioeconomic factors and the immunocompetence of the individual at the time of the infection (Table 4). Sex (52,70,75) and socioeconomic factors are also determinants in lymphomagenesis (4). Our studies on XLP, for example, suggest that male children with the defect can die of IM almost immediately following disappearance of maternal antibody. They are vulnerable to EBV infection and cannot prevent the life-threatening lymphoproliferation.

IM is a disease of middle-class individuals (22). Perhaps silent infection tends to occur in young children in lower-class families (23) because of the increased chance of exposure to EBV of an infant whose mother is pregnant and shedding; transient, physiologic immunodeficiency accompanies normal pregnancy (80). The number of offspring in middle- and upper-class families is limited, and the children are generally born with several years intervening between pregnancies. Hence, very young individuals in such families tend not to be exposed to their pregnant mothers. Hodgkin's disease follows socioeconomic patterns similar to IM.

HYPOTHESIS: MECHANISM OF POLYCLONAL CONVERSION TO MONOCLONAL EBV-INDUCED B-CELL PROLIFERATION

Klein (32) has postulated that three steps occur sequentially during Burkitt's lymphomagenesis: First, EBV infects and immortalizes B cells in a polyclonal fashion; second, malaria increases the proliferation of B cells, increasing the likelihood of a specific 8;14 translocation producing 14q+; and third, the 14q+ alteration endows the cell with the capacity to escape host regulatory mechanisms. This hypothesis is very attractive but difficult to test in tropical Africa. Moreover, Klein has not mentioned the possibility that immune deficiency may allow B-cell proliferation to continue unabated. For example, Burkitt's lymphoma emerges approximately two and a half years after primary infection (7). In our opinion, African children at increased risk for Burkitt's lymphoma have multiple factors rendering them mildly immunodeficient to EBV: maleness, malnutrition, measles virus infection, and parasitism. All of these factors, including malaria, can be immunosuppressive (53).

The high-risk patient with XLP or the RTR offers excellent opportunities to test the hypothesis that EBV can, in patients with immunoregulatory disturbances, produce both polyclonal lymphoproliferation and monoclonal malignancies. For example, our collaborative study with Hanto et al. (18) has revealed an apparent EBV-induced polyclonal B-cell lymphoproliferation converting to monoclonal malignancy during a nine-month course. Specific cytogenetic translocations between chromosomes 8, 14, 2, and 22 are critical in determining the Ig phenotype of Burkitt's lymphoma (76). Prospective karyotype studies of immune-deficient patients at high risk for lymphoma may further define the mechanisms of conversions from polyclonal to monoclonal lymphoma.

SUMMARY AND CONCLUSIONS

EBV is a ubiquitous virus uniquely infecting the human B cell. The immune system activates T-cell immunoregulatory cells to control acute EBV infection. Multiple immune defenses have developed and allow for harmonious coexistence of virus and host. However, individuals that inherit or acquire marked immunoregulatory disturbances are then at increased risk for developing a variety of lymphoproliferative diseases, including malignant B lymphoma. The immune competence of an individual probably governs the outcome of infection. Sex, socioeconomic level, and hereditary factors govern the immune responses. Study of immune deficient patients will assist in gaining insight into normal immune responses to EBV and will provide knowledge about the impact of cytogenetic translocation in clonal B-cell proliferating and rational bases for correcting and preventing immunoregulatory disorders to the virus.

ACKNOWLEDGMENTS

This work was supported in part by a grant from the National Institutes of Health (CA 30196-01) and by the Lymphoproliferative Research Fund.

REFERENCES

1. Anderson, J. L., Bieber, C. P., Fowles, R. E., and Stinson, E. B. (1978): Idiopathic cardiomy-opathy, age, and suppressor-cell dysfunction as risk determinants of lymphoma after cardiac transplantation. *Lancet*, 2:1174–1177.

2. Ballow, M., Seeley, K., Sakamoto, K., St. Onge, S., Rickles, R. F., and Purtilo, D. T. (1983): Familial chronic mononucleosis. *Ann. Intern. Med.*, 97:821–825.

2a. Berkel, A. I., Henle, W., Henle, G., Klein, G., Ersoy, F., and Sanal, O. (1979): Epstein-Barr virus-related antibody patterns in ataxia-telangiectasia. *Clin. Exp. Immunol.*, 35:196–201.

3. Borzy, M., Hong, R., Horowitz, S., Gilbert, E., Kaufman, D., DeMondonca, W., Oxelius, V.-A., Dictor, J., and Pachman, L. (1979): Fatal lymphoma after transplantation of cultured thymus in children with combined immunodeficiency disease. *N. Engl. J. Med.*, 301:565–568.

4. Cantor, K., and Fraumeni, J. (1980): Distribution of Non-Hodgkin's lymphoma in the United States between 1950 and 1975. *Cancer Res.*, 40:2654–2656.

5. Chaganti, R. S. K. (1983): The significance of chromosome change to neoplastic development. In: *Chromosome Breakage and Neoplasia*, edited by J. German. Alan R. Liss, New York *(in press)*.

5a. Cheesman, S. H., Henle, W., Rubin, R. H., Tolkoft-Rubin, N. E., Cosmi, B., Cantell, K., Winkle, S., Herrin, J. T., Black, P. H., Russell, P. S., and Hirsch, M. S. (1980): Epstein-Barr virus infection in renal transplant recipients. *Ann. Intern. Med.*, 93:39–42.

6. Correa, P., and O'Connor, G. T. (1973): Geographic pathology of lymphoreticular tumors: sum-mary of survey from the Geographic Pathology Committee of the International Union Against Cancer. *JNCI*, 50:1609–1617.

7. de-Thé, G., Geser, A., Day, N. E., Tukei, P. M., Williams, E. H., Beri, D. P., Smith, P. G., Dean, A. G., Bornkamm, G. W., Feorino, P., and Henle, W. (1978): Epidemiological evidence for causal relationship between Epstein-Barr virus and Burkitt's lymphoma from Ugandan pro-spective study. *Nature*, 274:756–761.

8. Edington, G. M., and Gilles, H. M. (1969): *Pathology in the Tropics*, pp. 412–447. Williams & Wilkins, Baltimore.

9. Fenoglio, C. M., Oster, M. W., and McDougall, J. (1982): Cytomegalovirus RNA in Kaposi's sarcoma. *Lab. Invest.*, 46:25a (abstr.).

10. Filipovich, A. H., Spector, B. D., and Kersey, J. (1980): Immunodeficiency in humans as a risk factor in the development of malignancy. *Prev. Med.*, 9:252–259.

11. Gershon, R. K., Cohen, P., Hencin, R. S., and Liebhaber, S. A. (1972): Suppressor T cells. *J. Immunol.*, 108:586–598.

12. Green, J. A., Dawson, A. A., and Valerio, D. (1979): Hodgkin's disease and infectious mono-nucleosis. *Semin. Hematol.*, 2:313–314.

13. Grundy, G. W., Creagan, E. T., and Fraumeni, J. F. (1973): Non-Hodgkin's lymphoma in child-hood: epidemiologic features. *JNCI*, 51:767–776.

14. Gutensohn, N., and Cole, P. (1981): Childhood social environment and Hodgkin's disease. *N. Engl. J. Med.*, 304:135–140.

15. Haliotis, T., Rodger, J., Klein, M., Ortaldo, J., Fauci, A. S., and Herberman, R. B. (1980): Chediak-Higashi gene in humans. *J. Exp. Med.*, 151:1039–1048.

16. Hamilton, J. K., Paquin, L. A., Sullivan, J. L., Maurer, H. S., Cruzi, P. G., Provisor, A. J., Steuber, C. P., Hawkins, E., Yawn, D., Cornet, J., Clausen, K., Finkelstein, G. Z., Landing, B., Grunnet, M., and Purtilo, D. T. (1980): X-linked lymphoproliferative syndrome registry report. *J. Pediatr.*, 96:669–673.

17. Hanto, D. W., Frizzera, G., Gajl-Peczalska, K. J., Purtilo, D. T., Klein, G., Simmons, R. L., and Najarian, J. S. (1981): The Epstein-Barr virus (EBV) in the pathogenesis of post-transplant lymphoma. *Transplant. Proc.*, 13:756–760.

18. Hanto, D. W., Frizzera, G., Gajl-Peczalska, K. J., Sakamoto, K., Purtilo, D. T., Balfour, H. H., Jr., Simmons, R. L., and Najarian, J. S. (1982): Epstein-Barr virus-induced B-cell lymphoma after renal transplantation: Acyclovir therapy and transition from polyclonal to monoclonal B-cell proliferation. *N. Engl. J. Med.*, 306:913–918.

19. Hanto, D. W., Frizzera, G., Purtilo, D. T., Sakamoto, K., Sullivan, J. L., Saemundsen, A. K., Klein, G., Simmons, R. L., and Najarian, J. S. (1981): Clinical spectrum of lymphoproliferative disorders in renal transplant recipients and evidence for the role of Epstein-Barr virus. *Cancer Res.*, 41:4253–4261.

20. Hanto, D. W., Sakamoto, K., Purtilo, D. T., Simmons, R. L., and Najarian, J. S. (1981): The Epstein-Barr virus in the pathogenesis of posttransplant lymphoproliferative disorders. *Surgery*, 90:204–213.

21. Harada, S., Sakamoto, K., Seeley, J. K., Lindsten, T., Rogers, G., Pearson, G., and Purtilo, D. T. (1982): Immune deficiency in the X-linked lymphoproliferative syndrome. I. Epstein-Barr virus-specific defects. *J. Immunol.*, 129:2532–2535.

21a. Henle, W., and Henle, G. (1973): Evidence for an oncogenic potential of the Epstein-Barr virus. *Cancer Res.*, 33:1419–1423.

21b. Henle, W., and Henle, G. (1980): Epidemiologic aspects of Epstein-Barr virus (EBV)-associated diseases. *Ann. NY Acad. Sci.*, 354:326–331.

22. Henle, W., Henle, G., and Lennette, T. (1979): The Epstein-Barr virus. *Sci. Am.*, 241:48–59.

23. Herberman, R. B., Djeu, J. Y., Kay, H. D., Ortaldo, J. R., Riccardi, C., Bonnard, G. D., Holden, H. T., Gagnani, R., Santoni, A., and Puccetti, P. (1979): Natural killer cells: characteristics and regulation of activity. *Immunol. Rev.*, 44:43–70.

24. Hutt, M. S. R., Lowenthal, M. N., and Fine, J. (1975): Histiocytic medullary reticulosis (malignant histiocytosis) in Zambia. *J. Trop. Med. Hyg.*, 78:239–242.

25. Hutteroth, T. H., Litwin, S. D., and German, J. (1975): Abnormal immune responses of Bloom's syndrome lymphocytes in vitro. *J. Clin. Invest.*, 56:1–7.

26. Hymes, K. B., Greene, J. B., Marcus, A., William, D. C., Cheung, T., Prose, N. S., Ballard, H., and Laubenstein, L. J. (1981): Kaposi's sarcoma in homosexual men: a report of eight cases. *Lancet*, 1:598–600.

27. Johnson, D. R., Wolfe, L. G., Klein, G., Levan, G., Ernberg, S., and Aman, P. (1983): Epstein-Barr virus (EBV) induced lymphoproliferative diseases in cotton-topped marmosets. *Int. J. Cancer*, 31:91–97.

28. Joncas, J. H., Rioux, E., Wastiaux, J. P., Levritz, M., Robillard, L., and Menezes, J. (1976): Nasopharyngeal carcinoma and Burkitt's lymphoma in a Canadian family. 1. HLA typing, EBV antibodies and serum immunoglobulins. *Can. Med. Assoc. J.*, 115:858–860.

29. Joncas, J., Seeley, J., Purtilo, D. T., Ghibu, F. M., Lichaa, H., Robillard, L., Alfieri, C., Rioux, E., and Montplatsir, S. (1982): Immunological defect in a family with multiple nasopharyngeal carcinoma and Burkitt's lymphoma. In: *Comparative Leukemia and Related Diseases*, edited by D. Yohn, pp. 561–562. Elsevier/North-Holland, New York.

30. Joncas, J. H., William, A., Reece, E., and Fox, Z. (1981): Epstein-Barr virus antibodies in patients with ataxia-telangiectasia and other immunodeficiency diseases. *Can. Med. Assoc. J.*, 125:845–849.

31. Kersey, J. H., Filipovich, A. H., Spector, B. D., and Frizzera, G. (1980): Lymphoma after thymus transplantation (letter). *N. Engl. J. Med.*, 302:301–302.

32. Klein, G. (1979): Lymphoma development in mice and humans: Diversity of initiation is followed by convergent cytogenetic evolution. *Proc. Natl. Acad. Sci. USA*, 76:2442–2446.

33. Korsmeyer, S. J., Elfenbein, G. J., Goldman, C. K., Marshall, S. I., Santos, G. W., and Waldman, T. A. (1982): B cell, helper T cell, and suppressor T cell abnormalities contribute to disordered immunoglobulin synthesis in patients following bone marrow transplantation. *Transplantation*, 33:184–190.

34. Krikorian, J. G., Burke, J. S., Rosenberg, S. A., and Kaplan, H. S. (1979): Occurrence of non-Hodgkin's lymphoma after therapy for Hodgkin's disease. *N. Engl. J. Med.*, 300:452–458.

35. Krueger, G., Bedoya, V., and Grimley, P. M. (1971): Lymphoreticular tissue lesions in Steinbrinck-Chediak-Higashi syndrome. *Virchows Arch. (Pathol. Anat.)*, 353:273–288.

36. Lee, J. C., and Ihle, J. N. (1983): Chronic immune stimulation is required for Moloney leukemia virus-induced lymphomas. *Nature (in press)*.

37. Levis, W. R., Dattner, A. M., and Shaw, J. S. (1978): Selective defects in T cell function in ataxia-telangiectasia. *Clin. Exp. Immunol.*, 37:44–49.

38. Lindsten, T. Seeley, J. K., Ballow, M., Sakamoto, K., St. Onge, S., Yetz, J., Aman, P., and Purtilo, D. T. (1982): Immune deficiency in the X-linked lymphoproliferative syndrome. II. Immunoregulatory T cell defects. *J. Immunol.*, 129:2536–2540.

39. Lipinski, M., Virelitzier, J.-L., Tursz, T., and Griscelli, C. (1980): Natural killer and killer cell activities in patients with primary immunodeficiencies or defects in immune interferon production. *Eur. J. Immunol.*, 10:246–249.

40. Look, A. T., Naegele, R. F., Calihan, T., Herrod, H. G., and Henle, W. (1981): Fatal Epstein-

Barr virus infection in a child with acute lymphoblastic leukemia in remission. *Cancer Res.*, 41:4280–4283.

41. Louie, S., and Schwartz, R. S. (1978): Immunodeficiency and the pathogenesis of lymphoma and leukemia. *Semin. Hematol.*, 15:117–138.

42. Masucci, M. G., Szigeti, R., Ernberg, I., Masucci, G., Klein, G., Chessels, J., Sieff, C., Lie, S., Glomstein, A., Businco, L., Henle, W., Henle, G., Pearson, G., Sakamoto, K., and Purtilo, D. T. (1981): Cellular immune defects to Epstein-Barr virus-determined antigens in young males. *Cancer Res.*, 41:4284–4291.

43. McBride, A., and Fennelly, J. J. (1977): Immunological depletion contributing to familial Hodgkin's disease. *Eur. J. Cancer*, 13:519–554.

44. Miller, G., Shope, T., Coope, D., Waters, L., Pagano, J., Bornkamm, G. W., and Henle, W. (1977): Lymphoma in cotton-topped marmosets after inoculation with Epstein-Barr virus: tumor incidence, histologic spectrum antibody responses, demonstration of viral DNA, and characterization of viruses. *J. Exp. Med.*, 145:948–967.

45. Miller, R. M. (1975): Overview: host factors. In: *Persons at High Risk of Cancer: An Approach to Cancer Etiology and Control*, edited by J. Fraumeni, pp. 121–128. Academic Press, New York.

46. Miller, R. M. (1981): Second malignancy in acute lymphocytic leukemia. *Am. J. Dis. Child*, 135:313–316.

47. Penn, I. (1981): Depressed immunity and the development of cancer. *Clin. Exp. Immunol.*, 46:459–474.

48. Perry, G. S., Spector, B. D., Schuman, L. M., Mandel, J. S., Anderson, V. E., McHugh, R. B., Hanson, M. R., Fahlstrom, S. M., Krivit, W., and Kersey, J. H. (1980): The Wiskott-Aldrich syndrome in the United States and Canada (1982–1979). *J. Pediatr.*, 97:72–78.

49. Plouffe, J. F., Silva, J., Schwartz, R. S., Callen, J. P., Kane, P., Murphy, L. A., Goldstein, I. J., and Fekety, R. (1979): Abnormal lymphocyte responses in residents of a town with a cluster of Hodgkin's diseases. *Clin. Exp. Immunol.*, 35:163–170.

50. Purtilo, D. T. (1976): Hypothesis: pathogenesis and phenotypes of an X-linked recessive lymphoproliferative syndrome. *Lancet*, 2:882–885.

51. Purtilo, D. T. (1976): Malignancies in the tropics. In: *Pathology of Tropical and Extraordinary Disease*, edited by C. H. Binford and D. H. Connors. Armed Forces Institute of Pathology, Washington, D.C.

52. Purtilo, D. T. (1977): Opportunistic non-Hodgkin's lymphoma in X-linked recessive immunodeficiency and lymphoproliferative syndromes. *Semin. Oncol.*, 4:335–343.

53. Purtilo, D. T. (1980): Epstein-Barr virus-induced oncogenesis in immune deficient individuals. *Lancet*, 1:300–303.

54. Purtilo, D. T. (1980): Immune deficiency predisposing to Epstein-Barr virus-induced lymphoproliferative diseases: the X-linked lymphoproliferative syndrome as a model. *Adv. Cancer Res.*, 34:279–312.

55. Purtilo, D. T. (1980): Immunopathology of infectious mononucleosis and other complications of Epstein-Barr virus infections. *Pathol. Annu.*, 15(1):253–299.

56. Purtilo, D. T. (1981): Malignant lymphoproliferative disease induced by EBV in immunodeficient patients, including X-linked cytogenic and familial syndromes. *Cancer Genet. Cytogenet.*, 4:251–268.

57. Purtilo, D. T., Bechtold, T., Harada, S., Yetz, J., Rogers, G., Saemundsen, A. K., and Meuwissin, H. (1983): Epstein-Barr virus in a family with the Wiskott-Aldrich Syndrome. (Submitted for publication.)

58. Purtilo, D. T., and Connor D. H. (1975): Fatal infections in protein-calorie malnourished children with thymolymphatic atrophy. *Arch. Dis. Child.*, 50:149–152.

59. Purtilo, D. T., DeFlorio, D., Hutt, L. M., Bhawan, J., Yang, J. P. S., Otto, R., and Edwards, W. (1977): Variable phenotypic expression of an X-linked recessive lymphoproliferative syndrome. *N. Engl. J. Med.*, 297:1077–1081.

60. Purtilo, D. T., Hallgren, H., and Yunis, E. J. (1972): Depressed maternal lymphocyte response to phytohemagglutinin in human pregnancy. *Lancet*, 1:769–777.

61. Purtilo, D. T., Hutt, L. M., Allegra, S., Cassel, C., Yang, J. P. S., and Rosen, F. S. (1978): Immunodeficiency to the Epstein-Barr virus in the X-linked recessive lymphoproliferative syndrome. *Clin. Immunol. Immunopathol.*, 9:147–156.

62. Purtilo, D. T., Liao, S. A., Sakamoto, K., Snyder, L. M., DeFlorio, D., Bhawan, J., Paquin, L. A., Yang, J. P. S., Hutt-Fletcher, L. M., Muralidharan, K., Raffa, P., Saemundsen, A. K.,

and Klein, G. (1981): Diverse familial malignant tumors and Epstein-Barr virus. *Cancer Res.*, 41:4248–4251.

63. Purtilo, D. T., Paquin, L. A., DeFlorio, D., Virzi, F., and Sukhuja, R. (1979): Immunodiagnosis and immunopathogenesis of the X-linked recessive lymphoproliferative syndrome. *Semin. Hematol.*, 16:309–343.

64. Purtilo, D. T., Riggs, R. S., Evans, R., and Neafie, R. C. (1976): Humoral immunity of parasitized malnourished children. *Am. J. Trop. Med. Hyg.*, 25:229–232.

65. Purtilo, D. T., and Sakamoto, K. (1982): Reactivation of Epstein-Barr virus in pregnant women: social factors; and immune competence as determinants of lymphoproliferative diseases—a hypothesis. *Med. Hypotheses*, 8:401–408.

66. Purtilo, D. T., Sakamoto, K., Barnabei, V., Seeley, J., Bechtold, T., Rogers, G., Yetz, J., and Harada, S. (1982): Epstein-Barr virus-induced diseases in males with the X-linked lymphoproliferative syndrome (XLP). *Am. J. Med.*, 73:49–56.

67. Purtilo, D. T., Sakamoto, K., Harada, J., Rogers, G., and Ochs, H. D. (1983): Deficient Epstein-Barr virus (EBV)-specific antibody responses in patients with primary immunodeficiency syndromes (IDS). 13th International Cancer Congress, Seattle, Washington.

68. Purtilo, D. T., Sakamoto, K., Saemundsen, A. K., Sullivan, J. L., Synnerholm, A.-C., Anvret, M., Pritchard, J., Sloper, C., Sieff, C., Pincott, J., Pachman, L., Rich, K., Cruzi, F., Cornet, J. A., Collins, R., Barnes, N., Knight, J., Sandstedt, B., and Klein, G. (1981): Documentation of Epstein-Barr virus infection in immunodeficient patients with life-threatening lymphoproliferative diseases by clinical, virological, and immunopathological studies. *Cancer Res.*, 41:4226–4236.

69. Purtilo, D. T., and Sullivan, J. L. (1979): Immunological bases for superior survival of females. *Am. J. Dis. Child.*, 133:1251–1253.

70. Purtilo, D. T., Yang, J. P. S., Cassel, C. K., Harper, P., Stephenson, S. R., Landing, B. H., and Vawter, G. F. (1975): X-linked recessive progressive combined variable immunodeficiency (Duncan's disease). *Lancet*, 1:935–950.

71. Purtilo, D. T., Zelkowitz, L., Harada, S., Brooks, C. D., Bechtold, T., Saemundsen, A. K., Lipscomb, H. L., Yetz, J., and Rogers, G. (1983): Detection of X-linked lymphoproliferative syndrome (XLP) and evolving red cell aplasia, infectious mononucleosis, and progressive hypogammaglobulinemia phenotypes *(submitted for publication)*.

72. Reece, E. R., Gartner, J. G., Seemayer, T. A., Joncas, J. H., and Pagano, J. S. (1981): Epstein-Barr virus in a malignant lymphoproliferative disorder of B-cells occurring after thymic epithelial transplantation for combined immunodeficiency. *Cancer Res.*, 41:4243–4247.

73. Reid, M. M., Craft, A. W., and Cox, J. R. (1981): Immunoglobulin concentrations in children receiving treatment for acute lymphoblastic leukaemia. *J. Clin. Pathol.*, 34:479–482.

74. Reinherz, E. L., O'Brien, C., Rosenthal, P., and Schlossman, S. F. (1980): The cellular basis for viral-induced immunodeficiency: analysis by monoclonal antibodies. *J. Immunol.*, 125:1269–1274.

75. Rosenberg, S. A., Diamond, H. D., Jaslowitz, B., and Craver, L. F. (1961): Lymphosarcoma: A review of 1269 cases. *Medicine*, 40:31–84.

76. Rowley, J. D. (1982): Identification of the constant chromosome regions involved in human hematologic malignant disease. *Science*, 216:749–751.

77. Saemundsen, A. K., Purtilo, D. T., Sakamoto, K., Sullivan, J. L., Synnerholm, A. C., Hanto, D., Simmons, R., Anvret, M., Collins, R., and Klein, G. (1981): Documentation of Epstein-Barr virus infection in immunodeficient patients with life-threatening lymphoproliferative diseases by Epstein-Barr virus complementary RNA/DNA and viral DNA/DNA hybridization. *Cancer Res.*, 41:4237–4242.

78. Sakamoto, K., Aiba, M., Katayama, I., Sullivan, J. L., Humphreys, R. E., and Purtilo, D. T. (1981): Antibodies to Epstein-Barr virus-specific antigens in patients with hairy-cell leukemia. *Int. J. Cancer*, 27:453–458.

79. Sakamoto, K., Freed, H., and Purtilo, D. T. (1980): Antibody responses to Epstein-Barr virus in families with the X-linked lymphoproliferative syndrome. *J. Immunol.*, 125:921–925.

80. Sakamoto, K., Greally, J., Gilfillan, R., Sexton, J., Seeley, J., Barnabei, V., O'Dwyer, E., Bechtold, T., and Purtilo, D. T. (1982): Reactivation of Epstein-Barr virus in normal pregnant women. *Am. J. Reprod. Immunol.*, 2:217–221.

81. Sakamoto, K., Greally, J., Sexton, J., and Purtilo, D. T. (1982): Reactivation of Epstein-Barr

virus in pregnant women. In: *Comparative Leukemia and Related Diseases*, edited by D. Yohn, pp. 569–570. Elsevier/North-Holland, New York.

82. Sakamoto, K., Seeley, J. K., Lindsten, T., Sexton, J., Yetz, J., Ballow, M., and Purtilo, D. T. (1982): Abnormal anti-Epstein-Barr virus antibodies in carriers of the X-linked lymphoproliferative syndrome and in females at risk. *J. Immunol.*, 128:904–907.

83. Schubach, W. H., Hackman, R., Neiman, P. E., Miller, G., and Thomas, E. D. (1982): A monoclonal immunoblastic sarcoma in donor cells bearing Epstein-Barr virus genomes following allogeneic marrow grafting for acute lymphoblastic leukemia. *Blood*, 60:180–187.

84. Schwaber, J. F., Klein, G., Ernberg, I., Rosen, A., Lazarus, H., and Rosen, F. S. (1980): Deficiency of Epstein-Barr virus (EBV) receptors on B lymphocytes from certain patients with common variable agammaglobulinemia. *J. Immunol.*, 124:2191–2196.

85. Seeley, J. K., Bechtold, T., Lindsten, T., and Purtilo, D. T. (1982): NK deficiency in X-linked lymphoproliferative syndrome. In: *Natural Cell Mediated Immunity*, edited by R. Herberman, pp. 1211–1218. Academic Press, New York.

86. Seeley, J. K., Lindsten, J., Ballow, M., Sakamoto, K., and Purtilo, D. T. (1982): Defective lymphocyte function in X-linked lymphoproliferative syndrome. In: *Comparative Leukemia and Related Diseases*, edited by D. Yohn, pp. 571–572. Elsevier/North-Holland, New York.

87. Seeley, J. K., Sakamoto, K., Ip, S., Hansen, P., and Purtilo, D. T. (1981): Abnormal subsets in the X-linked lymphoproliferative syndrome. *J. Immunol.*, 127:2618–2620.

88. Seeley, J. K., Sakamoto, K., Lindsten, T., Harada, S., Ballow, M., Yetz, J., and Purtilo, D. T. (1983): Detection of males at risk for the X-linked lymphoproliferative syndrome *(submitted for publication)*.

89. Serck-Hanssen, A., and Purchit, G. P. (1968): Histiocytic medullary reticulosis: report of 14 cases from Uganda. *Br. J. Cancer*, 22:506–512.

90. Sullivan, J. L., Byron, K., Brester, F., and Purtilo, D. T. (1980): Deficient natural killer cell activity in the X-linked lymphoproliferative syndrome. *Science*, 210:543–545.

91. Sullivan, J. L., Sakamoto, K., Byron, K. S., Brewster, F. E., and Purtilo, D. T. (1980): Prospective immunological and virological studies in a fatal case of the X-linked lymphoproliferative syndrome. *Clin. Res.*, 28:641A.

92. Templeton, A. C. (1981): Kaposi's sarcoma. *Pathol. Annu.*, 16:315–336.

93. Tosato, G., Magrath, I., Koski, I., Dooley, N., and Blaese, M. (1979): Activation of suppressor T cells during Epstein-Barr virus-induced infectious mononucleosis. *N. Engl. J. Med.*, 301:1133–1137.

94. Tosato, G., Steinberg, A. D., and Blaese, R. M. (1981): Defective EBV-specific suppressor T-cell function in rheumatoid arthritis. *N. Engl. J. Med.*, 305:1238–1243.

95. Zulman, J., Jaffe, R., and Talal, N. (1978): Evidence that the malignant lymphoma of Sjogren's syndrome is a monoclonal B cell neoplasm. *N. Engl. J. Med.*, 299:1215–1220.

Pathogenesis of Leukemias and Lymphomas:
Environmental Influences, edited by
I. T. Magrath, G. T. O'Conor, and B. Ramot.
Raven Press, New York © 1984.

Detection and Isolation of Epstein-Barr Virus in Lymphocytes from Patients with Chronic B-Lymphocytic Leukemia

*Gary Armstrong, **Dan Longo, *Alberto Faggioni, *Dharam Ablashi, †Gary Pearson, and ‡Susan Slovin

*Laboratory of Cellular and Molecular Biology, **Medicine Branch, National Cancer Institute, National Institutes of Health, Bethesda, Maryland 20205; †Mayo Clinic, Rochester, Minnesota 55901; and ‡Department of Pathology, Tufts University School of Medicine, Boston, Massachusetts 02111

The Epstein-Barr virus (EBV) has been implicated as a causative agent of infectious mononucleosis (5). It is also considered to be a factor in the etiology of at least two human cancers [African Burkitt's lymphoma (1) and nasopharyngeal carcinoma (8)]. Anti-EBV antibodies are elevated compared to control populations in a variety of disease states such as Guillain-Barré syndrome (3), Hodgkin's disease (7,10), and chronic lymphocytic leukemia (CLL) (9,11). Moreover, B-cell lymphomas have been reported in immunodeficient individuals (15); this may also be associated with EBV. A common factor in all these diseases is an immunological derangement, usually immunosuppression, as a consequence of which reactivation of herpesvirus is a logical event.

Recently, we noted serological changes in two patients followed for a year and a half who eventually developed CLL. The anti-EBV titers in these patients were elevated before the diagnosis of CLL. In one patient, the anti-viral capsid antigen (VCA) IgG titer increased from 640 to 5,120, anti-early antigen (EA) IgG rose from 240 to 320, and anti-VCA IgA increased from undetectable (<10) to 40. These findings led us to investigate the cause of the elevated anti-EBV antibodies, specifically to determine if there is either an increased pool of EBV-infected normal B cells or if EBV-containing tumor cells could be detected. This investigation is important because of a recent demonstration that polyclonal EBV-infected cells give rise to "lymphoma" in renal transplant recipients and a variety of other immunodeficient states (15).

The 11 patients in this study (Table 1) were diagnosed as having CLL on the basis of absolute peripheral blood lymphocytosis, and bone marrow aspirates and biopsies revealing an increase in the percentage of small lymphocytes (over 30%) and a histologic pattern of marrow involvement consistent with CLL (either an increase in lymphoid nodules or diffuse marrow infiltration with small lymphocytes).

TABLE 1. *EBV immunovirological investigation in CLL patients*

Patient	Age (years)	Sex	WBC[a] (×10³)	EBV titers					Reactivity with 2F5.6		
				VCA (IgG)	EA (IgG)	VCA (IgA)	EBNA	ADCC[b] titer	EBNA fresh cells	Fresh cells	EBV isolation from fresh PBL[c]
P.I.	70	F	51.3	40	20/40	<10	<10	ND	0	0	0
C.D.	71	F	62.0	20/40	<10	<10	<10	ND	0	0	0
R.L.	63	F	103.0	640	160	40	<10	≥3,840	4–5%	4%	+
H.E.	41	M	17.0	20	<10	<10	<10	≥3,840	0	0	0
G.M.	70	F	32.5	320	160	20	<10	7,680	4–6%	5%	0
B.B.	70	M	25.9	1,280	320	<10	<10	2,880	0	0	0
H.M.	56	F	30.6	320	<10	<10	<10	ND	0	0	0
F.N.	71	M	34.2	20	<10	<10	<10	240	3–4%	3%	0
B.G.	73	F	16.8	160	40	<10	<10	11,520	0	0	0
N.C.	52	F	28.2	160	40	10	<10	ND	17–19%	17%	+
W.C.	49	M	14.7	160	20	<10	<10	ND	0	0	0

[a]At time of collection.

[b]Antibody-dependent cell cytotoxicity: ≥3,840 = high, <3,840 = low, 7,680 and above = very high. ND = not determined. Antibody titers to the viral capsid antigen, both IgG and IgA classes, as well as early antigen (diffuse component) were determined by indirect immunofluorescence (6). Titers are represented as the reciprocal of the dilution of patients' sera capable of reacting with the appropriate cell substrates. For anti-EBNA antibody, the anti-complement immunofluorescence method of Reedman and Klein (14) was used. Using the method of Pearson and Orr (12), patients' sera were screened for activity in the antibody-dependent cell-mediated cytotoxicity reaction.

[c]Peripheral blood lymphocytes.

Evidence that these cells belong to the B-cell lineages was provided by detection of membrane markers of the IgM class. The patients were Rai stages II to IV and were diagnosed two to 12 years before blood sampling for this study, with two exceptions.

Peripheral blood leukocytes from the 11 CLL patients were separated by plasma gel, as described before (2), and were stained by indirect immunofluorescence with monoclonal antibody 2F5.6, which is directed against the 320K EBV-induced membrane glycoprotein (13). This antibody reacts only with cells producing transforming EBV (2,13). In addition, EB nuclear antigen (EBNA) slides from freshly isolated lymphocytes were prepared and stained (14). For virus isolation, cell-free filtrates were prepared from a freeze-thaw preparation of 2 to 3 ml of packed leukocytes, which were then clarified by low-speed centrifugation and filtered with a 0.45μ millipore filter. This filtrate was tested on human cord blood lymphocytes for immortalization into permanent cell lines (2). Plasma and/or serum was also tested for antibodies to EBV antigens, including VCA (4), EA (6), (EBNA) as previously described, and antibody-dependent lymphocyte cytotoxicity (ADCC) (12). The plasmas were tested for antibodies in both the IgG and IgA classes.

Table 1 presents the serological and virus isolation results. The sera of all these patients contained IgG antibodies to VCA, many at elevated levels. In addition, sera from seven of the 11 patients (63.6%) contained antibody directed toward EBV anti-EA complex. Most interestingly, the sera of three patients contained IgA antibodies to VCA. All sera had a titer of less than 10 for antibodies to EBNA. ADCC titers ranged from 240 to 11,520. More important, EBV antigens were detected in fresh peripheral blood lymphocytes from four of these patients (Table 1). The 2F5.6 monoclonal antibody reacted with membrane antigens in 4 to 17% of the peripheral blood lymphocytes from these patients, and 4 to 19% of these cells were also positive for EBNA. Furthermore, transforming virus was directly isolated from fresh peripheral blood lymphocytes from two of these patients at different intervals. Evidence for transformation was noted in these cultures within 14 days after inoculation by rapid cell growth, presence of colonies of transformed cells, and presence of EBNA-positive cells.

These findings extend those of published reports showing that some patients with CLL had elevated antibody titers to EBV antigens (9,11). The question still to be answered is whether the EBNA-positive cells were normal or leukemic lymphocytes. However, it can be concluded for the present that either there is an expanded pool of EBV-containing normal cells or some CLL cells are infected with EBV. The unlikely possibility that most of the cells are EBV-DNA-positive but lack EBNA might also be considered. Further studies to determine the nature of the EBNA-positive cells in CLL are under way.

ACKNOWLEDGMENTS

We would like to thank the nursing staff of Labor and Delivery, Shady Grove Hospital, Rockville, Maryland, for the collection of cord blood used throughout this study and Jeannine Wingire for typing the manuscript.

Supported by NIH Fellowship #AMO6188-02.

REFERENCES

1. de-Thé, G., Geser, A., Day, N. E., Tukei, P. M., Williams, E. H., Beri, D. P., Smith, P. G., Dean, A. G., Bornkamm, G. W., Feorino, P., and Henle, W. (1978): Epidemiological evidence for causal relationship between Epstein-Barr virus and Burkitt's lymphoma from Ugandan prospective study. *Nature*, 274:756–761.
2. Gerber, P., Ablashi, D., Magrath, I., Armstrong, G., Andersen, P., and Trach, L. (1982): Persistence of transforming and nontransforming Epstein-Barr virus in high passages of P₃HR-1 cell lines. *JNCI*, 69:585–589.
3. Grose, C., and Feorino, P. (1972): Epstein-Barr virus and Guillain-Barré syndrome. *Lancet*, 2:1285–1287.
4. Henle, G., and Henle, W. J. (1966): Immunofluorescence in cells derived from Burkitt's lymphoma. *Bacteriology*, 91:1248–1256.
5. Henle, W., and Henle, G. (1973): Epstein-Barr virus and infectious mononucleosis. *N. Engl. J. Med.*, 288:263–264.
6. Henle, W., Henle, G., Zajac, B., Pearson, G., Waubke, R., and Scriba, M. (1970): Differential reactivity of human serum with early antigens induced by Epstein-Barr virus. *Science*, 169:188–190.
7. Hesse, J., Anderson, E., Levine, P. H., Ebbeson, P., Halberg, P., and Reisher, J. J. (1973): Antibodies to Epstein-Barr virus and cellular immunity in Hodgkin's and chronic lymphocytic leukemia. *Int. J. Cancer*, 11:237–243.
8. Ho, J. H. C., Kwan, H. C., Ng, M. H., and de Thé, G. (1978): Serum IgA antibodies to Epstein-Barr virus capsid antigen preceding symptoms of nasopharyngeal carcinoma. *Lancet*, 1:436.
9. Johannson, B., Klein, G., Henle, W., and Henle, G. (1971): Epstein-Barr virus (EBV) associated antibody patterns in malignant lymphoma and leukemia. II. Chronic lymphocytic leukemia and lymphocytic lymphoma. *Int. J. Cancer*, 8:475–486.
10. Levine, P. H., Ablashi, D. V., Berard, C. W., Carbone, P. P., Waggoner, D. E., and Malan, L. (1971): Elevated antibody titers to Epstein-Barr virus in Hodgkin's disease. *Cancer*, 27:416–421.
11. Levine, P. H., Merrill, D. A., Bethlenfalvay, N. C., Dabich, L., Stevens, D. A., and Waggoner, D. E. (1971): A longitudinal comparison of antibodies to the Epstein-Barr virus and clinical parameters in chronic lymphocytic leukemia and chronic myelocytic leukemia. *Blood*, 38:479–481.
12. Pearson, G., and Orr, T. W. (1976): Antibody-dependent lymphocyte cytotoxicity against cells expressing Epstein-Barr virus antigen. *JNCI*, 56:485–488.
13. Qualtiere, L. F., Chase, R., Vroman, B., and Pearson, G. R. (1982): Identification of Epstein-Barr virus strain differences with monoclonal antibody to a membrane glycoprotein. *Proc. Natl. Acad. Sci. USA*, 79:616–620.
14. Reedman, B. M., and Klein, G. (1973): Cellular localization of an Epstein-Barr virus (EBV)-associated complement-fixing antigen in producer and non-producer lymphoblastoid cell lines. *Int. J. Cancer*, 11:499–520.
15. Saemundsen, A. K., Purtilo, D. T., Sakamoto, K., Sullivan, J. L., Synnerholm, A.-C., Hanto, D., Simmons, R., Anvret, M., Collins, R., and Klein, G. (1981): Documentation of Epstein-Barr virus infection in immunodeficient patients with life-threatening lymphoproliferative diseases by Epstein-Barr virus complementary RNA/DNA and viral DNA/DNA hybridization. *Cancer Res.*, 41:4237–4242.

Pathogenesis of Leukemias and Lymphomas:
Environmental Influences, edited by
I. T. Magrath, G. T. O'Conor, and B. Ramot.
Raven Press, New York © 1984.

Cytogenetic Abnormalities in Lymphoid Neoplasia

Avery A. Sandberg

Roswell Park Memorial Institute, Buffalo, New York 14263

An evaluation of cytogenetic findings in the various forms of human lymphoid neoplasia in relation to the major themes of this volume (i.e., influence of geography, race, sex, age, socioeconomic status, etc.) is hampered by a lack of sufficient karyotypic data in each of these areas. It is unfortunate that in large series of cases with various lymphomas (3,12,13,23,27), cytogenetic studies were not performed for a number of reasons, such as lack of interest, unavailability of a cytogenetic laboratory, the erroneous assumption that the same translocation is present in various forms of lymphoma (e.g., the erroneous assumption that all American Burkitt's lymphomas (BL) have an 8;14 translocation) (23), and, undoubtedly, technical difficulties. To assume *a priori* that all lymphomas of a particular type will have the same karyotypic change on the basis of limited experience and/or data based on established cell lines will only delay the definition of the various lymphomas cytogenetically. Had the same attitude been taken in leukemia, we would not be in a position, as we are now, to subclassify the various acute and chronic leukemias into specific categories with characteristic clinical, cytologic, prognostic, and possibly etiologic parameters (64,69,75). In fact, the chromosome features characterizing each subgroup of human lymphoid disorders are only now starting to emerge, as adequate data are being obtained in various countries. BL is a good example of a lymphoid disorder in which cytogenetic subcategories are emerging (discussed below). In addition, the lack of a uniform system for classifying the lymphoid disorders makes comprehensive comparison of and correlation between the cytogenetic findings concerning these disorders obtained in various clinics in the same country and between countries, in particular, a difficult and complicated task. However, recent attempts to correlate the various classification systems and the establishment of a relatively uniform approach to the histopathologic diagnosis of the lymphomas (4,50) should go a long way toward expediting a cytogenetic definition of these disorders.

BURKITT'S LYMPHOMA AND LEUKEMIA

BL, both the endemic and nonendemic varieties, and the related disease acute lymphoblastic leukemia of Burkitt type (ALL-L3) are probably histologically, clinically, and karyotypically the best defined subgroup of lymphoid neoplasia. Thus, it may be best to discuss the cytogenetic findings in this group of diseases in relation to some of the major aims of this volume.

The description by Manolov and Manolova (38) of an elongation of the long arms of one chromosome, number 14 (14q+), in established cultures of cells originating from BL tissues of endemic origin, was a notable contribution to the cytogenetics of BL. For several years it was thought that this was a specific karyotypic anomaly in BL. However, Zech and her co-workers (79) showed that the extra material on the long arm of chromosome 14 originated from the long arm of a chromosome 8 in biopsies and cell lines of BL studied. Thus, the translocation 8;14 was soon shown to characterize almost all of the BL established cell lines and thereafter directly on tissues obtained from patients with Burkitt-type diseases (8,10,28, 36,43,44,54,73). Such a translocation, i.e., t(8;14)(q24;q32), was soon shown to characterize not only the endemic disease but also that found in nonendemic areas, including such widely separated lands as France, Japan, and the United States (8,28,44). Thus, it soon became apparent that the translocation between chromosomes 8 and 14 characterized not only Burkitt's tumors and leukemias associated with Epstein-Barr virus (EBV), but also those not associated with evidence of EBV (42) (Figs. 1 to 3). These findings seem to indicate that the genesis of Burkitt-type disease was probably closely related to the appearance of t(8;14), whether EBV was present in the tumor or not (33).

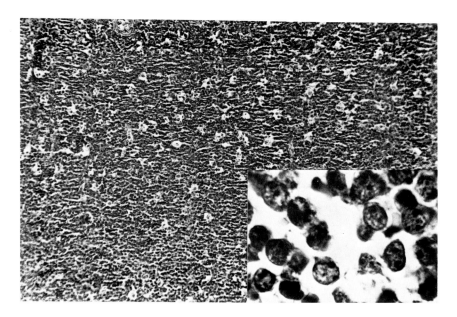

FIG. 1. Typical histologic appearance of a Burkitt-type lymphoma with the "starry sky" pattern in an American boy. The inset shows a higher magnification of cells with the characteristic appearance of Burkitt's cells (28).

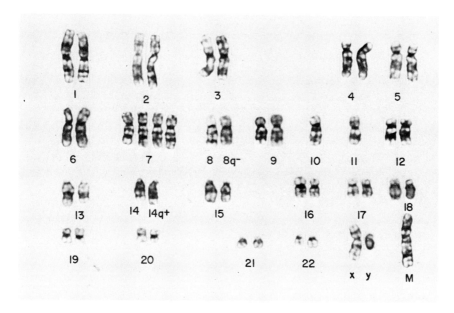

FIG. 2. G-banded karyotype of the tumor shown in Fig. 1, containing 47 chromosomes with the karyotype 47,XY, + 7, + 7, − 10, − 11,t(8;14)(q23;q32), + marker (M) (28). This karyotype demonstrates a rather common cytogenetic picture in BL, i.e., the translocation between chromosomes #8 and #14 *and* additional chromosomal changes.

The karyotypic findings in Burkitt-type diseases were further expanded and, thus, became more complicated when a variant translocation was described in a patient with typical BL involving chromosomes 2 and 8 and not 14, i.e., t(2;8)(p12;q24) (47) (Figs. 4 and 5), followed by the description of another variant translocation t(8;22) (7) (Figs. 6 and 7). Again, the translocation resulted from a break in band q24 of chromosome 8, pointing to the importance of the deletion of chromosome 8 in BL and related ALL-L3. Subsequently, nine other cases with the former and 10 with the latter variant translocation were reported from such diverse places as Belgium, Japan, Holland, Algeria, France, and the United States (Table 1). In addition, in each case the translocation appeared to involve the same band, particularly that of chromosome 8 (q24), and indicated that the key cytogenetic event in Burkitt-type disease may not be the 14q + but deletion of chromosome 8 at band q24 (9,19,74). Stress has been put on the possible significance of the deleted chromosome in the genesis of human neoplasia, rather than on the recipient chromosome (77) in conditions such as the Philadelphia chromosome (Ph[1]), i.e., t(9;22) in chronic myelocytic leukemia (CML) and t(8;21) in acute myeloblastic leukemia (64). Thus, at present there appears to be little doubt that the deletion of chromosome 8 is the *sine qua non* cytogenetic criterion for the diagnosis of Burkitt-type disease when translocations are present. That the story may be more complicated is borne out by the apparent lack of a specific translocation (although other changes were present) in some cases of Burkitt's diseases and the recent publication of a case of

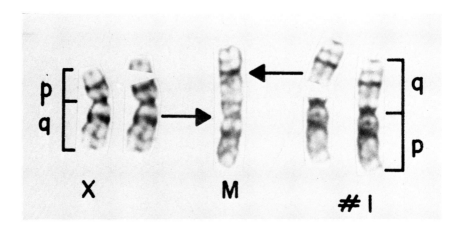

FIG. 3. Partial karyotype showing the genesis of the marker (M) of Fig. 2. It is caused by a translocation between the X and chromosome #1, i.e., t(X;1)(p21;q21) (28).

Burkitt-type leukemia (EBV-negative) in whose cells neither 8q − nor 14q + could be found (16).

The translocation t(8;14)(q24;q32) is a chromosomal change that characterizes the preponderant number of cases of Burkitt-type diseases irrespective of geographic location. With advances in the high resolution of chromosome sub-bands, it has recently been demonstrated that the breaks in chromosomes 8 and 14 occur in sub-bands q24.1 and q32.5, respectively (39,80). However, 20% or more of such cases may prove to have a variant translocation involving chromosome 8 and others, i.e., 2 and 22, with the deletion of chromosome 8 always involving the same band (33). Such translocations have been described from diverse places (Table 1).

An interesting feature of the variant translocations in Burkitt's diseases is related to the sex ratio of the affected individuals. BL and ALL-L3 are preponderantly diseases of young males, the incidence ranging from more than 60% to more than 75% in various series. Thus, the ratio of nine males to two females with t(8;22) is in keeping with that observed in patients with the usual translocation t(8;14). On the other hand, the patients with t(2;8) are evenly divided between males and females. Whether these differences have a significance in relation to the disease process will be settled when a much larger body of information has been gathered in this area.

The question naturally arises whether the diseases characterized by variant translocations in Burkitt's diseases are different, in any respect, from those with t(8;14). Unfortunately, the number of cases with variant translocations (a total of 21 to date)

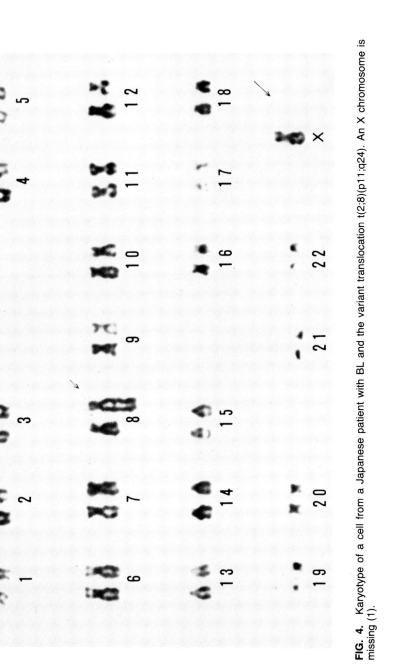

FIG. 4. Karyotype of a cell from a Japanese patient with BL and the variant translocation t(2;8)(p11;q24). An X chromosome is missing (1).

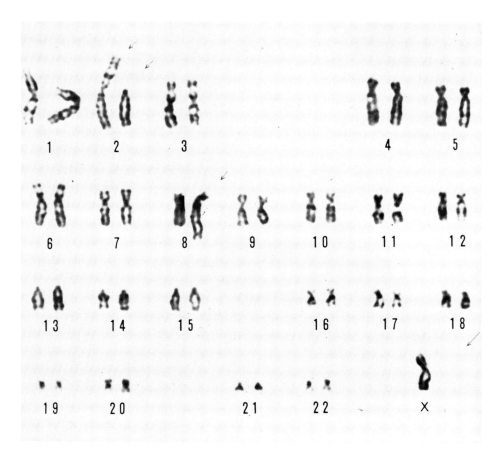

FIG. 5. Karyotype of another cell of the same patient of Fig. 4 containing the t(2;8) and missing X but also an additional anomaly of 2p+ (1).

is at present too small to draw conclusions; as more data are accumulated, a clearer picture may emerge of the significance of variant translocations in the clinical and biologic parameters of the diseases. A similar situation exists in CML in which variant Ph[1]-translocations do not appear to significantly affect various facets of the disease (64).

Specific translocations, particularly because they involve identical bands on involved chromosomes, have been postulated to be closely related to the primary event in the genesis of malignant process (26,66), whereas other karyotypic anomalies, considered secondary in nature, may be more closely related to the biologic behavior and phenotypic aspects of the disease. For example, it has been shown that heavy and light chain surface immunoglobulins expressed on Burkitt's cells may correlate with the karyotypic changes, i.e., tumors with t(2;8) expressing exclusively kappa and those with t(8;22) lambda chains (1,33); the loci for the genes for these immunoglobulins have been shown to be located on these chro-

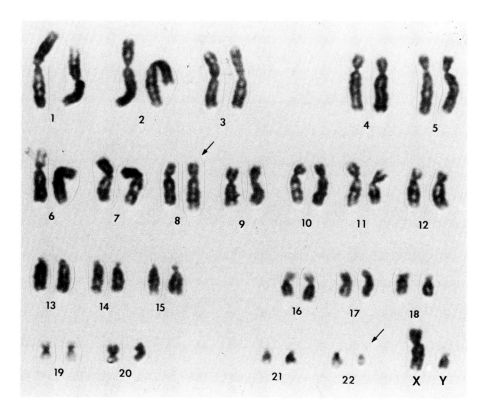

FIG. 6. Karyotype of a bone marrow cell from an American boy (2) with Burkitt-type leukemia (ALL-L3) with the variant translocation t(8;22) (q24;q12).

mosomes (18,37). The loci for the heavy chains have been shown to be on chromosome 14 (14,31). These considerations lead one to consider the possibility that malignancy, translocations, and the phenotypic expression of immunoglobulin chains may be related (24,32).

The secondary cytogenetic changes in Burkitt-type diseases are complex, although some evidence has been presented that involvement of chromosome 1 (Fig. 9), particularly partial trisomy of its long arm, may be more frequent than others (65), such as partial or total loss of chromosomes 15, 2, and 11. As a large volume of karyotypic data is obtained in Burkitt-type diseases, some of these changes may be shown to be related to certain clinical and phenotypic features, such as response to therapy, location of disease, manifestations, and prognosis. At present, it appears that the presence of secondary chromosome changes is often associated with a more progressive course of the disease than that in patients in whom the only karyotypic change in the affected cell is a specific translocation.

A number of cases with Burkitt-type disease have been described in which the only cytogenetic anomaly was a 14q+, with no evidence of a translocation (10,15). Other cases without a 14q+ or specific translocations have also been reported (73).

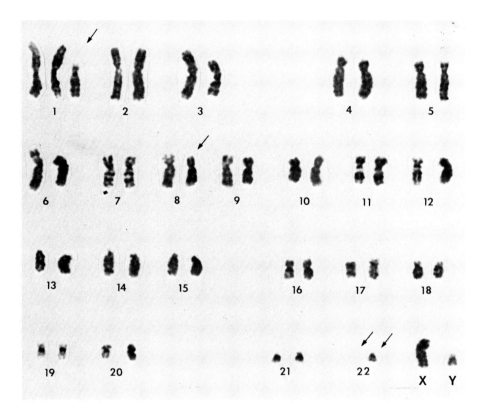

FIG. 7. Karyotype of a cultured blood cell of the same patient, Fig. 6 (1) containing the t(8;22) but also + del(1) and missing #22.

In most of these cases, the karyotypic changes were complex, a situation in which masking of translocations can readily occur and the presence of other subtle changes may not be readily ascertained. Thus, the possibility remains that translocations were also present in these cases but were not detectable because of the complexity of the karyotypic picture.

MALIGNANT NON-BURKITT'S LYMPHOMA

The cytogenetic findings in malignant lymphomas (ML) other than those of the Burkitt type have been reviewed recently (61,63). The findings are much more complex, variable, and protean than those described for Burkitt-type diseases (22, 29,30,40,57,58) (Figs. 8 and 9) (Tables 2 to 4). Chromosome #14 is frequently involved in translocations, but the donor chromosome as often as not is a chromosome other than 8 (Table 2, Fig. 8). Some of these translocations may characterize subtypes of lymphoma (Table 4). What appears clear is that as more karyotypic data are obtained in these disorders and as the classification of the lymphomas becomes more standardized and reliable, definite correlations will be and are being

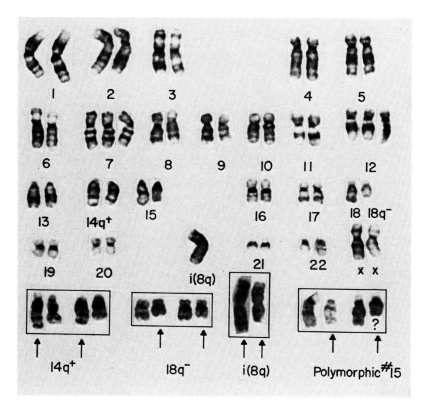

FIG. 8. C-banded karyotype of a lymphoma cell in the bone marrow with the karyotype 49,XX, + 7, + i(8q), + 12,?t(14;18) (29). The latter type of translocation is not uncommon in lymphoma. The boxed insets show chromosomes from other metaphases.

established among the chromosome findings, the type of disease, and other parameters (particularly immunologic).

A good example in this regard is a recently reported series of 55 patients with non-Hodgkin's lymphoma, in each of whom chromosomal changes were present, with the preponderant portion having clones of cells in the near-diploid range (34). About two-thirds of these lymphomas had the anomaly 14q +, the extra material a number 14 originating most often from chromosome 8 (30%), 18 (25%), and 1 (10%). Other frequent karyotypic changes were del(6)(q21-23); + 18;del(18)(q12-22);del(8)(q24);and + 4; in order of frequency. This study, which used an international Working Formulation, can already serve as a good example of progress being made in correlating chromosome findings in ML with the disease types when based on a comprehensive classification of the lymphomas.

The karyotypic changes in ML have been observed in various parts of the world, although the exact types differ with the nature of the lymphoma. Thus, 14q + in ML has been described from Japan, Australia, Europe, and the United States (41).

TABLE 1. Clinical and karyotypic findings of published Burkitt's lymphoma or leukemia (ALL-L3) cases with variant translocations: (2;8) or (8;22)

Patient's country	Age and sex	Survival (months)	EBV[a]	Source[b]	Karyotype	Reference
		Cases with t(2;8)				
Japan	29, M	8.0	+	BM	46,XY,t(2;8)(p12;q24)	Miyoshi et al. (47)
Belgium	4, F	5.5	NT[c]	LN	46,XX,t(2;8)(p12;q23)	Van Den Berghe et al (77)
West Germany	34, F	3.0	+	Cell line	46,XX,t(2;8)(p11;q24)	Bornkamm et al. (11)
United States	20, M	2.0	NT	PB	46,XY,t(2;8)(p13;q24)	Rowley et al. (62)
Japan	45, F	6.0	NT	PE,PB	45,X,−X,t(2;8)(p11;q24)	Abe et al. (1)
				BM	45,X,−X,−2,t(2;8)(p11;q24),+de r(2)t(2;der(8) t(2;8)(p11;q24))(p13;q21)	
Holland	7, F	2.0	−	BM,LN	46,X,Xp+,t(2;8)(p11;q24),lq−,7p+,17p−	Slater et al. (70)
France	22, M	7.0+	−	BM	46,XY,t(2;8)(p12;q24)	Berger et al. (7)
Kenya	13, M	—	+	Cell line	46,XY,t(2;8)(p12;q24),der(1) triplication (q22-q32)del(q42-qter)	Bernheim et al. (8)
Uganda	7, F	—	+	Cell line	46,XX,t(2;8)(p12;q24)	Bernheim et al. (8)
Algeria	8, M	4.0	+	Tumor	46,XY,t(2;8;9)(p11;q23;q31)	Philip et al. (54,55)

		Cases with t(8;22)				
Turkey-France	65, M	1.0	BM	—	46,XY,t(8;22)(q23;q12),t(1;6)(q21;qter)	Berger et al. (6)
France	7, M	6.0	BM	—	46,XY,t(8;22)(q23;q12)/46,XY,t(8;22)(q23;q12),−6,t(1;6)(q23;q26)	
France	19, M	6.0	LN,PB	+	46,XY,t(8;22)(q23;q11),14q+	
France (trip to Cameroon before diagnosis)	54, M		PE	probably neg.	45,X,−Y,t(1;14)(q22;q32),t(8;22) (q24;q11), 3q+,6q−,6q+,7q+,9p−,14q−,18q−	
Japan	29, F	5.0	Ascites	—	46,XX,t(8;22)(q24;q13)	Miyoshi et al. (46)
France	70, F	15.0	LN	NT	47,XX,t(8;22)(q24;q21),+8,t(11;21)(q14;q22), 4q+,6q+,others	Berger and Bernheim (5)
France	31, M	6.0	PB	—	46,XX,t(8;22)(q24;q11)	
France	13, M	6.0	BM	NT	47,XY,t(8;22)(q24;q11),t?22/47,XY,t(8;22) (q24;q11),+?22,dup(1)(q23,q24)	
United States	6, M	0.5	BM	NT	46,XY,t(8;22)(q24;q12)	Abe et al. (2)
Uganda	M	—	Cell line	+	46,XY,t(8;22)(q24;q11)	
Kenya	M	—	Cell line	+	46,XY,t(8;22)(q24;q11),t(4;5)(q22;q13),del(11)	Bernheim et al. (8)

[a]EBV antibodies present in serum.
[b]BM = bone marrow, LN = lymph node, PE = pleural effusion, PB = peripheral blood.
[c]NT = not tested.

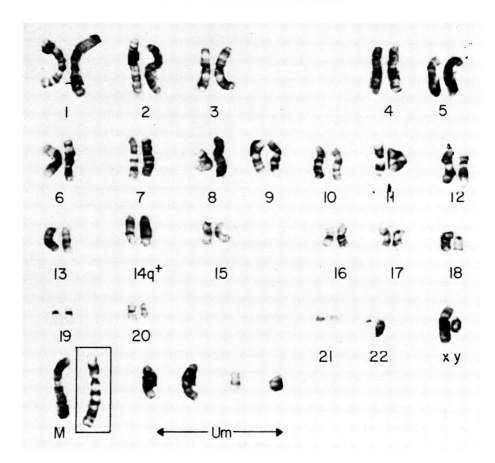

FIG. 9. G-banded karyotype of a lymphoma cell in the bone marrow, showing two 14q+ chromosomes, 18p−, and a marker (M) originating from chromosome 1 (29). Four other chromosomes of unknown origin (Um) are also shown.

TABLE 2. *Translocations involving chromosome 14 in non-Burkitt's lymphoma*

t(1;14)(q23;q32)
t(8;14)(q24;q32)
t(10;14)(q24;q32)
t(11;14)(q13;q32)
t(12;14)(q13;q32)
t(14;14)(q24;q32)
t(14;18)(q32;q21)
t(Y;14)(q12;q24?)

TABLE 3. *Common karyotypic changes in malignant lymphomas*

14q+
del(1)
del(3)
del(6)
+18
del(18)
del(8)
+7

TABLE 4. *Cytogenetic findings in some lymphomas*

Lymphoma	Cytogenetic findings
Small cell, lymphocytic	Pseudodiploid (46 chromosomes)
Follicular	47–48 chromosomes 14q+ t(14;18)(q32;q21-22)
Diffuse, large cell	48–50 chromosomes 14q+ t(8;14)(q24;q32)
Immunoblastic	del(6)(q21) t(8;14)(q24;q32)
Small cell, noncleaved	Pseudodiploid (46 chromosomes) 14q+ t(11;14)(q13;q32) +12

The anomaly 14q+ is prominent in ML of various types (41); the band involved frequently is q32, the same band as in BL. However, a group of cases with lymphoma involving band 14q13 has been described (20). Other chromosomes frequently involved in morphologic anomalies (not necessarily translocations) in ML are 1, 6, 3, 9, 11, 18, and 2, in order of frequency (65,71). Only after a uniform system of classifying lymphoid neoplasias has been universally established will it be possible to ascertain with certainty the significance of nonrandom or random changes in these diseases in relation to geography, sex, age, and other factors (Fig. 10).

ADULT T-CELL LEUKEMIA

Adult T-cell leukemia is more frequent in Japan than in the Western world (78). Chromosomal studies have been performed in several areas of Japan, particularly Okayama and Kyoto (45,48,76). The patients in Okayama have 14q+ and 6q− as the most common anomalies, whereas those in Kyoto seem to have anomalies of chromosome 7 (trisomy of 7 or 7q) as a frequent karyotypic change. Obviously,

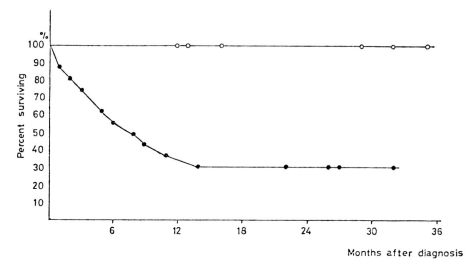

FIG. 10. Actuarial survival curves of patients with lymphoma (closed circles represent patients with markers of wholly or partly unknown origin; open circles represent patients without such markers) (30).

much more remains to be learned, including cytogenetically, about this disease entity before these apparent differences can be evaluated.

CHRONIC LYMPHOCYTIC LEUKEMIA

The karyotypic findings in chronic lymphocyte leukemia (CLL) have only recently been reported, primarily because of the inability in the past to obtain the leukemic cells in mitosis. The introduction of a number of B-cell stimulants made studies in CLL possible (21,49,63,68). Because CLL, at least in the Western world, is predominantly a B-cell disease, the use of these mitogenic agents is necessary to induce mitoses in the leukemic cells. To date, the cytogenetic data obtained in CLL indicate that trisomy 12 is the most common abnormality; 14q+ is present in a significant number but not the majority of patients (Fig. 11). Already some evidence is emerging on prognostic correlations between the karyotypic changes in CLL, survival, and course of the disease (25,59). In our group of patients, a correlation is apparent between the production of certain immunoglobulins, macroglobulin, and +12 (25). Undoubtedly, as more chromosomal data are obtained in this disease, further correlations will emerge between the karyotypic changes and such parameters as immunoglobulin production and the biologic behavior of the disease.

T-CELL DISEASES

The cytogenetic findings in T-cell diseases have been obtained primarily on patients with cutaneous T-cell lymphomas (Sézary syndrome and mycosis fungoides) and T-cell CLL (17,35,51–53). In the latter, a 14q+ has been found in a

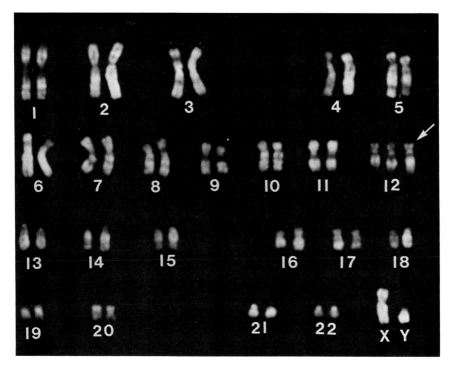

FIG. 11. Karyotype of a leukemic cell from a patient with CLL with the common karyotypic anomaly of trisomy 12 (arrow) (63).

few cases, as well as in an occasional case of T-cell lymphoma (51–53). In general, however, the karyotypic changes in these conditions are complex and to date have not been associated with the emergence of any nonrandom cytogenetic findings indicative of one condition or another.

HODGKIN'S DISEASE

Although Hodgkin's disease (HD) is a common disorder among the lymphomas, the karyotypic characteristics of this disease have not been well defined (60,67). Thus, a 14q+ anomaly has been found in a significant number of the cases (about one-third); the source of the extra material on the number 14 has been difficult to ascertain in most cases, and when caused by a translocation, the chromosomes involved (other than 14) have varied. In addition, technical difficulties and the cellular nature of HD tissues have presented obstacles in obtaining a large volume of reliable cytogenetic data on this disease. However, the karyotypic data unequivocally indicate that HD is a malignancy of lymphoid origin (60).

ACUTE LYMPHOBLASTIC LEUKEMIA

Cytogenetically, acute lymphoblastic leukemias (ALL) can now be subdivided into several categories, in which the chromosome findings are not only characteristic of the type of leukemia—e.g., L3-type of Burkitt's leukemia associated with t(8;14)—but also can serve as prognostic indicators (75) (Fig. 12). This has been made possible by the examination of a large body of data in ALL, which has led to a clearer definition, both cytogenetically and clinically, of subgroups of leukemias within ALL (Table 5).

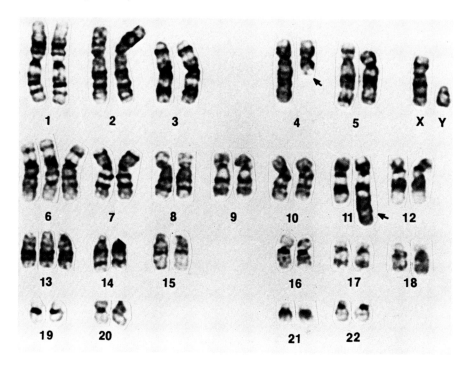

FIG. 12. Karyotype of a leukemic cell from a patient with ALL having extra chromosomes in groups 8 and 13 and a translocation between chromosomes 4 and 11 (64). The latter is associated with a rather poor survival (75).

TABLE 5. *Median survival and unique aspects of ALL as related to karyotypic changes*

Chromosome findings	Unique features	Approximate median survival (months)
t(8;14)	Burkitt-type ALL (L3)	5
t(4;11)	? Myeloid origin	8–10
t(9;22)	Ph¹-positive	12
Pseudodiploid	No morphologic abnormalities	>24
6q −	Also present in lymphoma	>36
Hyperdiploid or diploid	No morphologic abnormalities	>36

DISCUSSION

The possible role of cytogenetics in staging studies of lymphoma and in the histopathology of the diseases has been pointed out already (56,72). Parameters of lymphoma development related to the chromosome changes in this group of neoplasias have also received attention (32).

Even though more data are needed on the karyotypic changes in lymphoid neoplasias from other parts of the world, besides those from countries from which cytogenetic findings have already been published, as well as on other parameters (socioeconomic levels, sex distribution, histopathology), the chromosome findings appear to characterize the various lymphomas without regard, at least at this writing, to geography and other parameters. In other words, lymphomas of the same histopathology are accompanied by similar cytogenetic findings in various parts of the world, which may indicate that the cells involved and the causative parameters related to the lymphoma are universally similar, if not the same.

ACKNOWLEDGMENT

This work was supported in part by grant CA-14555 from the National Cancer Institute.

REFERENCES

1. Abe, R., Hayashi, Y., Sampi, K., and Sakurai, M. (1982): Burkitt's lymphoma with 2/8 translocation: A case report with special reference to the clinical features. *Cancer Genet. Cytogenet.*, 6:143–151.
2. Abe, R., Tebbi, C. K., Yasuda, H., and Sandberg, A. A. (1982): North American Burkitt-type ALL with a variant translocation t(8;22). *Cancer Genet. Cytogenet.*, 7:185–195.
3. Baroni, C. D., and Malchiodi, F. (1980): Histology, age and sex distribution, and pathologic correlations of Hodgkin's disease. *Cancer*, 45:1549–1555.
4. Berard, C. W., Greene, M. H., Jaffe, E. S., Magrath, I., and Ziegler, J. (1981): A multidisciplinary approach to non-Hodgkin's lymphomas. *Ann. Intern. Med.*, 94:218–235.
5. Berger, R., and Bernheim, A. (1982): Cytogenetic studies on Burkitt's lymphoma-leukemia. *Cancer Genet. Cytogenet.*, 7:231–244.
6. Berger, R., Bernheim, A., Bertrand, S., Fraisse, J., Frocrain, C., Tanzer, J., and Lenoir, G. (1981): Variant chromosomal t(8;22) translocation in four French cases with Burkitt lymphoma-leukemia. *Nouv. Rev. Fr. Hematol.*, 23:39–41.
7. Berger, R., Bernheim, A., Weh, H.-J., Flandrin, G., Daniel, M.-T., Brouet, J.-C., and Colbert, N. (1979): A new translocation in Burkitt's tumor cells. *Hum. Genet.*, 53:111–112.
8. Bernheim, A., Berger, R., and Lenoir, G. (1981): Cytogenetic studies on African Burkitt's lymphoma cell lines: t(8;14), t(2;8), and t(8;22) translocations. *Cancer Genet. Cytogenet.*, 3:307–315.
9. Bertrand, S., Berger, R., Philip, T., Bernheim, A., Bryon, P.-A., Bertoglio, J., Doré, J.-F., Brunat-Mentigny, M., and Lenoir, G. M. (1981): Variant translocation in a non-endemic case of Burkitt's lymphoma: t(8;22) in an Epstein-Barr virus negative tumour and in a derived cell line. *Eur. J. Cancer*, 17:577–584.
10. Biggar, R. J., Lee, E. C., Nkrumah, F. K., and Whang-Peng, J. (1981): Direct cytogenetic studies by needle aspiration of Burkitt's lymphoma in Ghana, West Africa. *JNCI*, 67:769–776.
11. Bornkamm, G. W., Kaduk, B., Kachel, G., Schneider, U., Fresen, K. O., Schwanitz, G., and Hermanek, P. (1980): Epstein-Barr virus-positive Burkitt's lymphoma in a German woman during pregnancy. *Blut*, 40:167–177.

12. Ciampi, A., Bush, R. S., Gospodarowicz, M., and Till, J. E. (1981): An approach to classifying prognostic factors related to survival experience for non-Hodgkin's lymphoma patients: Based on a series of 982 patients: 1967–1975. *Cancer*, 47:621–627.

13. Colby, T. V., Hoppe, R. T., and Warnke, R. A. (1981): Hodgkin's disease: A clinicopathologic study of 659 cases. *Cancer*, 49:1848–1858.

14. Croce, C. M., Shander, M., Martinis, J., Cicurel, L., D'Ancona, G. G., Dolby, T. W., and Koprowski, H. (1979): Chromosomal location of the genes for human immunoglobulin heavy chains. *Proc. Natl. Acad. Sci. USA*, 76:3416–3419.

15. Douglass, E. C., Magrath, I. T., Lee, E. C., and Whang-Peng, J. (1980): Cytogenetic studies in non-African Burkitt lymphoma. *Blood*, 55:148–155.

16. Douglass, E. C., Magrath, I. T., and Terebelo, H. (1982): Burkitt cell leukemia without abnormalities of chromosomes no. 8 and 14. *Cancer Genet. Cytogenet.*, 5:181–185.

17. Edelson, E. L., Berger, C. L., Raafat, J., and Warburton, D. (1979): Karyotype studies of cutaneous T cell lymphoma: Evidence for clonal origin. *J. Invest. Dermatol.*, 73:548–550.

18. Erikson, J., Martinis, J., and Croce, C. M. (1981): Assignment of the genes for human λ immunoglobulin chains to chromosome 22. *Nature*, 294:173–175.

19. Fraisse, J., Lenoir, G., Vasselon, C., Jaubert, J., and Brizard, C. P. (1981): Variant translocation in Burkitt's lymphoma: 8;22 translocation in a French patient with an Epstein-Barr virus-associated tumor. *Cancer Genet. Cytogenet.*, 3:149–153.

20. Fukuhara, S., Ueshima, Y., Shirakawa, S., Uchino, H., and Morikawa, S. (1979): 14q Translocations, having a break point at 14q13, in lymphoid malignancy. *Int. J. Cancer*, 24:739–743.

21. Gahrton, G., Robèrt, K.-H., Friberg, K., Zech, L., and Bird, A. G. (1980): Nonrandom chromosomal aberrations in chronic lymphocytic leukemia revealed by polyclonal B-cell-mitogen stimulation. *Blood*, 56:640–647.

22. Gödde-Salz, E., Schwarze, E.-W., Lennert, K., and Grote, W. (1981): T(Y;14)—A new type of 14q+ marker chromosome (Letter). *Cancer Genet. Cytogenet.*, 3:89–90.

23. Grogan, T. M., Warnke, R. A., and Kaplan, H. S. (1982): A comparative study of Burkitt's and non-Burkitt's "undifferentiated" malignant lymphoma: Immunologic, cytochemical, ultrastructural, cytologic, histopathologic, clinical and cell culture features. *Cancer*, 49:1817–1828.

24. Gunven, P., Klein, G., Klein, E., Norin, T., and Singh, S. (1980): Surface immunoglobulins on Burkitt's lymphoma biopsy cell from 91 patients. *Int. J. Cancer*, 25:711–719.

25. Han, T., Ozer, H., Sadamori, N., Gajera, R., Gomez, G., Henderson, E. S., Minowada, J., and Sandberg, A. A. (1982): Clinical significance of clonal chromosome changes in leukemic lymphocytes of chronic lymphocytic leukemia. *ASCO Abstr.*, 1:186.

26. Hecht, F., Kaiser-McCaw, B., and Sandberg, A. A. (1981): Chromosome translocations in cancer. *N. Engl. J. Med.*, 304:1493.

27. Herrmann, R., Barcos, M., Stutzman, L., Walsh, D., Freeman, A., Sokal, J., and Henderson, E. S. (1982): The influence of histologic type on the incidence and duration of response in non-Hodgkin's lymphoma. *Cancer*, 49:314–322.

28. Kakati, S., Barcos, M., and Sandberg, A. A. (1979): Chromosomes and causation of human cancer and leukemia. XXXVI. The 14q+ anomaly in an American Burkitt lymphoma and its value in the definition of lymphoproliferative disorders. *Med. Pediatr. Oncol.*, 6:121–129.

29. Kakati, S., Barcos, M., and Sandberg, A. A. (1980): Chromosomes and causation of human cancer and leukemia. XLI. Cytogenetic experience with non-Hodgkin, non-Burkitt lymphomas. *Cancer Genet. Cytogenet.*, 2:199–220.

30. Kaneko, Y., Abe, R., Sampi, K., and Sakurai, M. (1982): An analysis of chromosome findings in non-Hodgkin's lymphomas. *Cancer Genet. Cytogenet.*, 5:107–121.

31. Kirsch, I. R., Morton, C. C., Nakahara, K., and Leder, P. (1982): Human immunoglobulin heavy chain genes map to a region of translocations in malignant B lymphocytes. *Science*, 216:301–303.

32. Klein, G. (1979): Lymphoma development in mice and humans: Diversity of initiation is followed by convergent cytogenetic evolution. *Proc. Natl. Acad. Sci. USA*, 76:2442–2446.

33. Lenoir, G. M., Preud'homme, J. L., Bernheim, A., and Berger, R. (1982): Correlation between immunoglobulin light chain expression and variant translocation in Burkitt's lymphoma. *Nature*, 298:474–476.

34. Levine, E. G., Arthur, D. C., Frizzera, G., Gajl-Peczalska, K. J., Lindquist, L., Peterson, B. A., Hurd, D. D., and Bloomfield, C. D. (1982): Cytogenetic analysis of 55 cases of malignant lymphoma (ML): Correlation with histologic and immunologic phenotype. *AACR Abstr.*, 23:116.

35. Liang, J. C., Gaulden, M. E., and Herndon, J. H. (1980): Chromosome markers and evidence for clone formation in lymphocytes of a patient with Sézary syndrome. *Cancer Res.*, 40:3426–3429.

36. Magrath, I. T., Pizzo, P. A., Whang-Peng, J., Douglass, E. C., Alabaster, O., Gerber, P., and Freeman, C. B. (1980): Characterization of lymphoma-derived cell lines: Comparison of cell lines positive and negative for Epstein-Barr virus nuclear antigen. I. Physical, cytogenetic, and growth characteristics. *JNCI*, 64:465–476.

37. Malcolm, S., Barton, P., Bentley, D. L., Ferguson-Smith, M., Murphy, C., and Rabbitts, T. (1981): Assignment of a V Kappa locus for immunoglobulin light chain to the short arm of chromosome 2 (2 cen to 2 p13). In: *Human Gene Mapping Conference. VI.* National Foundation, White Plains, NY.

38. Manolov, G., and Manolova, Y. (1972): Marker band in one chromosome 14 from Burkitt lymphomas. *Nature*, 237:33–34.

39. Manolova, Y., Manolov, G., Kieler, J., Levan, A., and Klein, G. (1979): Genesis of the 14q + marker in Burkitt's lymphoma. *Hereditas*, 90:5–10.

40. Mark, J., Dahlenfors, R., and Ekedahl, C. (1979): Recurrent chromosomal aberrations in non-Hodgkin and non-Burkitt lymphomas. *Cancer Genet. Cytogenet.*, 1:39–56.

41. Mitelman, F. (1981): Marker chromosome 14q + in human cancer and leukemia. *Adv. Cancer Res.*, 34:141–170.

42. Mitelman, F., Andersson-Anvret, M., Brandt, L., Catovsky, D., Klein, G., Manolov, G., Manolova, Y., Mark-Vendel, E., and Nilsson, P. G. (1979): Reciprocal 8;14 translocation in EBV-negative B-cell acute lymphocytic leukemia with Burkitt-type cells. *Int. J. Cancer*, 24:27–33.

43. Miyamoto, K., Miyano, K., Miyoshi, I., Hamasaki, K., Nishihara, R., Terao, S., Kimura, I., Maeda, K., Matsumura, K., Nishijima, K., and Tanaka, T. (1980): Chromosome 14q + in a Japanese patient with Burkitt's lymphoma. *Acta Med. Okayama*, 34:61–65.

44. Miyamoto, K., Sato, J., Miyoshi, I., Nishihara, R., Terao, S., Hara, M., and Kimura, I. (1980): 8;14 Translocation in a Japanese Burkitt's lymphoma. *Acta Med. Okayama*, 34:139–142.

45. Miyamoto, K., Sato, J., Kitajima, K., Togawa, A., Suemaru, S., Sanada, H., and Tanaka, T. (1983): Adult T-cell leukemia: chromosome analysis of fifteen cases. *Cancer*, 52:471–478.

46. Miyoshi, I., Hamazaki, K., Kubonishi, I., Yoshimoto, S., Kitajima, K., Kimura, I., Miyamoto, K., Sato, J., Yorimitsu, S., Tao, S., Ishibashi, K., and Tokuda, M. (1981): A variant translocation (8;22) in a Japanese patient with Burkitt lymphoma. *Gann*, 72:176–177.

47. Miyoshi, I., Hiraki, S., Kimura, I., Miyamoto, K., and Sato, J. (1978): 2/8 Translocation in a Japanese Burkitt's lymphoma. *Experientia*, 35:742–743.

48. Miyoshi, I., Miyamoto, K., Sumida, M., Nishihara, R., Lai, M., Yoshimoto, S., Sato, J., and Kimura, I. (1981): Chromosome 14q + in adult T-cell leukemia. *Cancer Genet. Cytogenet.*, 3:251–259.

49. Morita, M., Minowada, J., and Sandberg, A. A. (1981): Chromosomes and causation of human cancer and leukemia. XLV. Chromosome patterns in stimulated lymphocytes of chronic lymphocytic leukemia. *Cancer Genet. Cytogenet.*, 3:293–306.

50. Non-Hodgkin's Lymphoma Pathologic Classification Project (1982): National Cancer Institute sponsored study of classifications of non-Hodgkin's lymphomas: Summary and description of a working formulation for clinical usage. *Cancer*, 49:2112–2135.

51. Nowell, P., Daniele, R., Rowlands, D., Jr., and Finan, J. (1980): Cytogenetics of chronic B-cell and T-cell leukemia. *Cancer Genet. Cytogenet.*, 1:273–280.

52. Nowell, P., Finan, J., Glover, D., and Guerry, D. (1981): Cytogenetic evidence for the clonal nature of Richter's syndrome. *Blood*, 58:183–186.

53. Nowell, P. C., Finan, J. B., and Vonderheid, E. C. (1982): Clonal characteristics of T cell lymphomas: Cytogenetic evidence from blood, lymph nodes, and skin. *J. Invest. Dermatol.*, 78:69–75.

54. Philip, T., Lenoir, G.-M., Brunat-Mentigny, M., Bertrand, S., Gentilhomme, O., Souillet, G., and Philippe, N. (1980): Individualisation pathogenique du lymphome de Burkitt en France. *Pediatrie*, 35:659–676.

55. Philip, T., Lenoir, G. M., Fraisse, J., Philip, I., Bertoglio, J., Ladjaj, S., Bertrand, S., and Brunat-Mentigny, M. (1981): EBV-positive Burkitt's lymphoma from Algeria, with a three-way rearrangement involving chromosomes 2, 8 and 9. *Int. J. Cancer*, 28:417–420.

56. Pierre, R. V., Dewald, G. W., and Banks, P. M. (1980): Cytogenetic studies in malignant lymphoma: Possible role in staging studies. *Cancer Genet. Cytogenet.*, 1:257–261.

57. Prieto, F., Badia, L., Herranz, C., Redón, J., Caballero, M., Artiges, E., and Báguena, J. (1978): Cromosoma marcador (14q +) y linfomas. *Rev. Esp. Oncol.*, 25:399–408.
58. Reeves, B. R., and Pickup, V. L. (1980): The chromosome changes in non-Burkitt lymphomas. *Hum. Genet.*, 53:349–355.
59. Robert, K.-H., Gahrton, G., Friberg, K., Zech, L., and Nilsson, B. (1982): Extra chromosome 12 and prognosis in chronic lymphocytic leukaemia. *Scand. J. Haematol.*, 28:163–168.
60. Rowley, J. D. (1982): Chromosomes in Hodgkin's disease. *Cancer Treat. Rep.*, 66:59–63.
61. Rowley, J. D., and Fukuhara, S. (1980): Chromosome studies in non-Hodgkin's lymphomas. *Semin. Oncol.*, 7:255–266.
62. Rowley, J. D., Variakojis, D., Kaneko, Y., and Cimino, M. (1981): A Burkitt-lymphoma variant translocation (2p − ;8q +) in a patient with ALL, L3 (Burkitt type). *Hum. Genet.*, 58:166–167.
63. Sadamori, N., Han, T., Minowada, J., Henderson, E. S., Ozer, H., and Sandberg, A. A. (1981): Clonal chromosome changes in stimulated lymphocytes of CLL. *Blood*, 58(Suppl. 1):151a.
64. Sandberg, A. A. (1980): *The Chromosomes in Human Cancer and Leukemia.* Elsevier/North-Holland, New York.
65. Sandberg, A. A. (1981): Chromosome changes in the lymphomas. *Hum. Pathol.*, 12:531–540.
66. Sandberg, A. A. (1982): Chromosomal changes in human cancer: Specificity and heterogeneity. In: *Tumor Cell Heterogeneity: Origins and Implications*, Vol. 4, edited by A. H. Owens, Jr., P. S. Coffey, and S. B. Baylin, pp. 367–397. Academic Press, New York.
67. Schaadt, M., Diehl, V., Stein, H., Fonatsch, C., and Kirchner, H. H. (1980): Two neoplastic cell lines with unique features derived from Hodgkin's disease. *Int. J. Cancer*, 26:723–731.
68. Schröder, J., Vuopio, P., and Autio, K. (1981): Chromosome changes in human chronic lymphocytic leukemia. *Cancer Genet. Cytogenet.*, 4:11–21.
69. Second International Workshop on Chromosomes in Leukemia (1980). *Cancer Genet. Cytogenet.*, 2:89–113.
70. Slater, R. M., Behrendt, H., and van Heerde, P. (1982): Cytogenetic studies on four cases of non-endemic Burkitt lymphoma. *Med. Pediatr. Oncol.*, 10:71–84.
71. Slavutsky, I., de Vinuesa, M. L., Dupont, J., Mondini, N., and Brieux de Salum, S. (1981): Abnormalities of chromosome No. 1: Two cases with lymphocytic lymphomas. *Cancer Genet. Cytogenet.*, 3:341–346.
72. Spiers, A. S. D., Neiman, R. S., Lord, K. E., Deal, D. R., Spiers, A. S. D., Jr., and Schneider, L. I. (1979): Cytogenetics—An aid to histopathology in malignant lymphomas. *JAMA*, 241:1227–1228.
73. Stewart, S. E., Lovelace, E., Whang, J. J., and Ngu, V. A. (1965): Burkitt tumor: Tissue culture, cytogenetic and virus studies. *JNCI*, 34:319–327.
74. Tanzer, J., Frocrain, C., Alcalay, D., and Desmarest, M. C. (1980): Pleuropericardite a cellules de Burkitt chez un poitevin. Chromosome 14q + par translocation (1;14), association a une translocation (8;22), a la perte de l'y et a de nombreuses autres anomalies. *Nouv. Rev. Fr. Hematol.* (Suppl.) 22:CVII (abs).
75. Third International Workshop on Chromosomes in Leukemia (1981): *Cancer Genet. Cytogenet.*, 4:94–142.
76. Ueshima, Y., Fukuhara, S., Hattori, T., Uchiyama, T., Takatsuki, K., and Uchino, H. (1981): Chromosome studies in adult T-cell leukemia in Japan: Significance of trisomy 7. *Blood*, 58:420–425.
77. Van Den Berghe, H., Parloir, C., Gosseye, S., Englebienne, V., Cornu, G., and Sokal, G. (1979): Variant translocation in Burkitt lymphoma. *Cancer Genet. Cytogenet.*, 1:9–14.
78. Watanabe, S., Shimosato, Y., Shimoyama, M., Minato, K., Suzuki, M., Abe, M., and Nagatani, T. (1980): Adult T cell lymphoma with hypergammaglobulinemia. *Cancer*, 46:2472–2483.
79. Zech, L., Haglund, U., Nilsson, K., and Klein, G. (1976): Characteristic chromosomal abnormalities in biopsies and lymphoid-cell lines from patients with Burkitt and non-Burkitt lymphomas. *Int. J. Cancer*, 17:47–56.
80. Zhang, S., Zech, L., and Klein, G. (1982): High-resolution analysis of chromosome markers in Burkitt lymphoma cell lines. *Int. J. Cancer*, 29:153–157.

*Pathogenesis of Leukemias and Lymphomas:
Environmental Influences*, edited by
I. T. Magrath, G. T. O'Conor, and B. Ramot.
Raven Press, New York © 1984.

Burkitt-Type Lymphoma: EBV Association and Cytogenetic Markers in Cases from Various Geographic Locations

*Gilbert M. Lenoir, **Thierry Philip, and *Roger Sohier

*International Agency for Research on Cancer, 69372 Lyons cedex 08, France; and
**Centre Léon-Bérard, Pediatric Oncology Department, 69374 Lyons cedex 08, France

Following the initial clinical description by D. Burkitt in 1958 of "a lymphoma involving the jaw in African children" (7), the term "Burkitt's lymphoma" (BL) has been extended by a UICC Recommendation (45) to a well-defined pathological entity initially described in East Africa (36,50) and later detailed by a WHO Working Group Memorandum (2). It appeared possible, on the basis of this clear pathological definition, to initiate a broad spectrum of studies not only in the so-called endemic African areas but also in other parts of the world where this lymphoma has been recognized (14,39,51).

Unfortunately, confusion set in rapidly, particularly during the 1970s, because of the peculiar epidemiological and clinical features of the African tumor. Thus, the pathological definition came to be ignored by authors who emphasized one or another characteristic of the tumor, such as its viral association, its clinical presentation, and its epidemiological features. The situation was worsened by the fact that the term BL did not appear in some major histopathological classifications (28) or was included only in imprecise groups, such as "undifferentiated lymphoma" (44).

African BL has been studied extensively and is well characterized from the epidemiological, clinical, and laboratory points of view; whereas only limited and scattered information is available on this lymphoma outside endemic areas. For this reason, an international collaborative project was initiated at the International Agency for Research on Cancer (IARC) to study and compare BL cases from various geographic locations, with special emphasis on the etiological role of the Epstein-Barr virus (EBV) and of cytogenetic abnormalities.

We report and discuss here the results of our ongoing investigations of BL cases originating in central Africa, North Africa, and Europe (mainly France). However, before we present and discuss these data, we review briefly the studies that have been conducted in Africa, from the time this lymphoma was described to the present, that allowed a clear pathological definition of Burkitt-type lymphoma to be made and that point to the etiological importance of EBV.

283

HOW THE AFRICAN BURKITT'S LYMPHOMA
WAS CHARACTERIZED

It may be helpful to distinguish two decades in the history of BL. The story starts at the end of the 1950s, when Burkitt reported a high frequency of lymphosarcomas, predominantly involving the jaw, in young East African children (7). The epidemiological features of this lymphoma, which occurs mainly in tropical areas (Africa and also New Guinea) (46) under certain conditions of altitude and rainfall (with time-space clustering of cases), were such that an infectious agent was suspected of playing a role in its etiology (8). The isolation of EBV from continuous lymphoid lines obtained from cases of BL (16) and, later, evidence of the presence of the viral genome within the tumor cells strongly supported this hypothesis (56). By the end of the 1960s, then, BL was considered to be mainly an African lymphoma [the most common childhood cancer in tropical regions (38)] with a predominant jaw localization, and it was suspected to have a viral etiology.

During the second decade, from the 1970s to the present, a more detailed analysis of African BL confirmed the main characteristics just described but brought to light some corrections and additions. Epidemiological studies [see also review by de-Thé (12)] set the annual incidence of BL at 2.2 to 3.8 per 100,000 of the child population (20), but time-space clustering was questioned (47). Further, a decline in incidence was documented on several occasions (6,35). It was shown that this highly chemosensitive tumor, which affects predominantly boys (male-female ratio 2:1) not only has a jaw localization but also frequently shows an abdominal presentation. This clinical characteristic had been reported in Burkitt's early articles; however, the impressive picture of children with massive jaw swellings that he presented at that time put the other clinical presentations in the shade.

Laboratory investigations showed that BL was the consequence of a monoclonal proliferation (17) of lymphoid cells belonging to the B-cell subset (1). Virological laboratory studies indicated that EBV can transform human B lymphocytes *in vitro* (19) and can induce fatal lymphoproliferative diseases when injected into new world primates (32). Much later, it was demonstrated that this virus can cause polyclonal lymphoproliferative disorders in human immunocompromised individuals that are difficult to classify pathologically (see D. Purtilo et al., *this volume*).

A seroepidemiological prospective survey strengthened the probable causative role of EBV in BL (13,21). It was shown, however, that the EBV/BL association (based on the detection of viral markers within tumor cells), although detected in the great majority of cases, was not consistent: 4% of the cases of African BL were found not to be EBV-associated (23). The virus thus appeared to be only one of the possible causative agents of BL. Furthermore, even for EBV-associated BL, a multifactorial etiology has been proposed; malaria infection is suspected of playing an important role as a cofactor (9,37).

A major breakthrough came when cytogenetic investigations showed that the BL cell is characterized by nonrandom cytogenetic changes—a 14q+ marker (30), later shown to result from a reciprocal translocation between chromosomes 8 and 14, t(8;14) (53) (reviewed in detail by A. A. Sandberg, *this volume*).

The initial description is still considered valid from the pathological and cytological viewpoints. BL is a malignant lymphoma comprising a monomorphic outgrowth of undifferentiated lymphoid cells with little variation in size and shape, an amphophilic cytoplasm with clear vacuoles, and a noncleaved nucleus containing two to five basophilic nucleoli (2,36). At low magnification, a "starry sky" pattern is usually observed, which is caused by macrophage infiltration of this rapidly growing tumor.

A study is being done by the IARC to evaluate if it is possible to define the overall characteristics of lymphomas that have similar histopathologic features and that arise outside endemic African regions and to define more precisely their virological and cytogenetic features. The results of this study are summarized below.

BURKITT'S LYMPHOMA OUTSIDE ENDEMIC AFRICAN AREAS

Literature Survey

First of all, in 1980, a literature survey was done to find out if the disease had been identified worldwide. Although perhaps incomplete, this survey provided interesting data (Table 1 and Fig. 1). The very heterogeneous data show that this cancer has been reported on all continents. It is mainly a childhood disease—most cases arise in patients under the age of 15. However, the data from the American BL registry (27) indicate that adult cases are not exceptional in that series; 24.5% of the cases occur in people more than 20 years old. A male predominance was observed in most series (male-female ratio about 2:1) except in North Africa, although the number of patients there was very limited. Abdominal masses were reported as a very frequent clinical presentation, and it may be that the high proportion of jaw tumors reported from Asia are simply the consequence of preferential reporting of cases with maxillary involvement.

One must be very cautious in analyzing data obtained from this literature survey, because, with the exception of the nationwide American BL registry, in which the pathology of all cases was carefully reviewed, the data come from scattered reports. These data do not allow estimation of either the incidence of BL outside the endemic African region or the relative proportion of BL among malignant non-Hodgkin's lymphomas within a given area. Furthermore, most reports were clinically oriented, and very few of them included virologic or cytogenetic data. The impossibility of drawing valid conclusions from this extensive literature survey led the IARC to conduct a collaborative study.

Preliminary Results of the IARC Study

Most of the cases included in the study originated in France or Algeria—in France, through a large collaborative study with the major cancer treatment centers, and in Algeria with C.H.U. Mustapha, Alger (Professor Aboulola). This approach

TABLE 1. Summary of 1980 literature survey of cases of Burkitt's lymphoma[a]

Geographical area	Number of published cases	Age									Sex					Site of primary localization						
		<8		9–15		16–19		>20		Total[b]	Males		Females		Total	Jaw		Abdomen		Other		Total[b]
		No.	%	No.	%	No.	%	No.	%		No.	%	No.	%		No.	%	No.	%	No.	%	
North America	269	116	43.1	59	21.9	28	10.4	66	24.5	269	179	66.5	90	33.5	269	13	4.8	104	38.7	152	56.5	269
Central America	1			1	100.0					1			1		1					1		1
South America	47	33	80.5	5	12.2	1	2.4	2	4.9	41	29	61.7	18	38.3	47	16	48.5	16	48.5	1	3.0	33
Asia	45	27	60.0	14	31.1	1	2.2	3	6.7	45	32	71.1	13	28.9	45	23	51.1	17	37.8	5	11.1	45
Australia	2			2						2	1		1		2	1		1				2
Europe	181	82	49.1	57	34.1	17	10.2	11	6.6	167	133	73.5	48	26.5	181	24	14.6	97	59.1	43	26.2	164
Middle East	86	70	81.4	10	11.6	4	4.7	2	2.3	86	52	60.5	34	39.5	86	7	10.1	56	81.2	6	8.7	69
North Africa	9	8	88.9	1	11.1					9	4	44.4	5	55.6	9	2	22.2	7	77.8			9

[a]References available on request to R. Sohier, IARC.
[b]Number of cases for which information was available (when less than the number of published cases, insufficient information was available on each parameter).

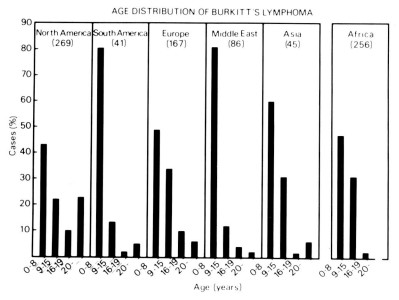

AGE DISTRIBUTION OF BURKITT'S LYMPHOMA

FIG. 1. Age distribution of Burkitt's lymphoma cases collected in 1980 literature survey. For comparison, data from Africa are included from Olweny's study (40) on Ugandan cases.

made it possible to collect formalin-fixed pathological specimens for the evaluation of the relative frequency of BL among malignant non-Hodgkin's lymphomas and to collect specimens for virological, cytogenetic, immunological, and tissue culture studies.

Relative Frequency of BL Among Non-Hodgkin's Lymphomas

Through a retrospective pathological analysis of 87 cases of childhood lymphoma (42), we were able to show that Burkitt-type lymphomas are far from being a rare disease and represent at least one-third of malignant childhood non-Hodgkin's lymphoma in France. This conclusion agrees well with those of previous reports, especially those of Cossman and Berard (10) for the United States. Therefore, BL cannot be considered a rare disease in Europe; cases do not occur in a sporadic manner. We suggest that the so-called "endemic" areas (Central Africa, New Guinea) be designated "high-incidence" areas, whereas the other areas be considered to have a "low incidence."

What does a "low incidence" of BL mean in France, for example? One can extrapolate from the relative frequency: if BL represent 30% of malignant childhood non-Hodgkin's lymphoma, then they comprise about 3% of childhood cancers, i.e., an incidence of about 0.2 per 100,000 per year. This figure is about 20- to 40-fold lower than that reported from the West Nile district of Uganda (12). The clinical data available in our retrospective analysis of French cases (42) indicate a male-female ratio of 3.7:1; however, the age distribution was very similar to that reported for African cases (peak incidence between the ages of six and nine). Most of the cases (68%) presented with abdominal masses, whereas jaw localization was rare (4%). As reported from all other areas (54), the tumor shows a very marked sensitivity to chemotherapy: the cure rate of localized disease is now 80%, and that for widespread disease 65% (41).

A similar study is under way in North Africa, but no definitive data are yet available, for instance to evaluate the relative frequency of BL in these countries. However, as in Europe and the United States, the disease has a predominantly abdominal presentation.

Association with Epstein-Barr Virus

The presence of EBV viral markers (EBV-DNA or EB nuclear antigen) within the malignant cells proves the association of EBV with a BL case. Another indication of the association is elevated anti-EBV antibody titers in patients' sera as compared with those of controls. These include anti-viral capsid antigen (VCA) titers and the presence of antibodies against the R subtype of the early antigens (EA). In high-incidence areas, the percentage of BL tumors associated with EBV has been well established (22): an analysis of more than 100 tumors by molecular hybridization showed that 96% contained copies of the EBV genome, whereas the remaining 4% were free of viral markers, even though in most cases serological studies showed a past EBV infection.

Outside the high-incidence areas, only limited information is available. Several isolated cases of EBV-associated tumors have been reported; however, no precise estimate is available for a given country or population. In the best documented series of cases, studied in the United States (55), only about 10% contained the EBV genome. This suggests that, outside the high-incidence areas, the frequency of EBV-associated cases may be very low.

Our study included 42 North African cases. All but one had elevated EBV serology (anti-VCA≥320), with detectable anti-EA antibodies, usually of the R subtype. EB viral markers were detected in all 15 cases for which tumor material was available. This unexpected finding suggests that in Algeria, an African country where BL is not considered to occur with high frequency, the EBV/BL association may be as common as it is in the so-called "endemic" Central African region. In a given population, then, the level of the EBV/BL association may be related not to the incidence of the tumor but to socioeconomic level and, consequently, to age at primary infection.

The results of our investigations with regard to the French Caucasian BL cases indicate that, as reported in the United States, only a minority are EBV-associated. The pathological review of our cases is still in progress, but only nine EBV-associated cases were proved in a series of about 80 cases. EBV-associated cases therefore may represent only about 10% of all BL cases in France.

Cytogenetic Investigations

When our project was initiated, a characteristic nonrandom cytogenetic anomaly, the t(8;14) translocation, was recognized to be a frequent marker for BL cells (3,31). It was later suggested that other variant translocations may be found in BL cases outside Africa. These are of two types, t(2;8) and t(8;22) (4,34,49).

By a careful analysis of BL material originating from central Africa, Bernheim et al. (5) showed clearly that these variant translocations are also found in EBV-associated cases from high-incidence areas. Our ongoing chromosome analysis of 50 BL cases (mainly through a collaboration with R. Berger, Hôpital Saint-Louis, Paris) indicates that (a) the nonrandom cytogenetic anomalies so far observed in BL are of only three types, t(8;14), t(2;8), or t(8;22); (b) they are not associated with EBV, are independent of clinical presentation, and are found in Burkitt-type lymphomas as well as in Burkitt-type leukemias; and (c) they are not specific to certain populations—we have observed the three types of translocation in cases from France, North Africa, Central Africa, and Japan. Miyoshi also observed all three types in Japanese cases (33).

Are these translocations specific and constant markers of BL? Anomalies of chromosome 14, such as 14q+ markers, have been reported frequently in other malignant diseases, mainly lymphoproliferative disorders; however, specific t(8;14), t(8;22), and t(2;8) are found almost exclusively in BL tumors. No Burkitt tumor in our series was without one of these translocations. They can thus be considered reliable, constant markers of BL, even though some BL without chromosomal changes have been reported as exceptions in the literature (15,48). In our study of 50 cases, 36 presented with a t(8;14), four with a t(2;8), and 10 with a t(8;22), representing 72%, 8%, and 20%, respectively.

In Vitro Cell Culture

The pioneer work of Pulvertaft (43) and of Epstein et al. (16) in the early 1960s showed that malignant BL cells can be cultured *in vitro* and propagated as continuous lymphoid cell lines. The rate of establishment of permanent cultures was reported to be very high when using African biopsy material, and the preparations required only a standard tissue culture medium such as RPMI 1640 supplemented with fetal calf serum. African BL can thus be considered an exceptional tumor, because an unlimited amount of malignant material can be obtained relatively easily by *in vitro* culture. We decided to establish whether this was also true for cases originating from low-incidence areas, especially cases where malignant cells did not harbor the EBV genome, which is considered to be a very good *"in vitro* mitogenic factor."

In the course of our study, 50 new BL lines were established spontaneously, about half (24) from EBV-genome-negative tumors. This confirmed the great similarity among BL cases and showed that the ability to grow *in vitro* is a characteristic associated with Burkitt cells and not with the presence of viral DNA. It is clear, however, that the presence of the EBV genome within malignant lymphoid cells confers on them an important growth advantage. For example, only a few weeks are required to establish EBV-genome-positive Burkitt's lines, whereas months (two to four) are needed to establish EBV-genome-negative Burkitt's lines. Furthermore, the growing capacity of the latter depends greatly on the quality and concentration of the fetal calf serum used. Nevertheless, the relative ease with which these cells can be cultured provides a unique opportunity for conducting cytogenetic, immunological, and biochemical investigations.

Immunological Markers

As reported by others, we found that all our BL cases involved proliferation of lymphocytes of the B-cell subset, all of which synthesized heavy chain immunoglobulins predominantly of the μ subtype: In our series, only two tumors were

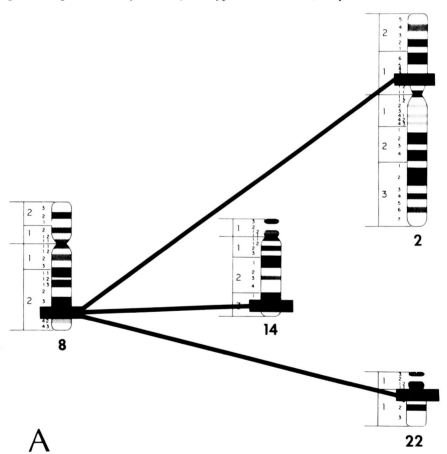

A

FIG. 2. A, Schematic representation of the chromosomal breaks observed in three types of Burkitt translocations: t(8;14), t(2;8) and t(8;22). **B,** Hatched areas represent regional localization of immunoglobulins. H = heavy-chain genes, K = kappa light chain genes, and λ = lambda light chain genes.

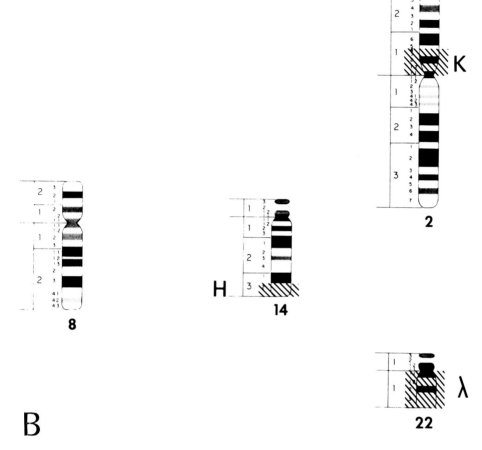

gamma producers and only one was alpha. As reported by Magrath et al. (29) in a study of North American BL cases, EBV-genome-positive and -negative BL may differ slightly with regard to markers of immunological differentiation. An in-depth comparative study of our cell lines is in progress to resolve this question.

CONCLUSION AND PROSPECTS

This ongoing project and many previous studies clearly indicate that BL can be considered as a prototype of lymphoid malignancy, the etiological basis of which can be evaluated by pathological, clinical, epidemiological, and laboratory investigations. It is thought currently that chromosomal translocations may represent crucial events in the genesis of a malignant cell clone. In this B-cell malignancy, the nonrandom cytogenetic anomalies that are detected always involve chromosome 8 (a segment designated q24) and one of the three chromosomes bearing immunoglobulin genes: 14 (heavy-chain clusters), 2 (light-chain kappa), or 22 (light-chain lambda). As shown in Fig. 2, the breakpoints on chromosomes 2 and 22 correspond precisely to the location of the immunoglobulin genes (24,25), and it was shown recently that there is a functional correlation between the type of variant translocation and the type of light chain expressed in BL (26). This suggests that the malignant state in BL might result from the transposition of a DNA segment from chromosome 8 to an active chromosome segment within the immunoglobulin loci. Recent data, as yet unpublished, support this hypothesis not only in human BL but also in an animal model, namely, mouse plasmacytoma. The availability of numerous Burkitt lines offers a unique source of material for dissecting this molecular puzzle.

Even though chromosomal rearrangement may prove to be the final and crucial step in the malignant process, the role of EBV cannot be ignored. Epidemiological studies have indicated that it may be a causative agent, acting most probably as an initiating factor. But how does it initiate? What aspect of the viral infection is the risk factor? Is it the very early infection stage, as proposed by de-Thé (11)? In North Africa, where most BL cases are EBV-associated, is the viral infection a risk factor, as in central Africa? Many questions remain to be elucidated through careful epidemiological surveys. It must not be forgotten that outside the so-called endemic areas, 80 to 90% of BL cases are not EBV-associated. What is the initiator in these cases? Is it a virus or other factors that activate B-lymphocyte proliferation? This question remains totally open.

The studies that have been done on BL in a limited number of countries must be extended on a worldwide basis. For a better understanding of lymphoid malignancy, other non-Hodgkin's lymphomas should be studied using a similar approach: on the basis of the precise cytological, immunological, and clinical definition of a lymphoid neoplasia, the epidemiological characteristics of the disease should be investigated in order to define etiological factors. Findings in oncovirology and cytogenetics that have arisen from the BL study have also led to fruitful discoveries in respect to other lymphoid malignancies, as shown by the recent discovery of retroviruses in T leukemias (18) and by the recent indication that most malignant lymphoid cell types have their particular chromosomal rearrangement (52).

ACKNOWLEDGMENTS

We are grateful to Ms. Chantal Fuchez and Elizabeth Heseltine for their expert assistance in the preparation of this manuscript.

REFERENCES

1. Béchet, J. M., Fialkow, P., Nilsson, K., and Klein, G. (1974): Immunoglobulin synthesis and glucose-6-phosphate dehydrogenase as cell markers in human lymphoblastoid cell lines. *Exp. Cell Res.*, 89:275–282.
2. Berard, C., O'Conor, G. T., Thomas, L. B., and Torloni, H. (1969): Histopathological definition of Burkitt's tumour. *Bull. WHO*, 40:601–607.
3. Berger, R., Bernheim, A., Brouet, J. C., Daniel, M. T., and Flandrin, G. (1979): t(8;14) Translocation in a Burkitt's type of lymphoblastic leukaemia (L3). *Br. J. Haematol.*, 43:87–90.

4. Berger, R., Bernheim, A., Weh, H. J., Flandrin, G., Daniel, M. T., Brouet, J. C., and Colbert, N. (1979): A new translocation in Burkitt tumor cells. *Hum. Genet.*, 53:111–112.
5. Bernheim, A., Berger, R., and Lenoir, G. (1981): Cytogenetic studies on African Burkitt's lymphoma cell lines: t(8;14), t(2;8) and t(8;22) translocations. *Cancer Genet. Cytogenet.*, 3:307–315.
6. Biggar, R. J., Nkruma, F. K., Neequaye, J., and Levine, P. H. (1981): Changes in presenting tumour site of Burkitt's lymphoma in Ghana, West Africa, 1965–1978. *Br. J. Cancer*, 43:632–636.
7. Burkitt, D. (1958): A sarcoma involving the jaws in African children. *Br. J. Surg.*, 46:218–223.
8. Burkitt, D. (1962): A children's cancer dependent on climatic factors. *Nature*, 194:232–234.
9. Burkitt, D. (1969): Etiology of Burkitt's lymphoma, an alternative to a vectored virus. *JNCI*, 42:19–28.
10. Cossman, J., and Berard, C. W. (1980): Histopathology of childhood non-Hodgkin's lymphomas. In: *Non-Hodgkin's Lymphomas in Children*, edited by J. Graham pole, p. 13. Masson, New York.
11. de-Thé, G. (1977): Is Burkitt's lymphoma related to perinatal infection by Epstein-Barr virus? *Lancet*, 1:335–338.
12. de-Thé, G. (1979): The epidemiology of Burkitt's lymphoma: Evidence for a causal association with Epstein-Barr virus. *Am. J. Epidemiol.*, 1:32–54.
13. de-Thé, G., Geser, A., Day, N. E., Tukei, P. M., Williams, E. H., Beri, D. P., Smith, P. G., Dean, A. G., Bornkamm, G. W., Feorino, P., and Henle, W. (1978): Epidemiological evidence for causal relationship between Epstein-Barr virus and Burkitt's lymphoma from Ugandan prospective study. *Nature*, 274:756–761.
14. Dorfman, R. F. (1965): Childhood lymphosarcoma in St. Louis, Missouri, clinically and histologically resembling Burkitt's tumor. *Cancer*, 18:418–430.
15. Douglass, E. C., Magrath, I. T., and Terebelo, H. (1982): Burkitt cell leukemia without abnormalities of chromosomes no. 8 and 14. *Cancer Genet. Cytogenet.*, 5:181–185.
16. Epstein, M. A., Achong, B. G., and Barr, Y. N. (1964): Virus particles in cultured lymphoblasts from Burkitt's lymphoma. *Lancet*, 1:702–703.
17. Fialkow, P. J., Klein, G., Gartler, S. N., and Clifford, P. (1970): Clonal origin for individual Burkitt tumours. *Lancet*, 1:384–386.
18. Gallo, R. C., and Wong-Staal, F. (1982): Retroviruses as etiologic agents of some animal and human leukemias and lymphomas and as tools for elucidating the molecular mechanism of leukemogenesis. *Blood*, 60:545–557.
19. Gerber, P., Whang-Peng, J., and Monroe, J. H. (1970): Lymphoproliferative effect of Epstein-Barr virus on normal human lymphocytes in culture. *Bibl. Haematologica*, 36:739–750.
20. Geser, A., Brubaker, G., and Olwit, G. W. (1980): The frequency of Epstein-Barr virus infection and Burkitt's lymphoma at high and low altitudes in East Africa. *Rev. Epidemiol. Santé Publique*, 28:307–321.
21. Geser, A., de-Thé, G., Lenoir, G., Day, N. E., and Williams, E. H. (1982): Final case reporting from the Ugandan prospective study of the relationship between EBV and Burkitt's lymphoma. *Int. J. Cancer*, 29:397–400.
22. Geser, A., Lenoir, G. M., Anvret, M., Bornkamm, G. W., Klein, G. Williams, E. H., Wright, D. H., and de-Thé, G. (1983): Epstein-Barr virus markers in a series of Burkitt's lymphomas from the West Nile District, Uganda. *Eur. J. Cancer (in press)*.
23. Klein, G. (1974): Studies on the Epstein-Barr virus genome and the EBV-determined nuclear antigen in human malignant disease in tumor viruses. *Cold Spring Harbor Symp. Quant. Biol.*, 39:783–796.
24. Klein, G. (1981): The role of gene dosage and genetic transpositions in carcinogenesis. *Nature*, 294:313–318.
25. Klein, G., and Lenoir, G. (1982): Translocations involving Ig-locus-carrying chromosomes: a model for genetic transposition in carcinogenesis. *Adv. Cancer Res.*, 37:381–387.
26. Lenoir, G. M., Preud'homme, J. L., Bernheim, A., and Berger, R. (1982): Correlation between immunoglobulin light chain expression and variant translocation in Burkitt's lymphoma. *Nature*, 298:474–476.
27. Levine, P. H., Kamaraju, L. S., Connelly, R. R., Berard, C. W., Dorfman, R. F., Magrath, I., and Easton, J. M. (1982): The American Burkitt's Lymphoma registry: Eight years' experience. *Cancer*, 49:1016–1022.

28. Lukes, R. J., and Collins, R. D. (1974): Immunologic characterization of human malignant lymphomas. *Cancer*, 34:1488–1503.
29. Magrath, I. T., Freeman, C. B., Pizzo, P., Gadek, J., Jaffe, E., Santaella, M., Hammer, C., Frank, M., Reaman, G., and Novikovs, L. (1980): Characterization of lymphoma-derived cell lines: Comparison of cell lines positive and negative for Epstein-Barr virus nuclear antigen. II. Surface markers. *JNCI*, 64:477–483.
30. Manolov, G., and Manolova, Y. (1972): Marker band in one chromosome 14 in Burkitt's lymphoma. *Nature*, 237:33–34.
31. McCaw, B. K., Epstein, A. L., Kaplan, H. S., and Hecht, F. (1977): Chromosome 14 translocation in African and North American Burkitt's lymphoma. *Int. J. Cancer*, 19:482–486.
32. Miller, G. (1974): The oncogenicity of Epstein-Barr virus. *J. Infect. Dis.*, 130:187–205.
33. Miyoshi, I., Hamasaki, K., Miyamoto, M., Nagase, K., Narahara, K., Kitajima, K., Kimura, I., and Sato, J. (1981): Chromosome translocations in Burkitt's lymphoma. *N. Engl. J. Med.*, 304:734.
34. Miyoshi, I., Hiraki, S., Kimura, I., Miyamoto, K., and Sato, J. (1979): 2/8 Translocation in a Japanese Burkitt's lymphoma. *Experientia*, 35:742–743.
35. Morrow, R. H., Kisuule, A., Pike, M., and Smith, P. G. (1976): Burkitt's lymphoma in the Mengo districts of Uganda: Epidemiological features and their relationship to malaria. *JNCI*, 56:479–482.
36. O'Conor, G. T. (1961): Malignant lymphoma in African children. II. A pathological entity. *Cancer*, 14:270–283.
37. O'Conor, G. T. (1970): Persistent immunologic stimulation as a factor in oncogenesis, with special reference to Burkitt's tumor. *Am. J. Med.*, 48:279–285.
38. O'Conor, G. T., and Davies, J. N. P. (1960): Malignant tumors in African children with special reference to malignant lymphoma. *J. Pediatr.*, 56:526–535.
39. O'Conor, G. T., Rappaport, H., and Smith, E. B. (1965): Childhood lymphoma resembling "Burkitt tumor" in the United States. *Cancer*, 18:411–417.
40. Olweny, C., Katungole-Mbidde, E., Otir, D., Lwanga, S., Magrath, I. T., and Ziegler, J. L. (1980): Long term experience with Burkitt lymphoma in Uganda. *Int. J. Cancer*, 26:261–267.
41. Patte, C., Benz-Lemoine, E., Philip, T., Demeocq, F., Bernard, A., Rodary, C., Caillou, B., and Lemerle, J. (1982): Aggressive treatment of B-cell non Hodgkin lymphoma (NHL)—A protocol of the French Pediatric Oncology Society—Preliminary results on 60 patients. *Eur. J. Cancer*, 18:1052.
42. Philip, T., Lenoir, G. M., Bryon, P. A., Gerard-Marchant, R., Souillet, G., Philippe, N., Freycon, F., and Brunat-Mentigny, M. (1982): Burkitt-type lymphoma in France among non-Hodgkin malignant lymphomas in Caucasian children. *Br. J. Cancer*, 45:670–678.
43. Pulvertaft, R. J. V. (1965): A study of malignant tumours in Nigeria by short-term tissue culture. *J. Clin. Pathol.*, 18:261–273.
44. Rappaport, H. (1966): Malignant Lymphomas in Tumors of the Hematopoietic System, pp. 101–130. The Armed Forces Institute of Pathology, Washington, D.C.
45. F. C. Roulet, editor (1963): *The Lymphoreticular Tumours in Africa. A Symposium Organized by the International Union Against Cancer.* S. Karger, Paris.
46. Seldam, T., Cooke, R., and Atkinson, L. (1966): Childhood lymphoma in the territories of Papua and New Guinea. *Cancer*, 19:437–446.
47. Siemiatycki, J., Brubaker, G., and Geser, A. (1980): Space-time clustering of Burkitt's lymphoma in East Africa: analysis of recent data and a new look at old data. *Int. J. Cancer*, 25:197–203.
48. Slater, R. M., Behrendt, H., and van Heerde, P. (1982): Cytogenetic studies on four cases of non-endemic Burkitt lymphoma. *Med. Pediatr. Oncol.*, 10:71–84.
49. Van Den Berghe, H., Parloir, C., Gosseye, S., Englebienne, V., Cornu, G., and Sokal, G. (1979): Variant translocation in Burkitt lymphoma. *Cancer Genet. Cytogenet.*, 1:9–14.
50. Wright, D. H. (1963): Cytology and histochemistry of the Burkitt lymphoma. *Br. J. Cancer*, 17:50–55.
51. Wright, D. H. (1966): Burkitt's tumour in England. A comparison with childhood lymphosarcoma. *Int. J. Cancer*, 1:503–514.
52. Yunis, J. J., Oken, M. M., Kaplan, M. E., Ensrud, K. M., Howe, R. R., and Theologides, A. (1982): Distinctive chromosomal abnormalities in histologic subtypes of non-Hodgkin's lymphoma. *N. Engl. J. Med.*, 107:1231–1236.
53. Zech, L., Haglund, V., Nilsson, K., and Klein, G. (1976): Characteristic chromosomal abnor-

malities in biopsies and lymphoid cell lines from patients with Burkitt and non-Burkitt lymphomas. *Int. J. Cancer*, 17:47–56.

54. Ziegler, J. L. (1981): Burkitt's lymphoma. *N. Engl. J. Med.*, 305:735–743.
55. Ziegler, J. L., Andersson, M., Klein, G., and Henle, W. (1976): Detection of Epstein-Barr virus DNA in American Burkitt's lymphoma. *Int. J. Cancer*, 17:701–706.
56. Zur Hausen, H., Schultz-Holthausen, H., Klein, G., Henle, W., Henle, G., Clifford, P., and Santesson, L. (1970): EBV DNA in biopsies of Burkitt's tumors and anaplastic carcinomas of the nasopharynx. *Nature*, 228:1056–1058.

Pathogenesis of Leukemias and Lymphomas:
Environmental Influences, edited by
I.T. Magrath, G.T. O'Conor, and B. Ramot.
Raven Press, New York © 1984.

Epidemiology and Pathogenesis of Leukemias and Lymphomas: Summary and Comments

David Purtilo

Department of Pathology and Laboratory Medicine, Pediatrics and Eppley Institute for Research in Cancer and Allied Diseases, University of Nebraska Medical Center, Omaha, Nebraska 68105

This section of this volume concerns etiological and pathogenetic factors in lymphomagenesis and leukemogenesis. Among topics discussed are the impact of ionizing radiation, drugs, immune deficiency, and Epstein-Barr virus (EBV) infections in lymphomas and leukemias, and the significance of cytogenetic aberrations in these disorders. R. W. Miller (Chapter 24) emphasizes the importance of case reports, which provide the initial clues to etiology and pathogenesis of leukemia and lymphoma. Among the examples he cites are leukemia in patients with chromosomal instability, including patients with ataxia telangiectasia, Bloom's syndrome, Fanconi anemia, and neurofibromatosis. Moreover, the incidence of leukemia in patients with trisomy 21 (Down's syndrome) is approximately three times that in the normal age-matched population. Malignant lymphomas occur at higher frequency in individuals with cellular immune deficiencies. Miller recounts that 15 years ago he proposed, based on these observations, that chromosomal breakage predisposed to acute myelogenous leukemias, whereas defects in cellular immunity predisposed to malignant lymphomas.

Miller also stresses the marked differences in the frequency of various lymphoproliferative malignancies in Japan and the United States. For example, he notes that chronic lymphocytic leukemia accounts for 2% of all cases of adult leukemia in Japan, compared to 30% in the United States. Non-Hodgkin's follicular lymphomas comprise 6% of lymphomas in Japan and 35% in the United States. In Japan, Hodgkin's disease is found predominantly in elderly persons. When graphed, this appears as a late peak (Mt. Fuji), whereas in North America, the profile is bimodal (Grand Tetons). Miller notes the markedly increased frequency of autoimmune disturbances in Japan and points out the apparent reciprocal relationship between incidence of autoimmunity and malignant lymphomas. He concludes that genetic host factors are extremely important in determining the type and frequency of leukemias and lymphomas in various countries.

S. C. Finch (Chapter 25) discusses the impact of ionizing radiation and drugs in the pathogenesis of lymphoid neoplasias. Important considerations in evaluating the likelihood of neoplasia arising after exposure to radiation include dose, timing of exposure, and host resistance. Important host factors include age at exposure, sex, genotype, and various organ susceptibility. Predictable periods occur chronologically after exposure to radiation, i.e., prodromal→latent→bone marrow depression and recovery periods. Finch reports the continuing confusion regarding the role of low-dose radiation (i.e., less than 100 rads), remains unclarified at this time.

The age of the individual when exposed to radiation is important in determining the type of leukemia the individual may develop. For example, individuals exposed before they are 20 years old tend to develop acute lymphocytic leukemia, whereas those exposed after 20 years of age often develop acute granulocytic leukemia. Comparison of the results of studies done on victims of the atomic bomb explosions in Hiroshima and Nagasaki has shed light on the impact of radiation type in carcinogenesis. Individuals from Hiroshima have continued through the 1970s to be at increased risk of developing leukemia, whereas the risk has disappeared in survivors living in Nagasaki.

Results of studies of patients treated for ankylosing spondylitis with irradiation corroborate the observations of increased incidence of leukemia and malignancies in victims of atomic bomb explosions. These patients, as well as individuals exposed to thorotrast injections, are at increased risk of developing leukemia.

Finch notes that the risk of leukemia has diminished with time following exposure at Hiroshima and Nagasaki. But other cancers have appeared during the past decade. There has been a slight increase in frequency of malignant lymphomas in individuals exposed to more than 100 rads. Also, myeloma has increased 2.5-fold among individuals who were 20 to 59 years old when exposed to the atomic bomb.

Regarding drug-induced leukemia and lymphoma, Finch emphasizes that alkylating agents such as chlorambucil predispose to acute myelogenous leukemia. When alkylating agents are coupled with radiation, individuals with Hodgkin's disease also have an increased risk of developing acute myelogenous leukemia. Seven of 25 cardiac allograft recipients who received Cyclosporin A have developed immunoblastic sarcoma of B cells (H. Kaplan, *personal communication*).

A. H. Filipovich et al. (Chapter 26) and D. Purtilo et al. (Chapter 27) discuss the role of immune deficiency in lymphomagenesis. Filipovich reports that the Immune Deficiency Cancer Registry at the University of Minnesota has registered 385 patients with primary immune deficiency and cancer, and 1,275 renal and other transplant patients have developed malignancies. She compares the frequency of malignant lymphoma in these two populations. In primary immune deficiency patients, 51% of patients with cancer have malignant lymphoma, whereas in transplant recipients 20% were lymphomas.

The specific types of cancers occurring in the immune-deficient patients provide possible clues to etiological factors in their development: Hodgkin's disease was markedly underrepresented (7% of all malignant lymphomas) in individuals with primary immune deficiencies. Renal transplant recipients do not frequently develop Hodgkin's disease, but often B-cell lymphomas are found. Similarly, carcinomas are markedly underrepresented.

Wiskott-Aldrich syndrome (WAS) is discussed in detail. Among 62 WAS patients with cancer, 44 (71%) have developed non-Hodgkin's lymphoma. This is 100-fold above age-matched controls. These patients averaged 7.9 years of age when cancer was diagnosed.

Filipovich notes a transitional or gray zone between classical malignant lymphoma and a quasimalignant lymphoma in renal transplant recipients. Five of seven malignant lymphomas studied at the University of Minnesota showed polyclonal surface marker characteristics. These collaborative studies were performed with G. Klein and D. Purtilo. All seven of these cases contained EBV genome in transplant patients.

Purtilo discusses immunoregulatory defects and EBV-associated lymphoid disorders, including fatal and chronic infectious mononucleosis, agammaglobulinemia, aplastic anemia, and malignant B-cell lymphoma. The X-linked lymphoproliferative syndrome (XLP) has served as a model for testing the hypothesis that the variable phenotypic expression following EBV infection is related to individual differences in function of subsets of T and B cells. Indeed, patients with XLP show a variety of T-cell defects. After EBV infection, the patients often show increased numbers of suppressor T cells. However, lymphocyte functional assays must be done. This allows for interpretation of the significance of abnormal numbers of subsets of T cells. The patients with XLP show defective helper function in pokeweed-mitogen-stimulated assays; i.e., immunoglobulin (Ig) secretion *in vitro* is decreased. The patients show defects in response to ϕX174: they fail to switch from IgM to IgG antibody response to secondary challenge. The patients show progressive immune attrition. Before EBV infection, natural killer (NK) cell activity is normal. After infection by the virus, NK defects are found. EBV-specific antibody responses are defective, especially against anti-EB nuclear-associated antigen. The patients show T-cell-specific defects in the autologous B-cell outgrowth assay.

Patients with acquired immune deficiencies, such as renal transplant recipients, are at increased risk of lymphomagenesis. Young patients who are immune-suppressed before EBV infections tend to show low-titer antibody responses to virus and have a short incubation before emergence of lymphoproliferative disorders. They often show a fatal infectious mononucleosis phenotype, whereas elderly patients reactivate virus and show high-antibody titers, long incubation periods, and a tendency toward malignant lymphomas. These malignant lymphomas are chiefly polyclonal, and all that have been examined thus far have contained EBV genome. One patient appeared to convert from polyclonal to monoclonal B-cell proliferation.

The results of these studies indicate that an individual's immune response to EBV may govern the clinical and pathological expression of the disease. Methods for detecting EBV in immune-deficient individuals have been developed that may allow attempts to prevent these life-threatening lymphoproliferative disorders by providing immunotherapy or antiviral therapy.

Armstrong and associates have described potential roles for EBV in chronic lymphocytic leukemia in Chapter 28. They have noted elevated anti-VCA IgG titers. Three of the cases they investigated had IgA titers. EA antibodies were often reactivated. In contrast, anti-EBNA, perhaps reflecting a T-cell defect, was absent. They also used newly developed monoclonal antibody (2F5 6) and had identified EBNA positive cells in several cases. In addition, they were able to get spontaneous outgrowth from peripheral blood in two patients. Further studies are indicated to define whether EBV infects the leukemic B-cell or whether the immune deficiency accompanying CLL leads to reactivation of the virus.

A. A. Sandberg (Chapter 29), discusses cytogenetic abnormalities in lymphoid neoplasia. An apparent bias against performing cytogenetic studies prevails in many current investigations of leukemia and lymphoma despite significant advances in techniques of banding and interpretation. Moreover, Sandberg indicates that specific cytogenetic aberrations are useful for prognosis. For example, individuals with chronic myelogenous leukemia and the Philadelphia chromosome have an average survival of 12 months. Persons with acute leukemia with t(4;11) survive eight to ten months, and individuals with t(8;14) and Burkitt lymphoma five months. More effective therapy may alter these associations.

Sandberg stresses the importance of the deleted portion of the chromosome as a determinant in carcinogenesis. For example, the deleted portion of chromosome 22 is important in chronic myelogenous leukemia. Similarly, deletion of a portion of the long arm of chromosome 8, i.e., 8q −, is found in individuals with Burkitt lymphomas.

Sandberg concludes that specific cytogenetic aberrations in lymphomas and leukemias were caused by a primary change that might be related to a specific etiological agent or, alternatively, the changes might be epiphenomena. Nevertheless, he stresses that the cytogenetic aberrations of the cell may be determinants in the biology of the cancer.

G. Lenoir et al. (Chapter 30) describe EBV association and karyotypic abnormalities in Burkitt's lymphoma (BL) in tropical, subtropical, and temperate climates. The frequency of BL in Lyon, France is 10% of that in tropical Africa. They note that patients from Algeria show marked association with EBV: 39 of 40 cases of BL have shown elevated viral capsid antibody titers, and all 12 biopsies examined for EBV genome have contained the virus. In contrast, nine of 80 cases of French Caucasian patients from Lyon have contained EBV genome. Age and socioeconomic factors are apparently important in Burkitt's lymphomagenesis.

Lenoir et al. discuss cytogenetic aberrations in BL, including three related translocations: t(8;14), t(2;8), and t(8;22). The breakpoint in chromosome 8 (i.e., q24) appears to be the same. Breakpoints in chromosomes 14 (i.e., q32), 2 (i.e., q13), and 22 (i.e., q11) are at sites where loci code for Ig. For example, the breakpoint on chromosome 14 is the locus for the heavy chain of Ig; the breakpoint on chromosome 2 is the site of kappa light chain genes; and the breakpoint on chromosome 22 is where the gene of the lambda chain resides.

Evaluation of the type of light chain expressed in Burkitt's lymphoma thus far has revealed gene products consistent with a specific breakpoint on these chromosomes. Finally, Lenoir et al. report on the correlation between karyotype and the Ig secreted by cells with the variant translocations; the BL with a t(2;8) secrete kappa light chains, and all seven tumors with an 8;22 translocation secrete lambda light chains. These translocations may be causally related to the malignant transformation of the cells. One hypothesis now being investigated is that transpositions of DNA from one chromosome to another may result in activation of previously quiescent genes. This could either be because of movement of quiescent genes into an actively transcribed region (e.g., 8;14) or because of movement of promotor sequences into a previously quiescent region (e.g., 14;8). Thus, an Ig promotor region, if translocated to chromosome 8, might activate an oncogene, whereas an oncogene translocated into an active chromosomal region on chromosomes 14, 2, or 22 might be transcribed inappropriately.

In summary, environmental factors, including radiation, chemicals, and EBV, combined with host factors such as immune deficiency and susceptibility to chromosomal breakage, are determinants of lymphomagenesis.

Pathogenesis of Leukemias and Lymphomas:
Environmental Influences, edited by
I. T. Magrath, G. T. O'Conor, and B. Ramot.
Raven Press, New York © 1984.

"Molecular" Epidemiology of Human Lymphomas and Leukemias: Implications of Nonproducer Retrovirus-Induced Avian and Mammalian Lymphomas

Henry S. Kaplan

Department of Radiology, Cancer Biology Research Laboratory, Stanford University
School of Medicine, Stanford, California 94305

Interest in the possible retroviral etiology of human lymphomas and leukemias has been stimulated by an extensive body of evidence identifying type C retroviruses as the etiologic agents of such neoplasms in a broad spectrum of avian and mammalian species, including chickens, mice, rats, guinea pigs, cats, cattle, sheep, and gibbon apes (46). The argument that these viruses may also play an important role in the induction of the corresponding types of human tumors gains in plausibility from the fact that the morphologic spectrum and clinical manifestations of the lymphomas of cats, cattle, and gibbon apes closely resemble those in humans (45). It is therefore relevant to review briefly some of the distinctive features of the life cycle of retroviruses and their known or postulated molecular mechanisms of oncogenesis, placing particular emphasis on the highly sophisticated methods required to reveal retrovirus "footprints" in apparently virus-negative, nonproducer lymphomas. These facts have important implications with respect to the types of evidence that may need to be sought to establish the retroviral etiology of human lymphomas and leukemias.

MORPHOLOGY AND CLINICAL MANIFESTATIONS

T- and B-cell lymphoblastic lymphomas and pleomorphic "histiocytic" or "undifferentiated" (usually B-cell) lymphomas are the most common types seen in laboratory mice, but myeloid and erythroblastic leukemias and plasmacytomas also occur in certain inbred strains (45). The T-lymphoblastic lymphomas typically arise in the thymus (44) and rapidly disseminate; their morphology, thymic origin, and pattern of dissemination closely resemble those of human convoluted T-cell lymphoblastic lymphomas. Murine B-cell neoplasms, including the pleomorphic "histiocytic" lymphomas, typically arise in the spleen, mesenteric nodes, Peyer's patches, and/or peripheral nodes and tend to spread more slowly (36). Long-lived lymphomatous mice may develop high peripheral white blood cell and absolute lymphocyte counts and increased numbers of circulating blast forms.

In cats, T-lymphoblastic lymphomas of thymic origin are prevalent in young animals, whereas older animals are more likely to develop lymphomas (presumably of B-cell origin) involving the gastrointestinal tract and mesenteric nodes or disseminated neoplasms with marrow involvement and frank leukemia. Infrequently, feline lymphomas may localize in other sites, such as the central nervous system, the skin, the eye, and/or the kidney (16,17).

Lymphomas of cattle are classified into juvenile (calf and thymic), adult, and cutaneous forms (85). The adult form, which is usually widely disseminated when diagnosed, may occur enzootically in selected herds, but sporadic cases are also observed. Most adult bovine lymphomas, as well as those induced in sheep by the bovine leukemia virus, are of B-cell origin. The cutaneous form resembles human mycosis fungoides in its evolution from multiple urticarial lesions through phases of tumor formation, ulceration, and necrosis, and secondary spread to lymph nodes and visceral organs. The few gibbon ape lymphomas and leukemias described to date have been quite heterogeneous with respect to clinical manifestations and sites of involvement at autopsy (41).

RETROVIRUS STRUCTURE, LIFE CYCLE, AND TRANSMISSION

The mammalian type C retroviruses are spherical particles with a diameter of about 100 to 115 nM, a density of 1.15 to 1.16 g/ml, a centrally placed nucleoid, a core shell, and an outer envelope (7,19). There are no known intracellular precursors; instead, newly formed particles characteristically bud from the plasma membranes of their host cells and then appear singly or in clusters in extracellular fluids and spaces. Each replication-competent virus particle contains an approximately 70S RNA dimer composed of two approximately 35S RNA monomers, each with a molecular weight of approximately 3×10^6 daltons (6,21,87).

The virions contain several structural proteins (78,80,89): a major internal core protein (p30) with a molecular weight ranging from 24,000 (bovine) to 30,000 (murine) daltons; an envelope glycoprotein (gp70) with a molecular weight of about 70,000 daltons; and smaller polypeptides with molecular weights of about 10,000, 12,000, and 15,000 daltons (p10, p12, and p15). The p30 and gp70 have both been shown to bear type-specific, group-specific, and interspecies antigenic determinants (78,80).

A distinctive feature of all retroviruses is the presence within the virions of the enzyme RNA-dependent DNA polymerase, or "reverse transcriptase" (3,84). When a retrovirus particle infects a permissive cell and becomes uncoated, this enzyme synthesizes a complementary (minus) DNA strand on the viral RNA template. The viral RNA is then degraded, and a second (plus) strand of DNA is synthesized, yielding the provirus, a double-stranded DNA copy of the viral RNA genome. In the provirus, there is a duplication of both ends of sequences represented separately at the 5' and 3' ends of the viral RNA, thus forming distinctive "long terminal repeats" (LTRs). These confer a transposon-like structure on the provirus and apparently contain sequences essential for its integration into host cell DNA and for the control of viral gene expression (82,83).

Replication-competent retroviral genomes contain three genes (Fig. 1); proceeding from the 5' LTR, these are *gag*, which codes for a polyprotein (Pr65 *gag*) which is secondarily cleaved to yield the p15, p12, p30, and p10 polypeptides; *pol*, which codes for the reverse transcriptase; and *env*, which codes for the envelope glycoprotein (13). Avian sarcoma viruses contain an additional gene, *src*, which appears to be essential for neoplastic transformation (76). However, retroviruses that are leukemogenic or lymphomagenic do not bear an additional gene similar to *src*. Instead, other molecular alterations in their genomes appear to be correlated with the oncogenicity of these viruses. In the acute defective leukemia viruses of chickens and in the Abelson murine leukemia virus, two genomic species of viral RNA are found: a full-length replication-competent species containing the *gag*, *pol*, and *env* genes, and a shorter species in which variable segments of these genes have been deleted and replaced by other genes variously known as *myc*, *erb*, *abl*, *myb*, etc. (generically termed *onc*), which are essential to their oncogenicity (22). The shorter genomes are replication-defective because they lack the ability to produce the polymerase, p30, and/or gp70; their replication thus requires the presence of the full-length "helper" virus genome. The *src* and *onc* genes are now known to be homologous to, and apparently derived from, cellular genes (c-*src*, c-*onc*) that have been packaged into virions after recombination with proviral DNA (22,77). These cellular genes are normal genes that are strongly conserved in the DNA of many avian and mammalian species. Their oncogenicity after integration into viral genomes is attributed to their having come under the control of promotor sequences in the viral LTRs (8,83). Thus, it is clear that retroviruses are not intrinsically

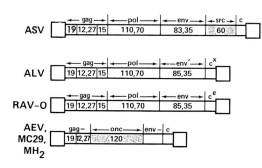

FIG. 1. Diagrammatic representation of the genomic structure of four avian retrovirus proviral DNAs. The boxes at the 5' and 3' ends of each provirus represent the LTRs. RAV-0 is an endogenous, replication-competent, nononcogenic chicken virus. Avian leukosis virus (ALV) is an exogenous, replication-competent virus that induces B-cell lymphomas in chickens. It differs from RAV-0 mainly at its 3' end, in a noncoding region designated *c* and in the adjacent U3 segment of the LTR. In contrast, the replication-competent avian sarcoma viruses (ASV) have a genome about 15% longer than that of RAV-0, because of the acquisition of an additional gene, *src*, which is responsible for their oncogenicity. Finally, the group of rapidly oncogenic viruses diagrammed on the bottom line are all defective, because of the insertion of various *onc* genes in place of part or all of the *pol*, *gag*, and/or *env* genes. The *src* and *onc* genes are homologous to and apparently derived from highly conserved normal cellular genes.

oncogenic; instead, they acquire oncogenicity secondarily by recombining with and acting as transducing vectors for cellular genes under conditions that substitute viral for normal cellular control of the expression of those genes. The products of the *onc* genes (transforming proteins) have not been identified in all instances; however, with only rare exceptions to date, those identified have shared one significant attribute: they are protein kinases that preferentially phosphorylate proteins at tyrosine rather than serine or threonine residues (15,88).

The term *endogenous* is used to describe retroviruses whose intact unaltered genomes are represented in the DNA of all normal cells of the host species. Endogenous viruses are transmitted "vertically" through the germ cells and the fetus from one generation to the next (34,40). Although they are replication-competent, their expression may be repressed in some host species. No endogenous retrovirus has to date been shown to be oncogenic. Instead, during the course of replication, different types of endogenous retroviruses are likely to undergo recombinational interactions that generate altered, *exogenous* retroviruses, some of which thus acquire oncogenicity (1,12,23,25). Thus, all known oncogenic retroviruses are recombinants; however, not all recombinant retroviruses are oncogenic. Exogenous recombinant retroviruses are transmitted "horizontally," i.e., by contagion.

The permissiveness of cells of a given species (and inbred strain, in the case of mice) is determined by both genetic factors and the differentiated phenotype. Mice of inbred strains homozygous for one of two alleles, n or b, of the Fv-1 gene, are nonpermissive for the replication of retroviruses of the nonhomologous tropism; thus, B-tropic viruses replicate preferentially in cells of Fv-1^{bb} genotype, N-tropic viruses in cells of Fv-1^{nn} genotype (66). Even within cells of homologous tropism, however, retroviruses may exhibit striking selectivity with respect to cell type; some are thymotropic (able to replicate well in thymocytes *in vivo*) but not fibrotropic (unable to replicate well on fibroblasts), whereas others have the opposite pattern of cytotropism (20). In mice, retroviruses that have the capacity to induce thymic T-cell lymphomas are all thymotropic but vary with respect to fibrotropism. Retroviruses differ strikingly in the target cell specificity of their oncogenic effects; some infect and transform only T lymphocytes (9,70), others only B or pre-B cells (4,70), and still others only erythroblastic or myeloid cell precursors (81).

RETROVIRAL ETIOLOGY OF NON-PRODUCER LYMPHOMAS AND LEUKEMIAS

About 25 to 30% of feline lymphomas and lymphatic leukemias do not express either feline leukemia virus (FeLV) or the antigens of its structural proteins (27,37). It would be logical to conclude that such lymphomas and leukemias are of nonviral etiology. Yet growing evidence now suggests that these tumors are indeed caused by FeLV despite their failure to produce virus or to express viral structural antigens. First, cats raised under conditions in which they are never exposed to FeLV develop neither producer nor nonproducer lymphomas and leukemias (37). Second, epidemiologic studies of multiple-cat households in which FeLV is endemic reveal that the risk of developing a nonproducer lymphoma, relative to that in the general feline population, is increased to about the same extent (approximately 40-fold) as that of developing an FeLV-positive lymphoma (28,37). Finally, the feline oncornavirus cell membrane antigen, which is expressed on cells transformed by FeLV or by the related feline sarcoma virus, is consistently present on the cells of nonproducer lymphomas (79).

Bursal (B-cell) lymphomas of chickens are induced by the avian leukosis virus (ALV). Unlike the acute defective leukemia viruses of chickens, ALV is a replication-competent exogenous virus; careful mapping of its genome reveals no cell-derived *onc* gene and only minor differences, mainly in and near the U3 region at its 3' end, from the genome of the endogenous, nonlymphomagenic virus RAV-0 (14,18,75,86). It was postulated that these differences in the U3 region might confer two new properties on the virus: the capacity to integrate into the DNA of target cells preferentially at or near the site of one or more cellular homologs of viral *onc* genes, and amplified promotor activity of its LTR, which would thus be expected to take over control of and augment the expression of the affected cellular gene. Strong support for this "promoter insertion" hypothesis has recently been reported (38,60,64); however, the site of viral LTR insertion in some tumors is downstream, instead of upstream, from the c-*myc* gene, suggesting that mechanisms other than simple amplification of promoter activity may be involved. Particularly relevant, however, is the fact that in many of the lymphomas studied with the aid of specific molecular probes, all virus-related sequences other than the LTR had been deleted (64). The restriction nuclease fragments containing the LTR were identical in size in the DNA of all of the nonproducer lymphoma cells from different tissues of any one bird (60), indicating that the tumors were monoclonal in origin and that LTR insertion had occurred before transformation.

C57BL/Ka mice exposed to fractionated whole-body X-irradiation develop a high incidence of T-cell lymphomas of thymic origin (47). Despite the fact that viral antigens are undetectable during the preneoplastic latent period and even in most of the fully developed lymphomas, cell-free extracts prepared from such lymphomas in the autochthonous host (55) or following serial transplantation into syngeneic hosts (52) or supernatant culture fluids harvested at various intervals after such nonproducer lymphomas are placed in culture (54) have been shown to contain a family of thymotropic, lymphomagenic (T + L +) retroviruses, called radiation leukemia virus (RadLV). Mapping of molecularly cloned and uncloned proviral DNA of these and related viruses indicates that RadLV is an exogenous, recombinant virus (35). Most important, some radiogenic lymphoma cell lines that have been permanently devoid of viral antigens or virus production have yielded T + L + progeny virus after injection by a related T − L − virus, suggesting the "rescue" of replication-defective oncogenic viral information from these nonproducer lymphomas (53). In a small number of RadLV-induced lymphomas studied to date, the EcoR1 restriction nuclease fragments containing sequences homologous to a cloned U3 region probe have varied greatly in length, at variance with the predictions of the promotor insertion hypothesis. However, as in the case of the avian B-cell lymphomas, these and other murine T-cell lymphomas appear to be monoclonal in origin, as indicated in the RadLV-induced tumors by the consistent presence of an additional 1.5 kb KpnI fragment containing recombinant viral sequences (35).

The bovine leukemia virus (BoLV) can be isolated when lymphomas from adult cattle of enzootically affected herds are placed in culture (10,24). When inoculated into sheep (50,62) or goats (63), BoLV has been shown to induce lymphoma of similar morphology and clinical behavior. Yet most of the juvenile and cutaneous forms of bovine lymphoma are apparently virus-negative. Molecularly cloned BoLV probes are now available to undertake more critical searches for replication-defective, subgenomic oncogenic viral sequences in such nonproducer lymphomas. Recent studies (51) of a series of 17 bovine lymphomas, using specific subgenomic viral probes, failed to reveal evidence for the integration of BoLV in proximity to any specific region in the cellular DNA genome, or of expression at the RNA level of the LTR and proximate cellular sequences, as predicted by the promoter insertion hypothesis. Thus, it may be necessary to seek other molecular mechanisms for the lymphomagenic activity of retroviruses in mammalian species.

IMPLICATIONS FOR THE EPIDEMIOLOGY OF HUMAN LYMPHOMAS AND LEUKEMIAS

Despite intensive and arduous efforts to detect them in large numbers of human lymphomas and leukemias, no really credible candidate human retroviruses were found until very recently (2,31). Part of the explanation may be that the expression of human retroviruses is strongly repressed. A type C retroviral isolate from the cultured cells of a myeloid leukemia patient, HL23 (29), after obligatory passage in subhuman primate and other cells, was found to have genomic and structural protein characteristics indistinguishable from those of the simian sarcoma virus complex, SSV-1/SSAV, and of the baboon endogenous virus (11,61). A retrovirus-like particle produced spontaneously by a human diffuse histiocytic lymphoma cell line, SU-DHL-1 (48,49), contained a reverse transcriptase and a 28,000-dalton core protein distantly related antigenically to those of SSV-1/SSAV (32,33) but was not infectious and did not yield enough high-molecular-weight RNA to permit its molecular cloning or genomic characterization.

Now, however, Gallo and his colleagues have published a series of papers (30,42,43,67–69,71–74) presenting evidence for the consistent association with cutaneous and other T-cell lymphomas and leukemias of a novel type C retrovirus, designated HTLV, and for the consistent presence of antibodies reactive with the p24 core protein of HTLV in the sera of patients with an unusual form of adult T-cell lymphoma/leukemia endemic to southern Japan. The sera of such patients were also reported (39) to react with a cell line, MT-1, established from such a Japanese adult T-cell lymphoma (58); a virus, designated ATLV, was subsequently isolated from such cultures, and normal cord blood lymphocytes cocultivated with such lymphomas were reported to undergo transformation (59). Recent studies by Gallo and his colleagues indicate that ATLV closely resembles or is identical to HTLV.

Although it is not unlikely that other retroviruses will soon be sporadically isolated from other types of human lymphomas and leukemias, most such neoplasms will probably remain virus-negative, as they have been in virtually all studies during the past decade. However, we are now finally in a position to apply the lessons learned from the nonproducer animal lymphomas described in the preceding section. Although conventional seroepidemiology has already yielded positive results for HTLV- (and ALTV-) related antigens in patients with a relatively rare type of T-cell lymphoma and in some normal individuals in the endemic area, negative responses were obtained with sera from patients with most other types of lymphomas (69,73,74). Such seemingly virus-negative human lymphomas may be caused by retroviruses that are defective and thus produce no viral antigens or infectious virus, or by retroviruses too distantly related to HTLV for their core proteins to share antigenic determinants. Nonetheless, it is reasonably likely that, when HTLV has been molecularly cloned, molecular hybridization studies with subcloned fragments of the viral genome will detect related viral genomic information in a much broader spectrum of human lymphomas and leukemias. Thus, the discovery of just one human lymphoma-associated retrovirus has now opened the possibility of a new kind of epidemiology, "molecular" or "genomic" epidemiology, using cloned probes of such remarkable specificity and sensitivity that they may well reveal the retroviral etiology of human lymphomas and leukemias where all classical epidemiologic and virologic approaches have failed. If so, experience with the prevention of murine and feline lymphomas (5,26,56,57,65) suggests that vaccines can be developed that will effectively protect human populations against the development of these neoplasms.

REFERENCES

1. Aaronson, S. A., Barbacid, M., Dunn, C. Y., and Reddy, E. P. (1981): Genetic approaches toward elucidating the mechanisms of type-C virus-induced leukemia. *Haematol. Blood Transfus.*, 26:455–459.
2. Aaronson, S. A., and Schlom, J. (1975): The search for RNA tumor viruses in human cancer. *Prog. Clin. Cancer*, 6:51–63.
3. Baltimore, D. (1970): RNA-dependent-DNA polymerase in virions of RNA tumor viruses. *Nature*, 226:1209–1211.
4. Baltimore, D., Rosenberg, N., and Witte, O. N. (1979): Transformation of immature lymphoid cells by Abelson murine leukemia virus. *Immunol. Rev.*, 48:3–22.
5. Basombrio, M. A., and Laguens, R. (1978): Active immunization against murine radiation-induced leukemia using a sarcoma virus pseudotype. *Int. J. Cancer*, 21:635–638.
6. Bender, W., Chien, Y.-H., Chattopadhyay, S., Vogt, P. K., Gardner, M. B., and Davidson, N. (1978): High-molecular-weight RNAs of AKR, NZB, and wild mouse viruses and avian reticuloendotheliosis virus all have similar dimer structures. *J. Virol.*, 25:888–896.
7. Bernhard, W. (1960): The detection and study of tumor viruses with the electron microscope. *Cancer Res.*, 20:712–727.
8. Bishop, J. M. (1981): Enemies within: the genesis of retrovirus oncogenes. *Cell*, 23:5–6.
9. Boniver, J., Decleve, A., Honsik, C., Lieberman, M., and Kaplan, H. S. (1981): Phenotypic characterization in mice of thymus target cells susceptible to productive infection by the radiation leukemia virus. *JNCI*, 67: 1139–1151.
10. Burny, A., Bex, F., Chantrenne, H., Cleuter, Y., Dekegel, D., Ghysdael, J., Kettmann, R., Leclercq, M., Leunen, J., Mammerickx, M., and Portetelle, D. (1978): Bovine leukemia virus involvement in enzootic bovine leukosis. *Adv. Cancer Res.*, 28:251–311.

11. Chan, E., Peters, W. P., Sweet, R. W., Ohno, T., Kufe, D. W., Spiegelman, S., Gallo, R. C., and Gallagher, R. E. (1976): Characterization of a virus (HL 23V) isolated from cultured acute myelogenous leukaemic cells. *Nature*, 260:266–268.

12. Chattopadhyay, S. K., Cloyd, M. W., Linemeyer, D. L., Lander, M. R., Rands, E., and Lowy, D. R. (1982): Cellular origin and role of mink cell focus-forming viruses in murine thymic lymphomas. *Nature*, 295:25–31.

13. Coffin, J. M. (1979): Structure, replication, and recombination of tumor virus genomes: some unifying hypotheses. *J. Gen. Virol.*, 42:1–26.

14. Coffin, J. M., Tsichlis, P. N., and Robinson, H. L. (1981): Genetics of leukemogenesis by avian leukosis viruses. In: *Modern Trends in Human Leukemia*. Vol. 4, edited by R. Neth, R. Gallo, J. Grof, K. Mannweiler, and K. Winkler, pp. 432–438. Springer-Verlag, Berlin.

15. Collett, M. S., and Erikson, R. L. (1978): Protein kinase activity associated with the avian sarcoma virus src gene product. *Proc. Natl. Acad. Sci. USA*, 75:2021–2024.

16. Cotter, S. M. (1976): Feline leukemia virus-induced disorders in the cat. *Vet. Clin. North Am.*, 6:367–378.

17. Crighton, G. W. (1969): Lymphosarcoma in the cat. *Vet. Rec.*, 84:329–331.

18. Crittenden, L. B., Hayward, W. S., Hanafusa, H., and Fadly, A. M. (1980): Induction of neoplasms by subgroup E recombinants of exogenous and endogenous avian retroviruses (Rous-associated virus type 60). *J. Virol.*, 33:915–919.

19. Dalton, A. J. (1972): RNA tumor viruses—terminology and ultrastructural aspects of virion morphology and replication. *JNCI*, 49:323–327.

20. Declève, A., Lieberman, M., Ihle, J. N., and Kaplan, H. S. (1976): Biological and serological characterization of radiation leukemia virus (RadLV). *Proc. Natl. Acad. Sci. USA*, 73:4675–4679.

21. Duesberg, P. H. (1968): Physical properties of Rous sarcoma virus RNA. *Proc. Natl. Acad. Sci. USA*, 60:1511–1518.

22. Duesberg, P. H. (1980): Transforming genes of retroviruses. *Biology*, 44:13–29.

23. Elder, J. H., Gautsch, J. W., Jensen, F. C., Lerner, R. A., Hartley, J. W., and Rowe, W. P. (1977): Biochemical evidence that MCF murine leukemia viruses are envelope (env) gene recombinants. *Proc. Natl. Acad. Sci. USA*, 74:4676–4680.

24. Ferrer, J. F., Cabradilla, C., and Gupta, P. (1980): Bovine leukemia: a model for viral carcinogenesis. In: *Viruses in Naturally Occurring Cancers*, edited by M. Essex, G. Todaro, and H. zur Hausen, pp. 887–899. Cold Spring Harbor Laboratory, Cold Spring Harbor, NY.

25. Fischinger, P. J., Frankel, A. E., Elder, J. H., Lerner, R. A., Ihle, J. N., and Bolognesi, D. P. (1978): Biological, immunological and biochemical evidence that HIX virus is a recombinant between Moloney leukemia virus and a murine xenotropic C type virus. *Virology*, 90:241–254.

26. Fish, D. C., Bare, R. M., Hill, P. R., and Huebner, R. J. (1979): Prevention of spontaneous leukemia in mice by oncornavirus immunization. *Int. J. Cancer*, 23:269–273.

27. Francis, D. P., Cotter, S. M., Hardy, W. D., Jr., and Essex, M. (1979): Comparison of virus-positive and virus-negative cases of feline leukemia and lymphoma. *Cancer Res.*, 39:3866–3870.

28. Francis, D. P., and Essex, M. (1980): Epidemiology of feline leukemia. In: *Feline Leukemia Virus*, edited by W. D. Hardy, Jr., M. Essex, and A. J. McClelland, pp. 127–131. Elsevier/North-Holland, Amsterdam.

29. Gallagher, R. E., and Gallo, R. C. (1975): Type cRNA tumor virus isolated from cultural human acute myelogenous leukemia cells. *Science*, 187:350–353.

30. Gallo, R. C. (1982): Regulation of human T-cell proliferation: T-cell growth factor, T-cell leukemias and lymphomas, and isolation of a new C-type retrovirus. In: *Malignant Lymphomas: Etiology, Immunology, Pathology, Treatment*, edited by S. A. Rosenberg and H. S. Kaplan, pp. 201–218. Academic Press, New York.

31. Gardner, M. B., Rasheed, S., Shimizu, S., Rongey, R. W., Henderson, B. E., McAllister, R. M., Klement, V., Charman, H. P., Gilden, R. V., Heberling, R. L., and Huebner, R. J. (1977): Search for RNA tumor virus in humans. In: *Origins of Human Cancer*, edited by H. H. Hiatt, J. D. Watson, and J. A. Winsten, pp. 1235–1251. Cold Spring Harbor Laboratory, Cold Spring Harbor, NY.

32. Goodenow, R. S., Brown, S., Levy, R., and Kaplan, H. S. (1980): Partial characterization of the virion proteins of a type-C RNA virus produced by a human histiocytic lymphoma cell line. In: *Viruses in Naturally Occurring Cancers*, edited by M. Essex, G. Todaro, and H. zur Hausen, pp. 737–752. Cold Spring Harbor Laboratory, Cold Spring Harbor, NY.

33. Goodenow, R. S., and Kaplan, H. S. (1979): Characterization of the reverse transcriptase of a

type C RNA virus produced by a human lymphoma cell line. *Proc. Natl. Acad. Sci. USA*, 76:4971–4975.

34. Gross, L. (1951): Pathologic properties, and "vertical" transmission of the mouse leukemia agent. *Proc. Soc. Exp. Biol. Med.*, 78:342–348.

35. Grymes, R. A., Scott, M. L., Kim, J. P., Fry, K. E., and Kaplan, H. S. (1983): Molecular studies of the radiation leukemia virus (RadLV) and related retroviruses of C57BL/Ka mice. *Prog. Nucleic Acid Res. Mol. Biol. (in press)*.

36. Haas, M., and Meshorer, A. (1979): Reticulum cell neoplasms induced in C57BL/6 mice by cultured virus grown in stromal hematopoietic cell lines. *JNCI*, 63:427–439.

37. Hardy, W. D., Jr., McClelland, A. J., Zuckerman, E. E., Snyder, H. W., Jr., MacEwen, E. G., Francis, D. P., and Essex, M. (1980): The immunology and epidemiology of feline leukemia virus non-producer lymphosarcomas. In: *Viruses in Naturally Occurring Cancers*, edited by M. Essex, G. Todaro, and H. zur Hausen, pp. 677–679. Cold Spring Harbor Press, Cold Spring Harbor, NY.

38. Hayward, W. S., Neel, B. G., and Astrin, S. W. (1981): Activation of a cellular *onc* gene by promoter insertion in ALV-induced lymphoid leukosis. *Nature*, 290:475–480.

39. Hinuma, Y., Nagata, K., Hanaoka, M., Nakai, M., Matsumoto, T., Kinoshita, K. I., Shirakawa, S., and Miyoshi, I. (1981): Adult T-cell leukemia: antigen in an ATL cell line and detection of antibodies to the antigen in human sera. *Proc. Natl. Acad. Sci. USA*, 78:6476–6480.

40. Jaenisch, R. (1976): Germ line integration and Mendelian transmission of the exogenous Moloney leukemia virus. *Proc. Natl. Acad. Sci. USA*, 73:1260–1264.

41. Johnsen, D. O., Wooding, W. L., Tanticharoenyos, P., and Bourgeois, C. H., Jr. (1971): Malignant lymphoma in the gibbon. *J. Am. Vet. Med. Assoc.*, 159:563–566.

42. Kalyanaraman, V. S., Sarngadharan, M. G., Bunn, P. A., Minna, J. D., and Gallo, R. C. (1981): Antibodies in human sera reactive against an internal structural protein of human T-cell lymphoma virus. *Nature*, 294:271–273.

43. Kalyanaraman, V. S., Sarngadharan, M. G., Poiesz, B., Ruscetti, F. W., and Gallo, R. C. (1981): Immunological properties of a type C retrovirus isolated from cultured human T-lymphoma cells and comparison to other mammalian retroviruses. *J. Virol.*, 38:906–915.

44. Kaplan, H. S. (1948): Comparative susceptibility of lymphoid tissues of strain C57 black mice to induction of lymphoid tumors by irradiation. *JNCI*, 8:191–197.

45. Kaplan, H. S. (1974): Leukemia and lymphoma in experimental and domestic animals. *Ser. Haematol.*, 7:94–163.

46. Kaplan, H. S. (1978): Etiology of lymphomas and leukemias: role of C-type RNA viruses. *Leuk. Res.*, 2:253–271.

47. Kaplan, H. S., and Brown, M. B. (1952): A quantitative dose-response study of lymphoid-tumor development in irradiated C57 black mice. *JNCI*, 13:185–208.

48. Kaplan, H. S., Goodenow, R. S., Epstein, A. L., Gartner, S., Declève, A., and Rosenthal, P. N. (1977): Isolation of a type C RNA virus from an established human histiocytic lymphoma cell line. *Proc. Natl. Acad. Sci. USA*, 74:2564–2568.

49. Kaplan, H. S., Goodenow, R. S., Gartner, S., and Bieber, M. M. (1979): Biology and virology of the human malignant lymphomas: 1st Milford D. Schulz Lecture. *Cancer*, 43:1–24.

50. Kenyon, S. J., Ferrer, J. F., McFeely, R. A., and Graves, D. C. (1981): Induction of lymphosarcoma in sheep by bovine leukemia virus. *JNCI*, 67:1157–1163.

51. Kettmann, R., Deschamps, J., Cleuter, Y., Couez, D., Burny, A., and Marbaix, G. (1982): Leukemogenesis by bovine leukemia virus: proviral DNA integration and lack of RNA expression of viral long terminal repeat and 3' proximate cellular sequences. *Proc. Natl. Acad. Sci. USA*, 79:2465–2469.

52. Lieberman, M., Declève, A., Gelmann, E. P., and Kaplan, H. S. (1977): Biological and serological characterization of the C-type RNA viruses isolated from the C57BL/Ka strain of mice. II. Induction and propagation of the isolates. In: *Radiation-Induced Leukemogenesis and Related Viruses*, edited by J. F. Duplan, pp. 231–246. North-Holland, Amsterdam.

53. Lieberman, M., Declève, A., Ihle, J. N., and Kaplan, H. S. (1979): Rescue of a thymotropic, leukemogenic C-type virus from cultured, nonproducer lymphoma cells of strain C57BL/Ka mice. *Virology*, 97:12–21.

54. Lieberman, M., Declève, A., Ricciardi-Castagnoli, P., Boniver, J., Finn, O. J., and Kaplan, H. S. (1979): Establishment, characterization, and virus expression of cell lines derived from radiation- and virus-induced lymphomas of C57BL/Ka mice. *Int. J. Cancer*, 24:168–177.

55. Lieberman, M., and Kaplan, H. S. (1959): Leukemogenic activity of filtrates from radiation-induced lymphoid tumors of mice. *Science*, 130:387–388.

56. Lieberman, M., and Kaplan, H. S. (1977): Vaccination against X-ray or radiation leukemia virus-induced thymic lymphoma development by inoculation of mice with syngeneic fibroblastic cells infected with an endogenous B-tropic nonleukemogenic virus. In: *Radiation-Induced Leukemogenesis and Related Viruses*, edited by J. F. Duplan, pp. 127–132. North-Holland, Amsterdam.

57. Mathes, L. E., Lewis, M. G., and Olsen, R. G. (1980): Immunoprevention of feline leukemia: efficacy testing and antigenic analysis of soluble tumor-cell antigen vaccine. In: *Feline Leukemia Virus*, edited by W. D. Hardy, Jr., M. Essex, and A. J. McClelland, pp. 211–216. Elsevier/North-Holland, Amsterdam.

58. Miyoshi, I., Kubonishi, I., Sumida, M., Kiraki, S., Tsubota, T., Kimura, I., Miyamoto, K., and Sato, J. (1980): A novel T-cell derived from adult T-cell leukemia. *GANN*, 71:155–156.

59. Miyoshi, I., Kubonishi, I., Yoshimoto, S., Akagi, T., Ohtsuki, Y., Shiraishi, Y., Nagata, K., and Hinuma, Y. (1981): Type C virus particles in a cord T-cell line derived by co-cultivating normal human cord leukocytes and human leukaemic T cells. *Nature*, 294:770–771.

60. Neel, B. G., Hayward, W. S., Robinson, H. L., Fang, J., and Astrin, S. M. (1981): Avian leukosis virus-induced tumors have common proviral integration sites and synthesize discrete new RNAs: oncogenesis by promoter insertion. *Cell*, 23:323–334.

61. Okabe, H., Gilden, R. V., Hatanaka, M., Stephenson, J. R., Gallagher, R. E., Gallo, R. C., Tronick, S. R., and Aaronson, S. A. (1976): Immunological and biochemical characterization of type C viruses isolated from cultured human AML cells. *Nature*, 260:264–266.

62. Olson, C., and Baumgartner, L. E. (1976): Pathology of lymphosarcoma in sheep induced with bovine leukemia virus. *Cancer Res.*, 36:2365–2373.

63. Olson, C., Kettmann, R., Burny, A., and Kaja, R. (1981): Goat lymphosarcoma from bovine leukemia virus. *JNCI*, 67:671–675.

64. Payne, G. S., Courtneidge, S. A., Crittenden, L. B., Fadly, A. M., Bishop, J. M., and Varmus, H. E. (1981): Analysis of avian leukosis virus DNA and RNA in bursal tumors: viral gene expression is not required for maintenance of the tumor state. *Cell*, 23:311–322.

65. Peters, R. L., Sass, B., Stephenson, J. R., Al-Ghazzouli, I. K., Hino, S., Donahoe, R. M., Kende, M., Aaronson, S. A., and Kelloff, G. J. (1977): Immunoprevention of X-ray-induced leukemias in the C57BL mouse. *Proc. Natl. Acad. Sci. USA*, 74:1697–1701.

66. Pincus, T., Hartley, J. W., and Rowe, W. P. (1971): A major genetic locus affecting resistance to infection with murine leukemia viruses. I. Tissue culture studies of naturally occurring viruses. *J. Exp. Med.*, 133:1219–1233.

67. Poiesz, B. J., Ruscetti, F. W., Gazdar, A. F., Bunn, P. A., Minna, J. D., and Gallo, R. C. (1980): Detection and isolation of type C retrovirus particles from fresh and cultured lymphocytes of patient with cutaneous T-cell lymphoma. *Proc. Natl. Acad. Sci. USA*, 77:7415–7419.

68. Poiesz, B. J., Ruscetti, F. W., Reitz, M. S., Kalyanaraman, V. S., and Gallo, R. C. (1981): Isolation of a new type C retrovirus (HTLV) in primary uncultured cells of a patient with Sézary T-cell leukaemia. *Nature*, 294:268–271.

69. Posner, L. E., Robert-Guroff, M., Kalyanaraman, V. S., Poiesz, B. J., Ruscetti, F. W., Fossieck, B., Bunn, P. A., Minna, J. D., and Gallo, R. C. (1981): Natural antibodies to the human T cell lymphoma virus in patients with cutaneous T cell lymphoma. *J. Exp. Med.*, 154:333–346.

70. Reddy, E. P., Dunn, C. Y., and Aaronson, S. A. (1980): Different lymphoid cell targets for transformation by replication-competent Moloney and Rauscher mouse leukemia viruses. *Cell*, 19:663–669.

71. Reitz, M. S., Poiesz, B. J., Ruscetti, F. W., and Gallo, R. C. (1981): Characterization and distribution of nucleic acid sequences of a novel retrovirus isolated from neoplastic human T-lymphocytes. *Proc. Natl. Acad. Sci. USA*, 78:1887–1891.

72. Rho, H. M., Poiesz, B., Ruscetti, F. W., and Gallo, R. C. (1981): Characterization of the reverse transcriptase from a new retrovirus (HTLV) produced by a human cutaneous T-cell lymphoma cell line. *Virology*, 112:355–360.

73. Robert-Guroff, M., Nakao, Y., Notake, K., Ito, Y., Sliski, A., and Gallo, R. C. (1982): Natural antibodies to human retrovirus HTLV in a cluster of Japanese patients with adult T cell leukemia. *Science*, 215:975–978.

74. Robert-Guroff, M., Ruscetti, F. W., Posner, L. E., Poiesz, B. J., and Gallo, R. C. (1981): Detection of the human T cell lymphoma virus p19 in cells of some patients with cutaneous T cell lymphoma and leukemia using a monoclonal antibody. *J. Exp. Med.*, 154:1957–1964.

75. Robinson, H. L., Pearson, M. N., DeSimone, D. W., Tsichlis, P. N., and Coffin, J. M. (1979): Subgroup-E avian-leukosis-virus-associated disease in chickens. *Cold Spring Harbor Symp. Quant. Biol.*, 4:1133–1142.
76. Stehelin, D., Guntaka, R. V., Varmus, H. E., and Bishop, J. M. (1976): Purification of DNA complementary to nucleotide sequences required for neoplastic transformation of fibroblasts by avian sarcoma viruses. *J. Mol. Biol.*, 101:349–365.
77. Stehelin, D., Varmus, H. E., Bishop, J. M., and Vogt, P. K. (1976): DNA related to the transforming gene(s) of avian sarcoma viruses is present in normal avian cells. *Nature*, 260:170–173.
78. Stephenson, J. R. (1980): Type C virus structural and transformation-specific proteins. In: *Molecular Biology of RNA Tumor Viruses*, edited by J. R. Stephenson, pp. 245–298. Academic Press, New York.
79. Stephenson, J. R., Kahn, A. S., Sliski, A. H., and Essex, M. (1977): Feline oncornavirus-associated cell membrane antigen (FOCMA): identification of an immunologically cross-reactive feline sarcoma virus coded protein. *Proc. Natl. Acad. Sci. USA*, 74:5608–5612.
80. Strand, M., and August, J. T. (1976): Structural proteins of ribonucleic acid tumor viruses. Purification of envelope, core, and internal components. *J. Biol. Chem.*, 251:559–564.
81. Tambourin, P. E., and Wendling, F. (1975): Target cell for oncogenic action of polycythaemia-inducing friend virus. *Nature*, 256:320–322.
82. Temin, H. M. (1981): Structure, variation and synthesis of retrovirus long terminal repeat. *Cell*, 27:1–3.
83. Temin, H. M. (1982): Function of the retrovirus long terminal repeat. *Cell*, 28:3–5.
84. Temin, H. M., and Mizutani, S. (1970): RNA-dependent DNA polymerase in virions of Rous sarcoma virus. *Nature*, 226:1211–1213.
85. Theilen, G. H., and Madewell, B. R. (1979): Leukemia-sarcoma disease complex. In: *Veterinary Cancer Medicine*, edited by T. H. Theilen and B. R. Madewell, pp. 204–288. Lea and Febiger, Philadelphia.
86. Tsichlis, P. N., and Coffin, J. M. (1980): Recombinants between endogenous and exogenous avian tumor viruses: role of the C region and other portions of the genome in the control of replication and transformation. *J. Virol.*, 33:238–249.
87. Tsuchida, N., and Green, M. (1974): Intracellular and virion 35S RNA species of murine sarcoma and leukemia viruses. *Virology*, 59:258–265.
88. Witte, O. N., Ponticelli, A., Gifford, A., Baltimore, D., Rosenberg, N., and Elder, J. (1981): Phosphorylation of the Abelson murine leukemia virus transforming protein. *J. Virol.*, 39:870–878.
89. Witte, O. N., Weissman, I. L., and Kaplan, H. S. (1973): Structural characteristics of some murine RNA tumor viruses studied by lactoperoxidase iodination. *Proc. Natl. Acad. Sci. USA*, 70:36–40.

Pathogenesis of Leukemias and Lymphomas:
Environmental Influences, edited by
I. T. Magrath, G. T. O'Conor, and B. Ramot.
Raven Press, New York © 1984.

Viral Etiology for Naturally Occurring Leukemias and Lymphomas

M. Essex

*Department of Microbiology, Harvard University School of Public Health,
Boston, Massachusetts 02115*

The first evidence that viruses, or "filterable agents," cause leukemia or lymphoma came about 75 years ago from the studies of Rous (65) and Ellerman and Bang (15) using chickens. About 45 to 50 years later, the first evidence that viruses could cause leukemia in mammals came from the work of Gross (33) using inbred mice. The first demonstration that viruses caused a naturally occurring leukemia or lymphoma in an outbred mammalian species came in 1964 from the work of Jarrett et al. using cats (44,45). During the next decade, it was shown that viruses caused leukemia and/or lymphoma in several other species under natural conditions. Table 1 lists the viruses involved in naturally occurring leukemias and lymphomas.

CHARACTERISTICS OF LEUKEMOGENIC VIRUSES

All the leukemogenic viruses thus far identified are either herpesviruses or retroviruses. The herpesviruses are DNA viruses that are lytic for most cells that they infect. Under some conditions, these agents establish latent infections in certain cells, where the DNA exists in an episomal form, and few viral proteins and almost no infectious virus are made. Retroviruses are RNA viruses that have a DNA proviral phase that is necessary for replication. The DNA provirus, which is made with

TABLE 1. *Viruses associated with leukemia and/or lymphoma*

Species	Neoplastic cell	Class of virus	Route of transmission	General reference
Chicken	T cell	Herpes (Marek's)	Airborne dander	55
Chicken	B cell	Retrovirus (ALV)	Egg albumin, droplets	56
Cat	T cell, others	Retrovirus (FeLV)	Saliva	20
Ox	B cell	Retrovirus (BLV)	Flies, colostrum	2
Gibbon	T cell, others	Retrovirus (GaLV)	Saliva	10
Man[a]	B lymphocyte	Herpes (Epstein-Barr)	Saliva	53
Man[a]	T lymphocyte	Retrovirus (HTLV)	Blood, others?	19

[a]Actual causative role not fully established.

virion reverse transcriptase, regularly integrates into the DNA of the host cell chromosomes. Retroviruses do not cause lysis in infected cells. Even when the cell produces large amounts of virus, the cell is not visibly damaged. The ability of a virus to establish a latent infection and to interact with the DNA of the cell is probably a requirement for oncogenic activity.

Viruses that cause leukemia under natural conditions are transmitted by a variety of routes, but all involve either horizontal transmission or the congenital transfer of infectious virus from mother to progeny. Many retroviruses have evolved to be genetically transmitted from parent to progeny as a regular part of the genetic complement of a given species. However, viruses in the latter category are not oncogenic under natural conditions in any species of animals. The only exceptions to this general rule are the viruses of AKR and C3H mice, but these are inbred strains that were selected for the phenotype of malignancy, a situation that obviously could not occur in nature.

Leukemogenic viruses of mammals are often transmitted by saliva, and such agents are generally ubiquitous in the population. In most cases a large proportion of the population becomes persistently infected, but relatively few develop leukemia or lymphoma. Even when the host does develop leukemia, the induction period is usually prolonged, varying from 10 to 50% or more of the normal life-span of that species. Animals that are infected with such viruses may also have an increased risk of developing nonneoplastic diseases. Some, such as anemias and glomeru-lonephritis, may occur without the assistance of any other agent(s). Other diseases, such as septicemia and pneumonia, may preferentially occur in leukemia virus-infected individuals because the leukemia virus depresses the immune response to a given cytopathic virus or bacterium, whereas an infection with that agent in a leukemia-free animal would be easily controlled.

In general, the severity of infection with the leukemia virus and the duration of the induction period are related to age at exposure and the dose of virus received. An animal that receives a large dose of leukemia virus at a young age is much more likely to develop a persistent infection and/or to develop leukemia. This could be because of a relatively inefficient immune response and/or because of the presence of a larger proportion of cells that have receptors for infection by the virus.

LEUKEMIA AND LYMPHOMA OF ANIMALS CAUSED BY VIRUSES

Feline Leukemia and Lymphoma

Perhaps the most complete understanding we have at present of how a naturally occurring mammalian leukemia may be caused by a virus is the case of feline leukemia. We have considerable knowledge about the feline leukemia virus (FeLV) and the general biology and epidemiology of the disease. Yet we know very little about either the molecular events that cause the target cell to become malignant or about the events that determine how this cell and its progeny interact with the host.

FeLV is typical of most retroviruses that exist in a variety of species. It has an RNA genome that contains three genes and goes through an obligatory DNA proviral stage for replication. It is during this proviral phase that integration into the host cell chromosomes occurs, latency may result, and interference with the regulation of certain host cell functions also occurs. The three genes encoded by the viral genome are *gag*, which make a polyprotein that is cleaved to form the virion core peptides designated p15c, p12, p30, and p10; *pol*, which encodes the reverse transcriptase that allows the RNA to become a DNA provirus; and *env*, which encodes for the peptides that occur at the virion surface, designated gp70 and p15e. At both ends of the proviral genome are stretches of several hundred nucleotides called the long terminal repeats (LTRs), which are involved in transcription and can also act as a promotor. These details have been reviewed elsewhere (23).

FeLV does not carry an *onc* gene and does not transform fibroblasts. It does have the potential to recombine with *onc* genes in the cells, as do most helper retroviruses (6). Once recombination has occurred, a feline sarcoma virus (FeSV) that contains an *onc* gene (e.g., *fes*) is produced. Such FeSVs cause polyclonal solid tumors when inoculated into cats and other species. Although useful for studying transformation and the induction of solid tumors, such viruses do not survive in nature because they are replication-defective.

Many different strains of FeLV are known. Some appear to be more highly leukemogenic than others. The strains have been divided into three subgroups based on patterns of interference and host range (43,68). These subgroups are designated A, B, and C. Although various suggestions for subgroup-related pathogenic effects have been made, they have been difficult to substantiate. A major reason for this is the fact that the B and C subgroups apparently never occur alone under natural conditions; they are dependent on A and when present are always co-isolated with A (42).

FeLVs cause several forms of lymphoproliferative neoplasia (27), including both lymphoid leukemia, a disease that appears similar to acute lymphoblastic leukemia in children (8), and several forms of lymphoma. One of the most common forms of lymphoma is the thymic form, which begins by a replacement of normal thymic tissue with malignant T lymphoblasts and occurs at the highest rates in younger animals. Other forms of lymphoma are the multicentric type, which originates in various lymph nodes and other abdominal tissues, and the alimentary form, which appears to originate in the lymphoid tissue along the wall of the gut. The relative rates of the different pathologic forms are known to differ greatly in different geographical areas. Although we might expect this variation to be directly related to variations in FeLV strains, no hard evidence to support this hypothesis is yet available. Only about 65 to 70% of the lymphoid tumors that occur in cats occur in animals that are viremic, and neither the peripheral blood nor the tumor cells have evidence of FeLV in the remaining 30 to 35% of cases. However, even in the latter cases it appears that a very small proportion of bone marrow cells are latently infected with FeLV (64).

FeLV is transmitted by contagion (35), primarily by the excretion of large amounts of infectious virus in saliva (28). Most cats that are exposed to an FeLV-excreter cat in a closed environment become infected within several months. If exposed to large doses of FeLV at a young age, the recipient cats are very likely to develop persistent viremia. Most cats exposed to lower doses of virus at an older age will not become viremic but will develop antibodies to one or more of the FeLV proteins. Although it was widely assumed that such exposed, nonviremic, antibody-positive cats were free of FeLV, it now appears possible that many become latent carriers for life, retaining the infection in a small population of bone marrow cells (64). The major immune response that allows the neutralization of free virus is the humoral response to gp70, the protein located most externally on the virus. However, we recently found that all the virion proteins occur at the surface of infected cells. It thus seems likely that a response to almost any of the virion antigens might limit the spread of infection *in vivo* by lysing cells that were actively making virus (51).

Feline lymphoma cells also express a tumor antigen at the cell surface, designated feline oncornavirus-associated cell membrane antigen (FOCMA) (17). FOCMA is distinct from the major virus structural proteins, and a humoral immune response to this antigen sometimes occurs even in the presence of a persistent viremia (18). An active humoral response to FOCMA appears to protect the animal from tumor development; FOCMA antibodies are lytic for tumor cells in the presence of cat complement (32).

For various reasons the induction period for development of leukemia following exposure to FeLV is long and variable. The length of the induction period, and whether or not leukemia develops at all, is related to age at the time of exposure, virus dose, virus strain, the various immune responses that can occur to both virus proteins and tumor cells, and presumably also to genetic factors of the host. The induction period for the "virus-negative" form of feline leukemia is longer than for the "virus-positive" form.

FeLV is also responsible for major health problems in cats by causing aplastic anemia (39) and by interfering with the normal immune response mounted to various infectious agents (22). As a result of the latter effect, cats that are persistently viremic with FeLV have elevated rates of peritonitis, septicemia, pneumonia, and various other infectious diseases (20). FeLV-infected cats also have higher rates of immune-complex glomerulonephritis (41).

Bovine Leukemia

Several forms of lymphoid neoplasia occur in cattle (2,24). The most common is a form designated enzootic bovine leukosis, which occurs as a multicentric-type disease in various lymph nodes as well as abdominal organs such as the spleen. This disease is caused by the bovine leukemia virus (BLV), a retrovirus. It occurs in adults, and the induction period is prolonged. Other forms of lymphoid neoplasia that occur in cattle are the thymic form, which occurs primarily in calves, and the generalized sporadic and skin forms, which occur primarily in adults. None of the latter forms have been associated with exposure to BLV.

BLV differs from most other mammalian retroviruses, including FeLV, in several ways (2,24). First, the major *gag* and *env* proteins are somewhat smaller than the comparable proteins of other mammalian retroviruses, about 24,000 daltons (p24) and 51,000 daltons (gp51), respectively. Second, none of the virus proteins show serologic cross-reactivity with comparable proteins of other mammalian retroviruses (except the human agent, see below), although the retroviruses of other species show considerable cross-reactivity with each other. Third, the BVL reverse transcriptase functions best in the presence of Mg^{2+} rather than Mn^{2+}. Finally, infected animals do not ordinarily contain detectable amounts of free virus in plasma as do many animals of other species infected with retroviruses.

Although free virus is not found in the plasma of BLV-infected animals, many cattle remain infected for life following first exposure, and lymphoid cells cultured from blood or bone marrow replicate complete virus when kept free of serum from infected animals. The lack of replication of the virus *in vivo*, and *in vitro* when exposed to serum from infected animals, is apparently because of a nonimmunoglobulin inhibitory factor (34). The existence of this factor was a major reason that the initial identification of BLV in infected cattle with enzootic bovine leukosis was so difficult.

The exact mechanism of transmission of BLV is unknown, but it is clear that the virus is transmitted in a horizontal manner and not genetically inherited. The means of transmission are thought to be flies and milk. The virus is highly cell-associated, and it is believed that transmission occurs with infected leukocytes rather than with free BLV (14). Although transmission does not appear to occur unless the animals are in direct contact, most animals that are in regular contact with infected cattle eventually become positive for antibodies to the agent (12). Although all antibody-positive cattle appear to carry the virus in latent form, less than 5% develop lymphoma (25). The role of the immune response in this situation is unclear.

The mechanism by which BLV causes disease at the molecular level is also unclear. Lymphoma cells taken from cattle with enzootic bovine leukosis have integrated BLV provirus at the same site in all cells of a single tumor but at different sites in different tumors. This strongly suggests that the viral genome plays an important role, because it must have been present before the malignant clone of cells appeared. However, attempts to explain this disease by the "promotor insertion" model through the demonstration of common species of mRNA or common integration sites have been unsuccessful (R. Kettmann and A. Burny, *personal communication*).

Although enzootic bovine leukosis is a monoclonal tumor, this disease is frequently preceded by a polyclonal phase of persistent lymphocytosis (2). Most of the cells of the polyclonal proliferation do not harbor BLV, suggesting that the response may be related to immune stimulation. However, both the proliferating polyclonal cells and the subsequent tumor cells do appear to be of B-cell lineage. Also, although many of the cattle with BLV-induced persistent lymphocytosis do not develop lymphoma, some cattle develop lymphoma without passing through a persistent lymphocytosis phase.

Avian Leukosis

Retroviruses cause a wide variety of malignancies, especially leukemias, in chickens. These virus-induced tumors can be divided into three classes. The first class consists of the "acute leukemias," such as myeloblastosis, erythoblastosis, and myelocytomatosis, which are caused by *onc*-gene-containing viruses that are defective for replication. The second class contains the solid tumors, especially gibrosarcomas, also caused by *onc*-containing viruses that are generally but not always defective for replication. The third class is the long-latent-period lymphoma or leukosis of B-cell origin, which is caused by a replication-competent virus that lacks an *onc* gene. The induction period of the first two groups of tumors, which are polyclonal in origin, is only a few weeks. The induction period for the leukosis of B cells is usually a minimum of six months and often longer (21). The B-cell disease occurs as a diffuse lymphoma of the abdominal viscera.

The avian leukemia viruses (ALVs) are transmitted both horizontally and by vertical means. The vertical transmission of leukogenic subgroups, however, is not genetic, but rather is limited to the congenital transmission of intact virus. The virus is in ovarian follicles and oviducts and thus often present in the eggs of young laying chickens (13). ALVs are also horizontally transmitted via oral secretions. Because of age at the time of acquisition, virus acquired by horizontal transmission is much less likely to persist in the bird and cause disease. When infected first as adults, chickens mount a subgroup-specific virus-neutralizing antibody response and eliminate most or all of the replicating virus. Conversely, chickens infected during embryonic development are likely to be immunologically tolerant to the virus and will probably remain viremic for life (66). Chickens in the latter category obviously have a much greater risk of developing leukosis.

ALVs have been divided into subgroups based on the major virus surface (envelope) glycoproteins. Chicken cells have subgroup-specific receptors, and genetic selection has apparently caused a situation where many cells are almost completely resistant to infection by one or more subgroups (73). Those ALVs that cause long-latent-period lymphomas are from the A and B subgroups. One subgroup, designated E or RAV-0, represents avian retroviruses that are genetically inherited. None of the agents in the latter group are oncogenic.

The target cell for oncogenesis by ALV is an IgM-positive B cell. Removal of the bursa of Fabricius, the primary source of B cells in young birds, will prevent lymphoma development.

Although the exact mechanism by which these monoclonal lymphomas emerge has not been established, it is in this system that substantial evidence was obtained for "downstream promotion" (56). Other studies have shown that the 3' LTR end of the viral genome is important for the retention of oncogenic activity (71). In many cases of ALV-induced lymphoma, the viral promoter appears to activate a specific conserved cellular *onc* gene *(myc)* and to cause a massive increase in the expression of this gene at the RNA level (56).

Marek's Disease

Marek's disease (MD) is a polyclonal growth of avian T cells that is caused by a herpesvirus, the Marek's disease agent (MDHV) (3). This disease was originally confused with ALV-induced lymphoma but is now easily distinguishable. Besides differences in clonality, class of agent, and cell type, MD and ALV-induced lymphoma also differ in pathologic type, mode of transmission, and immune control.

MD has a much shorter induction period and is usually manifested by paralysis of birds caused by the infiltration of nerve trunks with proliferating lymphoid cells (55). The virus is highly cell-associated. It does not ordinarily replicate from the altered lymphoid cells but rather from epithelial cells in the feather follicle (38). The virus produced from the latter source is transmitted efficiently by airborne dander.

Effective vaccines have been available for MD for about a decade (60). Two vaccines have been used. One represents an attentuated version of the MDHV that was passaged through chick kidney cells. The second represents a natural strain of a turkey herpesvirus that generates a cross-reactive immune response that will also protect against disease caused by the MDHV. The vaccines appear to prevent disease by preventing the development and/or expansion of pools of proliferating malignant T cells. It does not prevent infection with wild virulent MDHV. Successfully vaccinated birds can thus still become infected with MDHV and transmit the virus to others. Although the target cell for malignant alteration appears to be a T cell, it also appears that a cell-mediated immune response of cytolytic T cells is important for resistance to disease development (55). Genetic resistance is known to occur, but it is less clearly understood than the subgroup-specific resistance seen with the ALVs.

GIBBON APE LEUKEMIA

Gibbon ape leukemia viruses (GaLVs) have been repeatedly isolated from colonized gibbons from various locations, including California, Louisiana, Bermuda, and Thailand (10,48). This family of viruses has been found in association with, and has been used to induce, both lymphoid and myeloid forms of leukemia (41). The induction period for development of these diseases is prolonged, usually a year or more. The GaLVs are clearly transmitted in a contagious manner in colonized gibbons, and they are not inherited as a normal genetic component in this species (49). Related viruses have been found as genetically inherited xenotropic viruses in Asian mice (70). In gibbons these agents are transmitted in high levels in saliva, and the epidemiology of the agent in animals maintained in close contact appears very similar to the epidemiology of FeLV as observed in multiple-cat households. Most exposed gibbons are either persistently viremic with GaLV or positive for high levels of antibodies that react with antigens seen on cultured lymphoma cells (49). The genome of GaLVs lacks an *onc* gene and is similar in structure to FeLV. Little is known about the molecular events that lead to the development of GaLV-induced disease.

HUMAN LEUKEMIA AND LYMPHOMA

Burkitt's Lymphoma

Burkitt's lymphoma (BL) is one of two types of human lymphoid tumors that have been closely associated with a virus. BL is associated with the Epstein-Barr virus (EBV). The association between BL and an infectious agent was first suspected by Burkitt (1), when he observed that this peculiar type of lymphoma occurred at higher-than-expected rates in equatorial Africa. The tumor occurs primarily in young children, and shows a growth pattern often localized to the jaw. The tumor grows rapidly, and cases diagnosed at an early stage are quite sensitive to therapy. Because the tumor is primarily limited to lower lying areas where rainfall is abundant and holoendemic malaria is a major disease problem, various early investigators proposed that the suspected causative agent might be transmitted by mosquitoes (67). The possibility that *Plasmodium*-induced immunosuppression might act as a cofactor for BL has also been considered.

EBV is a cell-associated herpesvirus with a DNA genome of 10^8 daltons. It was first visualized by electron microscopy in cultures of lymphoid cells that were biopsied from a case of BL (16). Because the virus is so large and does not replicate very efficiently in cultured cells, the identification and characterization of the agent have been somewhat retarded. Most cells that grow in culture do not have receptors that will allow infection by the virus. This sensitivity appears to be limited to B lymphocytes of primates, because Burkitt's lymphoma is a monoclonal tumor of B-cell origin and EBV is able to immortalize human cord blood lymphocytes of the B lineage *in vitro*. EBV has also been epidemiologically linked to nasopharyngeal cancer in the Orient and has been proved to be the major cause of infectious mononucleosis (IM), a self-limiting polyclonal lymphoproliferative disease (36).

EBV has been seroepidemiologically studied through the use of several antigen-antibody systems as well as by nucleic acid hybridization. The EBV nuclear antigen is a basic protein that can be regularly detected in lymphoid cells that contain the EBV genome (61). It is not a virus structural protein but is present even when all virus structural proteins are absent. The early antigens are also nonstructural proteins of EBV that are found in some infected cells (37). The few lymphoid cells that make virus structural proteins may contain two additional antigens that have also been useful for seroepidemiological purposes, the viral capsid antigens in the cytoplasm of the cells and the virion envelope membrane antigens (MA) that occur at the cytoplasmic membrane surface (50). All of these antigens are immunogenic in EBV-infected people. The level and class of antibodies to a given protein have been used to determine the duration and magnitude of infection in a given individual and in some cases to provide prognostic information.

Seroepidemiologic studies have revealed that 90% or more of the human population in most of the world has not only been infected with EBV but remains persistently infected in a small proportion of B lymphocytes (53). In many areas of the world, including equatorial Africa, infection with EBV occurs in almost all of the population at a very young age (less than four years). It appears to be this type of infection that can lead to the development of BL when the appropriate cofactor(s) is present (11). In the case of IM, this disease apparently occurs only when first infection with EBV has been delayed until adulthood. Unlike BL, IM is a polyclonal disease, and many of the circulating lymphoid cells found in disease cases appear to be immune T lymphocytes that lack the EBV genome. These T cells may have been stimulated to proliferate by EBV-positive B cells (75). EBV is transmitted in saliva (5).

EBV is normally maintained in the lymphoid cells in episomal rather than integrated form, and cultured lymphoid cells may have up to 200 or more copies of the genome (76). Monoclonality in BL was demonstrated using isoenzyme markers (26).

Adult T-cell Leukemia/Lymphoma

Adult T-cell leukemia (ATL) and T-cell lymphoma are the most recent human tumors to be associated with a virus, in this case a virus recently isolated by Gallo and his colleagues and called the human T-cell leukemia virus (HTLV) (58). The disease that this virus has been associated with was recognized as a distinct clinical syndrome in Japan (72). The same disease, or variations of it, designated mycosis fungoides, Sézary syndrome, and lymphosarcoma cell leukemia, has also been described in various other areas of the world, especially the Caribbean basin (4). As described in southern Japan, particularly on the island of Kyushu (72), this disease occurs in middle-aged adults, follows an aggressive course, and has a poor prognosis. Characteristics of the disease are frequent cutaneous infiltration with malignant cells and the presence of hypercalcemia in a significant number of patients. Hepatomegaly, splenomegaly, and peripheral lymphadenopathy are frequent, but anemia is unusual.

The tumor cell represents a population of mature terminal-transferase-negative T cells of the OKT 4 helper-inducer phenotype (19). Despite the latter markers, the tumor cells show suppressor cell characteristics when added to *in vitro* assay systems, and patients frequently show a hypogammaglobulinemia. The tumor cells represent a monoclonal outgrowth (29,74). They are characterized by the presence of highly pleomorphic nuclei and show various cytogenetic abnormalities, including a 14 q + and/or a nonrandom trisomy of chromosome 7. The cells will grow only in the presence of T-cell growth factor; in fact, it was the discovery of this that led to the cultivation of such cells and the isolation of HTLV (30). However, some cells become constitutive producers of TCGF and can grow without the addition of exogenous growth factors.

The HTLV agent has a morphology characteristic of type C retroviruses (59). The virion RNA is the typical 70s. As with BLV, the reverse transcriptase of HTLV prefers Mg^{2+} to Mn^{2+} (63). HTLV is distinct from all other known mammalian retroviruses on the basis of both nucleic acid hybridization and serologic analysis of the major virion proteins (47,62). It was shown, however, that HTLV has a distant relationship to BLV, by demonstrating conservation in the amino acid sequences at the 5' end of the *gag* gene (57). Other characteristics that HTLV and BLV have in common are a major virus capsid protein (p24) that is smaller than that of other mammalian retroviruses, a major virus envelope protein that is also smaller (about 45,000 to 52,000 daltons), and an inability to replicate to sufficiently high titers to produce viremia *in vivo* (19). HTLV also has the ability to immortalize human lymphoid cells *in vitro* when irradiated infected donor cells are cocultivated with unexposed recipient cells (31). The cells that become immortalized have the same phenotype as biopsied tumor cells.

The epidemiology of HTLV bears a striking relationship to the occurrence of the ATL disease. Seroepidemiologic surveys conducted in various locations around the world have shown that the prevalence rate for antibodies to HTLV and/or HTLV-associated antigens is directly proportional to the relative rates of ATL-type diseases (19). The various antigens used for antibody screening have included p24, in a radioimmunoassay (46); ATLA, an antigen detected in the cytoplasm of cultured ATL lines by fixed-cell immunofluorescence (38); and HTLV-MA, an antigen detected at the membrane of living cultured ATL cells by immunofluorescence (N. Tachibana, M. F. McLane, T. H. Lee, C. Howe, V. S. Kalyanaraman, R. C. Gallo, and M. Essex, *in preparation*). Using these systems, 90% or more of the patients with characteristic ATL and/or T-cell lymphoma have been found to be positive for such antibodies. Also, up to 30 to 50% of the healthy relatives and household associates of cases were found to have such antibodies, as did a significant proportion of the general adult population in endemic areas. In regions of southern Japan, for example, up to 30% of the healthy adults may have such antibodies, whereas in the Caribbean basin the prevalence rate is 3 to 6% and in the northeastern United States and western Europe it is significantly less than 1%. Nevertheless, antibody-positive cases of ATL-type disease and occasional antibody-positive carriers have been found in various regions in the world.

Of considerable importance from the standpoint of transmission of the virus is the recognition that most or all antibody-positive people may be virus carriers (19,31). The seroepidemiologic finding that the proportion of antibody-positive healthy adults increases with age is compatible with this finding. The primary mechanism of the spread of HTLV is unknown. It appears likely that the virus could be transmitted in blood transfusions, but this would obviously be insufficient to account for the large proportion of infected people in endemic areas. It is clear that the virus is horizontally rather than genetically acquired (74; N. Tachibana et al., *in preparation*). Antibodies that react with the ATLA antigen have recently been found in some Japanese monkeys (54), but contact with these animals would be rare.

CONCLUSIONS

We still know relatively little about how viruses actually cause leukemia or lymphoma. It is clear that most virus-induced leukemias of animals, as well as most human leukemias and lymphomas, represent monoclonal populations of cells. In the case of animal leukemias caused by retroviruses, the provirus can be found at the same site in all the cells of a given tumor. This apparently is also the case for the provirus of HTLV in ATL tumor cells (74), which indicates that the virus was present before the tumor process began and makes a strong argument for the establishment of an etiological relationship (19). BL is also a monoclonal disease, but because EBV, like most herpesviruses, exists primarily in an episomal rather than an integrated form, it is difficult to establish whether or not the virus is present before the oncogenic process. Nevertheless, data supporting this position have been gained by seroepidemiologic means (11).

Even if such viruses really do cause these neoplastic diseases, we must recognize that the vast majority of infected people resist this process. Clearly, large segments of the given population experience latent infections with agents such as the animal retroviruses, EBV, and HTLV, whereas only a few get cancer. EBV and HTLV can immortalize human lymphoid cells in culture (B and T cells, respectively), but this process cannot of itself be equivalent to the development of leukemia, because vast numbers of people maintain comparable populations of virus-immortalized cells for prolonged periods *in vivo* without developing disease. In such cases, a "second insult," whereby one of the viral-genome-carrying cells grows out as a tumor, must be viewed as being of key importance, and we have yet to understand much about this event. Either way, we would have to consider viral oncogenesis as a multiple-stage process that involves a minimum of several key gene functions.

We also know relatively little about the role that the immune response might play in the development of such diseases. In the case of virus-induced leukemias in inbred mice, evidence shows that replicating murine retroviruses cause a first-stage type of lymphocyte proliferative expansion by continual antigenic stimulation (52). Such stimulated cells should be more prone to random mutagenic damage if only because of their increased rate of mitosis. As a variation on this theme, such antigenically stimulated cells should also release lymphokines, which in turn would stimulate many more cells (in this instance, in a polyclonal manner) and subsequently increase the risk of mutagenic damage in the latter population (40). Alternatively, because an efficient immune response is known to play a protective role in some retrovirus-induced tumors, we could also postulate that the tumor outgrowth is caused by an immunoselection event that results in a loss of expression of tumor cell antigen(s) at the cell surface.

When we consider nonimmunological explanations for the important "second event," one proposed mechanism that stands out is "promotor insertion" or "mutational insertion," whereby the LTR of a retrovirus integrates into the regulatory domain of a given *onc* gene. In the case of retrovirus-induced B-cell lymphomas of chickens, this cellular *onc* gene has been identified as *myc* in elegant studies by Neel et al., which demonstrated increased levels of c-*myc* expression in these tumors (56). Enthusiasm for a possible role for this gene recently increased, when it was shown that c-*myc* is contained on the arm of human chromosome number 8 that becomes translocated to chromosome 14 in B-cell tumors (9,69).

Recent studies in molecular genetics have also focused on the identification of putative "cancer genes" by the transfection of human tumor cell DNA to NIH 3T3 cells. Such studies have identified DNA sequences in several types of human tumor cells that have increased ability to transform NIH 3T3 target cells (7). Among the types of cancer that have been successfully identified in this manner are the leukemias and lymphomas. However, even in the case of ALV-induced B-cell lymphomas of chickens, where c-*myc* is found to be activated at the RNA level, the gene involved in transformation of NIH 3T3 cells by transfection is apparently not c-*myc*. Thus, if those genes that transform mouse fibroblasts are important in leukemogenesis, we must still postulate that at least two and perhaps more cellular genes are essential to the second-stage process.

REFERENCES

1. Burkitt, D. (1962): A children's cancer dependent on climatic factors. *Nature*, 194:232–234.
2. Burny, A., Bruck, C., Chantrenne, H., Cleuter, Y., Dekegel, D., Ghysdael, J., Kettman, R., Leclercq, M., Leunen, J., Mammerickx, M., and Portetelle, D. (1980): Bovine leukemia virus: Molecular biology and epidemiology. In: *Viral Oncology*, edited by G. Klein, pp. 231–290. Raven Press, New York.
3. Calnek, B. W. (1972): Effects of passive antibody on early pathogenesis of Marek's disease. *Infect. Immun.*, 6:193–198.
4. Catovsky, D., Greaves, M. F., Rose, M., Galton, D. A. G., Goolden, A. W. G., McClusky, D. R., White, J. M., Lampert, I., Bourikas, G., Ireland, R., Bridges, J. M., Blattner, W. A., and Gallo, R. C. (1982): Adult T-cell leukemia-lymphoma in Blacks from the West Indies. *Lancet*, 1:639–643.
5. Chang, R. S., and Golden, H. D. (1971): Transformation of human lymphocytes by throat washing from infectious mononucleosis patients. *Nature*, 234:359–360.
6. Coffin, J. M., Varmus, H. E., Bishop, J. M., Essex, M., Hardy, W. D., Jr., Martin, G. S., Rosenberg, N. E., Scolnick, E. M., Weinberg, R. A., and Vogt, P. K. (1981): A proposal for naming host cell-derived inserts in retrovirus genomes. *J. Virol.*, 40:953–957.
7. Cooper, G. M. (1982): Cellular transforming genes. *Science*, 217:801–806.
8. Cotter, S. M., and Essex, M. (1977): Animal model for human disease: Feline acute lymphoblastic leukemia and non-regenerative anemia. *Am. J. Pathol.*, 87:265–268.
9. Dalla-Favera, R., Bregni, M., Erikson, J., Patterson, D., Gallo, R. C., and Croce, C. M. (1982): The human c-*myc onc* gene is located on the region of chromosome 8 which is translocated in Burkitt lymphoma cells. *Proc. Natl. Acad. Sci. USA*, 79:7824–7827.
10. Deinhardt, F. (1980): Biology of primate retroviruses. In: *Viral Oncology*, edited by G. Klein, pp. 357–398. Raven Press, New York.
11. de-Thé, G., Geser, A., Day, N. E., Tukei, P. M., Williams, E. H., Beri, D. P., Smith, P. G., Dean, A. G., Bornkamm, G. W., Feorino, P., and Henle, W. (1978): Epidemiological evidence for casual relationship between Epstein-Barr virus and Burkitt's lymphoma from Ugandan prospective study. *Nature*, 274:756–761.
12. Devare, S. G., Stephenson, J. R., Sarma, P. S., Aaronson, S. A., and Chandler, S. (1976): Bovine lymphosarcoma: Development of a radioimmunologic technique for detection of the etiologic agent. *Science*, 194:1428–1430.
13. DiStefano, H. S., and Dougherty, R. M. (1966): Mechanisms for congenital transmission of avian leukosis virus. *JNCI*, 37:869–883.
14. Driscoll, D. M., Onuma, M., and Olson, C. (1977): Inhibition of bovine leukemia virus release by antiviral antibodies. *Arch. Virol.*, 55:139–144.
15. Ellerman, V., and Bang, O. (1908): Experimentelle Leukamie bei Huhnern. *Zentralbl. Bakteriol.*, 46:595–609.
16. Epstein, M. A., Achong, B. G., and Barr, Y. M. (1964): Virus particles in cultured lymphoblasts from Burkitt's lymphoma. *Lancet*, 1:702–703.
17. Essex, M. (1975): Horizontally and vertically transmitted oncornaviruses of cats. *Adv. Cancer Res.*, 21:175–248.

18. Essex, M. (1980): Feline leukemia and sarcoma viruses. In: *Viral Oncology*, edited by G. Klein, pp. 205–229. Raven Press, New York.
19. Essex, M. (1982): Adult T-cell leukemia/lymphoma: Role of a human retrovirus. *JNCI*, 69:981–985.
20. Essex, M. (1982): Feline leukemia: A naturally occurring cancer of infectious origin. *Epidemiol. Rev.*, 4:189–203.
21. Essex, M. (1982): Horizontal and vertical transmission of retroviruses. In: *Viruses Associated with Human Cancer*, edited by L. Phillips, pp. 553–582. Marcel Dekker, New York.
22. Essex, M., Hardy, W. D., Jr., Cotter, S. M., Jakowski, R. M., and Sliski, A. (1975): Naturally occurring persistent feline oncornavirus infections in the absence of disease. *Infect. Immun.*, 11:470–475.
23. Essex, M., and Worley, M. (1981): RNA tumor viruses of animals. In: *Virus Infections of Animals*, edited by E. Kurstak and C. Kurstak, pp. 545–590. Academic Press, New York.
24. Ferrer, J. F. (1980): Bovine lymphosarcoma. *Adv. Vet. Sci. Comp. Med.*, 24:1–68.
25. Ferrer, J. F., Piper, C. E., Abt, D. A., and Marshak, R. R. (1977): Diagnosis of bovine leukemia virus infection: Evaluation of serologic and hematologic tests by a direct infectivity detection assay. *Am. J. Vet. Res.*, 38:1977–1981.
26. Fialkow, P. J., Klein, E., Klein, G., Clifford, P., and Singh, S. (1973): Immunoglobulin and glucose-6-phosphate dehydrogenase as markers of cellular origin in Burkitt lymphoma. *J. Exp. Med.*, 138:89–101.
27. Francis, D. P., Cotter, S. M., Hardy, W. D., Jr., and Essex, M. (1979): Feline leukemia and lymphoma: Comparison of virus positive and virus negative cases. *Cancer Res.*, 39:3866–3870.
28. Francis, D. P., Essex, M., and Hardy, W. D., Jr. (1977): Excretion of feline leukemia virus by naturally infected pet cats. *Nature*, 269:252–254.
29. Gallo, R. C., Mann, D., Broder, S., Ruscetti, F. W., Maeda, M., Kalyanaraman, V. S., Robert-Guroff, M., and Reitz, M. S., Jr. (1982): Human T-cell leukemia-lymphoma virus (HTLV) is in T but not B lymphocytes from a patient with cutaneous T-cell lymphoma. *Proc. Natl. Acad. Sci. USA*, 79:5680–5683.
30. Gootenberg, J. E., Ruscetti, F. W., Mier, J. M., Gazdar, A., and Gallo, R. C. (1981): Human cutaneous T-cell lymphoma and leukemia cell lines produce and respond to T cell growth factor. *J. Exp. Med.*, 154:1403–1418.
31. Gotoh, Y.-I., Sugamura, K., and Hinuma, Y. (1982): Healthy carriers of a human retrovirus, adult T-cell leukemia virus (ATLV): Demonstration by clonal culture of ATLV-carrying T cells from peripheral blood. *Proc. Natl. Acad. Sci. USA*, 79:4780–4782.
32. Grant, C. K., Essex, M., Pedersen, N. C., Hardy, W. D., Jr., Cotter, S. M., and Theilen, G. H. (1978): Cat antisera and cat complement lyse feline lymphoblastoid cells. Correlation of lysis with detection of antibodies to feline oncornavirus-associated cell membrane antigen. *JNCI*, 60:161–166.
33. Gross, L. (1951): "Spontaneous" leukemia developing in C3H mice following innoculation in infancy, with A-K leukemic extracts, or AK embryos. *Proc. Soc. Exp. Biol. Med.*, 76:27–32.
34. Gupta, P., and Ferrer, J. (1982): Expression of BLV genome is blocked by a nonimmunoglobulin protein in plasma from infected cattle. *Science*, 215:405–407.
35. Hardy, W. D., Jr., Old, L. J., Hess, P. W., Essex, M., and Cotter, S. M. (1973): Horizontal transmission of feline leukemia virus in cats. *Nature*, 244:266–269.
36. Henle, G., Henle, W., and Diehl, V. (1968): Relation of Burkitt's tumor-associated herpes type virus to infectious mononucleosis. *Proc. Natl. Acad. Sci. USA*, 59:94–101.
37. Henle, G., Henle, W., Zajac, B., Pearson, G., Waubke, R., and Scriba, M. (1970): Differential reactivity of human serums with early antigens induced by Epstein-Barr virus. *Science*, 169:188–190.
38. Hinuma, Y., Nagata, K., Hanaska, M., Nakai, M., Matsumoto, T., Kinoshita, K.-I., Shirakawa, S., and Miyoshi, I. (1981): Adult T-cell leukemia: antigen in an ATL line and detection of antibodies to the antigen in human sera. *Proc. Natl. Acad. Sci. USA*, 78:6476–6480.
39. Hoover, E. A., Kociba, G. J., Hardy, W. D., Jr., and Yohn, D. S. (1974): Erythroid hypoplasia in cats inoculated with feline leukemia virus. *JNCI*, 53:1271–1276.
40. Ihle, J. N., Lee, J. C., Enjuanes, L., Cicurel, L., Horak, I., and Pepersack, L. (1980): Chronic immunostimulation as a possible mechanism in type C viral leukemogenesis. In: *Viruses in Naturally Occurring Cancer*, edited by M. Essex, G. J. Todaro, and H. zur Hausen, pp. 1049–1064. Cold Spring Harbor Press, Cold Spring Harbor, NY.

41. Jakowski, R. M., Essex, M., Hardy, W. D., Jr., Stephenson, J. R., and Cotter, S. M. (1980): Membranous glomerulonephritis in a household cluster of cats persistently viremic with feline leukemia virus. In: *Feline Leukemia and Sarcoma Viruses*, edited by W. D. Hardy, Jr., M. Essex, and A. J. McClelland, pp. 141–150. Elsevier/North-Holland, Amsterdam.

42. Jarrett, O., Hardy, W. D., Jr., Golder, M. C., and Hay, D. (1978): The frequency of occurrence of feline leukemia virus subgroups in cats. *Int. J. Cancer*, 21:334–337.

43. Jarrett, O., and Russell, P. H. (1978): Differential growth and transmission in cats of feline leukemia viruses of subgroups A and B. *Int. J. Cancer*, 21:466–472.

44. Jarrett, W. F. H., Crawford, E. M., Martin, W. B., and Davie, F. (1964): Leukaemia in the cat. A virus-like particle associated with leukaemia (lymphosarcoma). *Nature*, 202:567–568.

45. Jarrett, W. F. H., Martin, W. B., Crighton, G. W., Dalton, R. G., and Stewart, M. F. (1964): Leukaemia in the cat. Transmission experiments with leukaemia (lymphosarcoma). *Nature*, 202:566–567.

46. Kalyanaraman, V. S., Sarngadharan, M. G., Nakao, Y., Ito, Y., Aoki, T., and Gallo, R. C. (1982): Natural antibodies to the structural core protein (p24) of the human T-cell leukemia (lymphoma) retrovirus found in sera of leukemia patients in Japan. *Proc. Natl. Acad. Sci. USA*, 79:1653–1657.

47. Kalyanaraman, V. S., Sarngadharan, M. G., Poiesz, B., Ruscetti, F. W., and Gallo, R. C. (1981): Immunological properties of a type C retrovirus isolated from cultured human T-lymphoma cells and comparison to other mammalian retroviruses. *J. Virol.*, 38:906–915.

48. Kawakami, T. G., Sun, L., and McDowell, T. S. (1978): Distribution and transmission of primate type-C virus. In: *Advances in Comparative Leukemia Research 1977*, edited by P. Bentvelzen, J. Hilgers, and D. S. Yohn, pp. 33–36. Elsevier/North-Holland, Amsterdam.

49. Kawakami, T. G., Sun, L., and McDowell, T. S. (1978): Natural transmission of gibbon leukemia virus. *JNCI*, 61:1113–1115.

50. Klein, G., Clifford, P., Klein, E., and Stjernsward, J. (1966): Search for tumor-specific immune reactions in Burkitt's lymphoma patients by the membrane immunofluorescence reaction. *Proc. Natl. Acad. Sci. USA*, 55:1628–1635.

51. Lee, T. H., McLane, M. F., Essex, M., McCarty, J., and Grant, C. K. (1983): Feline leukemia virus proteins at the surface of cultured virus-producer cells. *Leuk. Rev.*, 1:93–94.

52. McGrath, M. S., Jerabek, L., Pillemer, E., Steinberg, R. A., and Weissman, I. L. (1981): Receptor mediated murine leukemogenesis: Monoclonal antibody induced lymphoma cell growth arrest. In: *Modern Trends in Human Leukemia, Vol. 4*, edited by R. Neth, R. C. Gallo, T. Graf, K. Mannweiler, and K. Winkler, pp. 360–364. Springer-Verlag, New York.

53. Miller, G. (1975): Epstein-Barr herpesvirus and infectious mononucleosis. *Prog. Med. Virol.*, 20:84–112.

54. Miyoshi, I., Yoshimoto, S., Fujishita, M., Taguchi, H., Kubonishi, I., and Niiya, K. (1982): Natural adult T-cell leukaemia virus infection in Japanese monkeys. *Lancet*, 2:658.

55. Nazerian, K. (1980): Marke's disease: A herpesvirus-induced malignant lymphoma of the chicken. In: *Viral Oncology*, edited by G. Klein, pp. 665–682. Raven Press, New York.

56. Neel, B. G., Hayward, W. S., Robinson, H. L., Fang, J., and Astrin, S. M. (1981): Avian leukosis virus-induced tumors have common proviral integration sites and synthesize discrete new RNAs: Oncogenesis by promoter insertion. *Cell*, 23:323–334.

57. Oroszlan, S., Sarngadharan, M. G., Copeland, T. D., Kalyanaraman, V. S., Gilden, R. V., and Gallo, R. C. (1982): Primary structure analysis of the major internal protein p24 of human type C T-cell leukemia virus. *Proc. Natl. Acad. Sci. USA*, 79:1291–1294.

58. Poiesz, B. J., Ruscetti, F. W., Gazdar, A. F., Bunn, P. A., Minna, J. D., and Gallo, R. C. (1980): Detection and isolation of type C retrovirus particles from fresh and cultured lymphocytes of a patient with cutaneous T-cell lymphoma. *Proc. Natl. Acad. Sci. USA*, 77:7415–7419.

59. Poiesz, B. J., Ruscetti, F. W., Reitz, M. S., Kalyanaraman, V. S., and Gallo, R. C. (1981): Isolation of a new type C retrovirus (HTLV) in primary uncultured cells of a patient with Sézary T-cell leukaemia. *Nature*, 294:268–271.

60. Purchase, H. G. (1976): Prevention of Marek's disease. *Cancer Res.*, 36:696–700.

61. Reedman, B. M., and Klein, G. (1973): Cellular localization of an Epstein-Barr virus (EBV)-associated complement-fixing antigen in producer and nonproducer lymphoblastoid cells of patients with infectious mononucleosis. *Int. J. Cancer*, 14:704–715.

62. Reitz, M. S., Poiesz, B. J., Ruscetti, F. W., and Gallo, R. C. (1981): Characterization and dis-

tribution of nucleic acid sequences of a novel type C retrovirus isolated from neoplastic human T lymphocytes. *Proc. Natl. Acad. Sci. USA*, 78:1887–1891.

63. Rho, H. M., Poiesz, B., Ruscetti, F. W., and Gallo, R. C. (1981): Characterization of the reverse transcriptase from a new retrovirus (HTLV) produced by a human cutaneous T-cell lymphoma cell line. *Virology*, 112:355–360.

64. Rojko, J. L., Hoover, E. A., Quackenbush, S. L., and Olsen, R. G. (1982): Reactivation of latent feline leukaemia virus infection. *Nature*, 298:385–388.

65. Rous, P. (1911): A sarcoma of the fowl transmissible by an agent separable from the tumor cells. *J. Exp. Med.*, 13:397–411.

66. Rubin, H., Fanshier, L., Cornelius, A., and Hughes, W. J. (1962): Tolerance and immunity in chickens after congenital and contact infection with an avian leukosis virus. *Virology*, 17:143–156.

67. Salaman, M. H., Wedderburn, N., and Bruce-Chwatt, L. J. (1969): The immunodepressive effect of a murine plasmodium and its interaction with murine oncogenic viruses. *J. Gen. Microbiol.*, 59:383–391.

68. Sarma, P. S., Log, J., Damine, J., Hill, P. R., and Huebner, R. (1975): Differential host range of viruses of feline leukemia-sarcoma complex. *Virology*, 64:438–446.

69. Taub, R., Kirsch, I., Morton, C., Lenoir, G., Swan, D., Tronick, S., Aaronson, S., and Leder, P. (1982): Translocation of the c-*myc* gene into the immunoglobulin heavy chain locus in human Burkitt's lymphoma and murine plasmacytoma cells. *Proc. Natl. Acad. Sci. USA*, 79:7837–7841.

70. Todaro, G. J. (1980): Interspecies transmission of mammalian retroviruses. In: *Viral Oncology*, edited by G. Klein, pp. 291–309. Raven Press, New York.

71. Tsichlis, P. N., and Coffin, J. M. (1980): Recombinants between endogenous and exogenous avian tumor viruses: Role of the C region and other portions of the genome in the control of replication and transformation. *J. Virol.*, 33:238–249.

72. Uchiyama, T., Yodoi, J., Sagawa, K., Takatsuki, K., and Uchino, H. (1977): Adult T-cell leukemia: Clinical and hematologic features of 16 cases. *Blood*, 50:481–492.

73. Vogt, P. K. (1967): Phenotypic mixing in the avian tumor virus group. *Virology*, 32:708–718.

74. Yoshida, M., Miyoshi, I., and Hinuma, Y. (1982): Isolation and characterization of retrovirus from cell lines of human adult T-cell leukemia and its implication in the disease. *Proc. Natl. Acad. Sci. USA*, 79:2031–2035.

75. zur Hausen, H. (1976): Biochemical approaches to detection of Epstein-Barr virus in human tumors. *Cancer Res.*, 36:678–680.

76. zur Hausen, H., Diehl, V., Wolf, H., Schulte-Holt-Hausen, H., and Schneider, U. (1972): Occurrence of the Epstein-Barr virus genomes in human lymphoblastoid cell lines. *Nature (New Biol.)*, 237:189–190.

Pathogenesis of Leukemias and Lymphomas:
Environmental Influences, edited by
I. T. Magrath, G. T. O'Conor, and B. Ramot.
Raven Press, New York © 1984.

A Retrovirus Associated with Human Adult T-cell Leukemia-Lymphoma

M. S. Reitz, Jr., M. Robert-Guroff, V. S. Kalyanaraman,
M. G. Sarngadharan, P. Sarin, M. Popovic, and R. C. Gallo

Laboratory of Tumor Cell Biology, National Cancer Institute, National Institutes of Health, Bethesda, Maryland 20205

When the causes of naturally occurring leukemia or lymphoma in different species have been identified, the primary agent has been a virus. In most cases, these viruses are retroviruses, or RNA tumor viruses. Species for which retroviruses appear to be the cause of most of these diseases include chickens, cats, wild mice, cattle, turkeys, and gibbon apes (3,35).

Retroviruses are characterized by, among other properties, an RNA genome existing as a dimer of two polyadenylated, approximately 8.4 Kb RNA molecules sedimenting at 70S, a reverse transcriptase that copies the RNA genome into a double-stranded DNA provirus, and a replication cycle that includes the integration of the provirus into the host cell DNA. Based on their natural route of transmission, two general types of retroviruses exist. Endogenous retroviruses are transmitted genetically as a provirus; are rarely expressed into viral DNA, protein, or particles; are found in the germ line of most or all members of their host species; and have not been associated with naturally occurring malignancy. Exogenous retroviruses, in contrast, are transmitted by infection with viral particles (although they may be very poorly infectious and have long latent periods). Infection can be congenital (by milk or intrauterine) or horizontal (from one individual to another). Exogenous viruses are frequently associated with or causative of leukemia and lymphoma. Age at the time of infection, virs dosage, and the host immune response all appear to be critical factors in determining whether or not disease will develop. (For a more critical discussion of the viral etiology of naturally occurring animal leukemias and lymphomas, see M. Essex, *this volume.*)

Until recently, no human retroviruses had been unequivocally demonstrated, although much suggestive data had been reported over the years. In retrospect, this was at least partly because of the inability to grow the appropriate types of cells *in vitro*. Our laboratory had long been interested in growing different specific types of hematopoietic cells. T cells were of obvious interest, because virus-induced leukemia in animals often involves T cells as targets for infection (15).

In 1976, we were able to identify a factor from short-term mitogen-stimulated cultures of peripheral blood lymphocytes from mixed donors that supported the long-term growth of human T cells (19,35). This was called the T cell growth factor (TCGF).

Using highly purified TCGF, T cells from normal people could be grown only after mitogen stimulation (16), indicating that TCGF is actually a second signal for T-cell growth. In using TCGF to culture T cells from patients with several neoplastic T-cell diseases, however, it was discovered that prior mitogen activation was not required, and long-term growth was achieved with TCGF alone (23). This seems to be caused by the constitutive expression of receptors for TCGF on the surface of T cells from these patients, but not from normal persons (8). Some of the biochemical markers of the cells from these neoplastic cultures, as well as their ability to respond directly to purified TCGF, suggested that the cultures consist, at least in part, of the malignant T cells.

IDENTIFICATION AND CHARACTERIZATION OF THE HUMAN T-CELL LEUKEMIA-LYMPHOMA VIRUS

Two T-cell lines (HUT-102 and CTCL-3), both derived from a patient (CR) with a highly malignant cutaneous lymphoma of mature T cells, were studied. Electron microscopy showed the presence of typical retrovirus particles in the cells (Fig. 1), and reverse transcriptase was demonstrated in the culture medium. This enzyme was associated with a particle that had a buoyant density of 1.16 g/cc in sucrose, characteristic of retrovirus (22). The virus, provisionally designated human T-cell leukemia-lymphoma virus (HTLV), was also shown to contain a polyadenylated 70S RNA, in common with other retroviruses (28).

In experiments with labeled cDNA prepared by reverse transcription of HTLV 70S RNA, no significant homology of HTLV DNA to any other animal retrovirus was observed (28). Similar findings were reported for two major core proteins, p24 (14) and p19 (31), and the reverse transcriptase (29), based on protein serology. The reverse transcriptase has several distinctive biochemical properties (29). They include a size somewhat larger (95,000 daltons) than that of reverse transcriptase from most type C retroviruses and a slight preference for Mg^{2+} over Mn^{2+} as the divalent cation. In these properties, as well as in the size of its core proteins, HTLV most closely resembles bovine leukemia virus, a leukemogenic virus of cattle. Consistent with this, Oroszlan et al. (21) have reported that the amino acid sequence of the p24 of HTLV shows a distant but significant relatedness to the p24 of BLV. It is, however, important to emphasize that conventional serologic and liquid nucleic acid hybridization assays do not show cross-reactivity between HTLV and BLV.

A second retrovirus was identified in the cultured T cells of a second patient (MB) with a similar disease that also exhibited a leukemic phase (24). This virus was shown to be very closely related or identical to HTLV by nucleic acid hybridization and protein serology. Viral proteins and proviral DNA were also detected in *uncultured* tissue from the same patient, virtually ruling out a laboratory contamination.

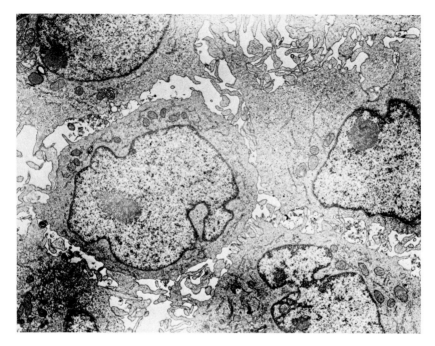

FIG. 1. HTLV particles in T-cell line CTC-16 from patient CR. Two HTLV particles are shown. ×30,000.

The absence of HTLV viral sequences in DNA from many samples of human cells and tissues tested in our laboratory indicated that HTLV is not an endogenous virus of man (28). The presence of HTLV provirus in some of the T cells of patient CR and its absence from other of the T cells, as well as from B cells derived from the same patient, indicate that CR acquired the virus via a postzygotic infection (6). HTLV is, therefore, like all of the leukemogenic retroviruses of other species, an exogenously transmitted virus.

PREVALENCE OF HTLV IN JAPANESE ADULT T-CELL LEUKEMIA

Since the first two patients from which HTLV was isolated were diagnosed as having mycosis fungoides (CR) or Sézary syndrome (MB), a number of serum samples were screened from patients with these diseases. Specific antibodies to both p24 and p19 were found in a few of these sera (12,27), as well as in the sera of the clinically normal spouse of CR (12). All other normal sera were negative, as were most of the sera obtained from patients with mycosis fungoides and/or Sézary syndrome. It seemed (and is now apparent) that most patients with antibodies against HTLV had similar clinical features, usually including a rapid disease course, hepatosplenomegaly, lymphoadenopathy, large and usually pleomorphic lympho-cytes with lobulated nuclei and mature T-cell surface phenotype markers (usually

OKT 4 +), and hypercalcemia. More than half of these patients have skin manifestations. Typical cells from a patient with this type of disease are shown in Fig.
2. This disease is similar or identical to a category of lymphoid neoplasm that has
been referred to as "diffuse peripheral T-cell lymphoma" (11).

A T-cell leukemia occurring in adults, which is endemic in southern Japan, had
been previously described by Takatsuki and his co-workers (33). The clinical symptoms of this disease, called adult T-cell leukemia (ATL), are very much like those
of the HTLV-positive cases in the United States (34,35). This prompted a survey
of Japanese ATL sera. It was soon evident that antibodies to the HTLV proteins
p24 and p19 were consistently present in these sera and were also found in sera
from some normal persons from the same geographical area (7,13,30). Consistent
with these findings, several laboratories in Japan have subsequently reported the
detection of retrovirus particles by electron microscopy in cultured T lymphocytes
from a few ATL patients and the presence of serum antibodies in almost all ATL
patients (and in approximately 26% of normal persons from the same region) specific
for determinants present on cells producing the retrovirus particles (10,18). The
similarity in the distribution of these antibodies and those against HTLV suggests
that the Japanese retrovirus is identical to HTLV. This has been verified by showing
that the virus produced by MT-1, a cell line used for the studies by Hinuma et al.
(10) and Miyoshi et al. (16), has antigenic determinants indistinguishable from

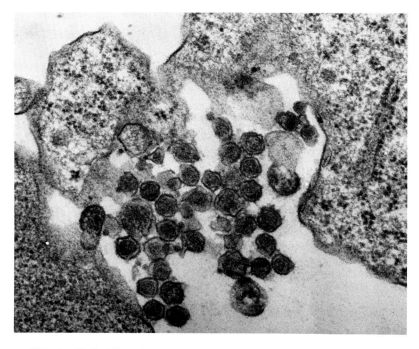

FIG. 2. Typical T cell from patient CR, showing indented nucleus. × 4,000.

HTLV p19 and p24 and that the viral mRNA and proviral DNA hybridize virtually completely to HTLV ^{3}H-cDNA (25).

Interestingly, cocultivation of cord blood T lymphocytes with a second cell line (MT-2) described in Miyoshi et al. (18) has resulted in the establishment of TCGF-independent cell lines of cord blood origin (17), which suggests that the MT-2 virus has acquired an oncogene, enabling it to directly transform human T cells. Infection of cord blood T cells with HTLV has, in our laboratory, routinely yielded several reproducible biological effects. These include a reduction in the requirement for TCGF, an abrogation of the crisis period that frequently prevents these cells from growing beyond six to eight weeks, and an acquisition of the ability to grow in soft agar (26). Moreover, in rare instances, TCGF independence and immortalization are obtained.

HTLV IN ATL IN THE CARIBBEAN

In collaboration with W. Blattner and his colleagues in the NCI Epidemiology Branch (W. A. Blattner et al., *this volume*) and D. Catovsky, M. Greaves, and D. Galton in London, our laboratory has identified the Caribbean as another region in which HTLV is unusually prevalent, for patients in this region with a similar T-cell neoplasm to that described above have antibodies against HTLV (2). In the Caribbean, as in southern Japan, incidence of this clinical entity appears to be relatively high (1), and as is true for the endemic region of Japan, some normal persons also are antibody-positive. We have isolated virus from cultured T cells of Caribbean and Japanese ATL patients, as well as of similar patients from the Boston area, Israel, Ecuador, Alaska, and the southeasten United States, and all appear very similar, if not identical (5). The extent of the geographical distribution of HTLV is not yet clear (except for Japan and the Caribbean basin), but the virus is probably present in other places not yet identified.

DISCUSSION

If HTLV is the primary causal agent in ATL, how might it induce the disease? One possibility is by insertion of a viral RNA polymerase promoter in a location where it could "turn on" cellular genes whose inappropriate expression would result in the transformed phenotype. There is good evidence that this is the main mechanism whereby avian retroviruses induce avian bursal lymphomas (9,20), and it has been termed "downstream promotion." It has been suggested that HTLV infection might cause the downstream promotion of the gene for TCGF, resulting in its constitutive expression and inappropriate T-cell expansion. Some, but not all, of the available evidence favors this model (4). It is obvious that HTLV infection alone does not suffice to cause ATL, because not only do many normal persons manifest persistent serum antibodies to HTLV (1,7,10,12,13,30) but in some cases they also harbor virus in their peripheral blood T cells (M. Robert-Guroff et al., *in preparation*). It has been estimated that only one of 2,000 infected persons develop ATL (see T. Suchi and K. Tajima, *this volume*). Host-specific or environmental factors, age at first infection, repetitive infections, route of infection, or other parameters may all play a role. HTLV might be involved in other diseases, including those of a nonneoplastic nature.

How is HTLV transmitted? If a substantial portion of the normal population in the endemic regions is indeed infected, a nonhuman reservoir of HTLV is not required. HTLV does not appear to be highly infectious and may require prolonged intimate contact for transmission. This could occur within families (mother's milk, sexual contact) or by blood transfusions or insect bites. Obviously, much remains to be determined. The identification of HTLV, however, in addition to providing new insights into a human neoplasm, raises the possibility of being able to better treat or even to prevent ATL in the future.

REFERENCES

1. Blattner, W. A., Kalyanaraman, V. S., Robert-Guroff, M., Lister, T. A., Galton, D. A. G., Sarin, P. S., Crawford, M. H., Catovsky, D., Greaves, M., and Gallo, R. C. (1982): The human type-C retrovirus, HTLV, in Blacks from the Caribbean region, and relationship to adult T-cell leukemia/lymphoma. *Int. J. Cancer*, 30:257–264.
2. Catovsky, D., Greaves, M. F., Rose, M., Galton, D. A. G., Golden, A. W. G., McCluskey, D. R., White, J. M., Lampert, I., Bourikas, G., Ireland, R., Bridges, J. M., Blattner, W. A., and Gallo, R. C. (1982): Adult T-cell lymphoma-leukaemia in Blacks from the West Indies. *Lancet*, 1:639–643.
3. Gallo, R. C. (1978): Leukemia, environmental factors and viruses. In: *Viruses and Environment*, edited by E. Kurstak and K. Maramorosch, pp. 43–78. Academic Press, New York.
4. Gallo, R. C. (1982): Regulation of human T-cell proliferation: T-cell growth factor, T-cell leukemias and lymphomas, and isolation of a new C-type retrovirus. In: *Malignant Lymphomas: Etiology, Immunology, Pathology, Treatment*, edited by H. S. Kaplan and S. A. Rosenberg, pp. 201–218. Academic Press, New York.
5. Gallo, R. C., Kalyanaraman, V. S., and Sarngadharanm, M. G. (1983): The human type-C retrovirus: association with a subset of adult T-cell malignancies. *Cancer Res. (in press)*.
6. Gallo, R. C., Mann, D., Broder, S., Ruscetti, F. W., Maeda, M., Kalyanaraman, V. S., Robert-Guroff, M., and Reitz, M. S., Jr. (1982): Human T-cell leukemia-lymphoma virus (HTLV) is in T- but not B-lymphocytes from a patient with cutaneous T-cell lymphoma. *Proc. Nat. Acad. Sci., U.S.A.*, 79:5680–5683.
7. Gallo, R. C., Robert-Guroff, M., Kalyanaraman, V. S., Ceccherini Nelli, L., Ruscetti, F. W., Broder, S., Sarngadharan, M. G., Ito, Y., Maeda, M., Wainberg, J., and Reitz, M. S. (1983): Human T-cell retrovirus and adult T-cell lymphoma and leukemia: Possible factors on viral incidence. In: *Biochemical and Biological Markers on Neoplastic Transformation*, edited by P. Chandra, pp. 503–513. Plenum Press, New York.
8. Gootenberg, J. E., Ruscetti, F. W., Mier, J. W., Gazdar, A. F., and Gallo, R. C. (1981): Human cutaneous T-cell lymphoma and leukemia cell lines produce and response to T-cell growth factor. *J. Exp. Med.*, 154:1403–1418.
9. Hayward, W. S., Neel, B. G., and Astrin, S. M. (1981): Activation of a cellular *onc* gene by promoter insertion in ALV-induced lymphoid leukosis. *Nature*, 290:475–480.
10. Hinuma, Y., Nagata, K., Misoka, J., Nakai, M., Matsumoto, T., Kinoshita, K. I., Shirakawa, S., and Miyoshi, I. (1981): Adult T-cell leukemia: Antigen in an ATL cell line and detection of antibodies to the antigen in human sera. *Proc. Natl. Acad. Sci. USA*, 78:6476–6480.
11. Jaffe, E. S. (1980): Non-Hodgkin's lymphomas as neoplasms of the immune system. *Ann. Intern. Med.*, 94:222–226.
12. Kalyanaraman, V. S., Sarngadharan, M. G., Bunn, P. A., Minna, J. D., and Gallo, R. C. (1981): Antibodies in human sera reactive against an internal structural protein of human T cell lymphoma virus. *Nature*, 294:271–273.
13. Kalyanaraman, V. S., Sarngadharan, M. G., Nakao, Y., Ito, Y., Aoki, T., and Gallo, R. C. (1982): Natural antibodies to the structural core protein (p24) of the human T-cell leukemia (lymphoma) retrovirus found in sera of leukemia patients in Japan. *Proc. Natl. Acad. Sci. USA*, 79:1653–1657.

14. Kalyanaraman, V. S., Sarngadharan, M. G., Poiesz, B. J., Ruscetti, F. W., and Gallo, R. C. (1981): Immunological properties of a type-C retrovirus isolated from cultured human T-lymphoma cells and comparison to other mammalian retroviruses. *J. Virol.*, 38:906–915.

15. Kaplan, H. (1974): Leukemia and lymphoma in experimental and domestic animals. *Sem. Hematol.*, 7:94–163.

16. Mier, J. W., and Gallo, R. C. (1980): Purification and some characteristics of human T-cell growth factor from phytohemagglutinin-stimulated lymphocyte conditioned media. *Proc. Natl. Acad. Sci. USA*, 77:6134–6138.

17. Miyoshi, I., Kubonishi, I., Sumida, M., Hiraki, S., Tsubota, T., Kimura, I., Miyamoto, K., and Sato, J. (1981): Transformation of normal human cord lymphocytes by co-cultivating with a lethally irradiated human T-cell line carrying type-C virus particles. *GANN*, 71:155–156.

18. Miyoshi, I., Kubonishi, I., Yoshimoto, S., Akagi, T., Ohtsuki, Y., Shiraiski, Y., Nagata, K., and Hinuma, Y. (1981): Type C virus particles in a cord T-cell line derived by co-cultivating normal human leukocytes and human leukemic T-cells. *Nature*, 294:770–771.

19. Morgan, D. A., Ruscetti, F. W., and Gallo, R. C. (1976): Selective *in vitro* growth of T-lymphocytes from normal human bone marrows. *Science*, 193:1007–1008.

20. Neel, B. G., Hayward, W. S., Robinson, H. L., Fang, J., and Astrin, S. M. (1981): Avian leukosis virus induced tumors have common proviral integration sites and synthesize discrete new RNAs: Oncogenesis by promotor insertion. *Cell*, 23:323–334.

21. Oroszlan, S., Sarngadharan, M. G., Copeland, T. D., Kalyanaraman, V. S., Gilden, R. V., and Gallo, R. C. (1982): Primary structure analysis of the major internal protein p24 of human type C T-cell leukemia virus. *Proc. Natl. Acad. Sci. USA*, 79:1291–1294.

22. Poiesz, B. J., Ruscetti, F. W., Gazdar, A. F., Bunn, P. A., Minna, J. D., and Gallo, R. C. (1980): Detection and isolation of type-C retrovirus particles from fresh and cultured lymphocytes of a patient with cutaneous T-cell lymphoma. *Proc. Natl. Acad. Sci. USA*, 77:7415–7419.

23. Poiesz, B. J., Ruscetti, F. W., Mier, J. W., Woods, A. M., and Gallo, R. C. (1980): T-cell lines established from human T-lymphocytic neoplasias by direct response to T-cell growth factor. *Proc. Natl. Acad. Sci. USA*, 77:6815–6819.

24. Poiesz, B. J., Ruscetti, F. W., Reitz, M. S., Kalyanaraman, V. S., and Gallo, R. C. (1981): Isolation of a new type C retrovirus (HTLV) in primary uncultured cells of a patient with Sézary T-cell leukaemia. *Nature*, 294:268–271.

25. Popovic, M., Reitz, M. S., Sarngadharan, M., Robert-Guroff, M., Kalyanaraman, V. S., Nakau, Y., Miyoshi, I., Minowada, J., Yoshida, M., and Gallo, R. C. (1982): The virus of Japanese T-cell leukemia is a member of the human T-cell leukemia group. *Nature*, 300:63–66.

26. Popovic, M., Sarin, P., Robert-Guroff, M., Kalyanaraman, V. S., Mann, D., Minowada, J., and Gallo, R. C. (1983): Isolation and transmission of human retrovirus (human T-cell leukemia virus). *Science*, 219:856–859.

27. Posner, L. E., Robert-Guroff, M., Kalyanaraman, V. S., Poiesz, B. J., Ruscetti, F. W., Bunn, P. A., Minna, J. D., and Gallo, R. C. (1981): Natural antibodies to the human T cell lymphoma virus in patients with cutaneous T cell lymphomas. *J. Exp. Med.*, 154:333–346.

28. Reitz, M. S., Poiesz, B. J., Ruscetti, F. W., and Gallo, R. C. (1981): Characterization and distribution of nucleic acid sequences of a novel type-C retrovirus isolated from neoplastic human T-lymphocytes. *Proc. Natl. Acad. Sci. USA*, 78:1887–1891.

29. Rho, H. M., Poiesz, B. J., Ruscetti, F. W., and Gallo, R. C. (1981): Characterization of the reverse transcriptase from a new retrovirus (HTLV) produced by a human cutaneous T-cell lymphoma cell line. *Virology*, 112:355–360.

30. Robert-Guroff, M., Nakao, Y., Notake, K., Ito, Y., Sliski, A., and Gallo, R. C. (1982): Natural antibodies to human retrovirus HTLV in a cluster of Japanese patients with adult T cell leukemia. *Science*, 215:975–978.

31. Robert-Guroff, M., Ruscetti, F. W., Posner, L. E., Poiesz, B. J., and Gallo, R. C. (1981): Detection of the human T cell lymphoma virus p19 in cells of some patients with cutaneous T cell lymphoma and leukemia using a monoclonal antibody. *J. Exp. Med.*, 154:1957–1964.

32. Ruscetti, F. W., Morgan, D. A., and Gallo, R. C. (1977): Functional and morphologic characterization of human T cells continuously grown *in vitro*. *J. Immunol.*, 119:131–138.

33. Takatsuki, K., Uchiyama, T., Sagawa, K., and Yodoi, J. (1977): Adult T-cell leukemia in Japan. In: *Topics in Hematology*, edited by S. Seno, F. Takaku, and S. Irino, pp. 73–77. Excerpta Medica, Amsterdam.

34. Takatsuki, K., Uchiyama, T., Ueshima, Y., and Hattori, T. (1979): Adult T-cell leukemia: Further

clinical observations and cytogenetic and functional studies of leukemic cells. *Jpn. J. Clin. Oncol.*, 9:317–324.

35. Uchiyama, T., Yohoi, J., Sagawa, K., Takatsuki, K., and Uchino, H. (1977): Adult T-cell leukemia: Clinical and hematologic features of 16 cases. *Blood*, 50:481–492.

36. Wong-Staal, F., and Gallo, R. C. (1982): Retroviruses and leukemia. In: *Leukemia*, edited by F. Gunz and E. Henderson, pp. 329–358. Grune & Stratton, New York.

Pathogenesis of Leukemias and Lymphomas:
Environmental Influences, edited by
I. T. Magrath, G. T. O'Conor, and B. Ramot.
Raven Press, New York © 1984.

Preliminary Epidemiologic Observations on a Virus Associated with T-cell Neoplasia in Man

*William A. Blattner, **Marjorie Robert-Guroff,
**V. S. Kalyanaraman, †Prem Sarin, ††Elaine S. Jaffe,
*Douglas W. Blayney, *Katharine A. Zener,
and †Robert C. Gallo

*Family Studies Section, Environmental Epidemiology Branch; †Laboratory of Tumor Cell Biology; and ††Laboratory of Pathology, National Cancer Institute, National Institutes of Health, Bethesda, Maryland 20205; and **Department of Cell Biology, Litton Bionetics, Inc., Kensington, Maryland 20895*

Human T-cell leukemia/lymphoma virus (HTLV) is the first retrovirus consistently isolated from patients with a specific disease (6,14,15). Earlier studies have shown that HTLV is distinct from any known animal retrovirus, and its proteins are not detectably related to any normal cellular protein (6,9,11,14,15,18–20). Recent studies of the amino acid sequence of HTLV p24 have shown a very distant relatedness to p24 of bovine leukemia virus (BLV) (13). However, the p24 and other major structural proteins are antigenically and structurally distinct from BLV proteins (9,11,18–20). HTLV proviral sequences are present in DNA of neoplastic T cells but not in DNA of uninfected cells, demonstrating that HTLV is an exogenous virus that must be acquired by infection (5,18).

We summarize here the current epidemiologic data on the distribution of HTLV and its association with certain malignancies. Our preliminary studies suggest that HTLV is associated with clusters of mature T-cell leukemia/lymphoma in restricted areas where HTLV infection is prevalent. Occasional patients from virus-nonendemic areas may have acquired their HTLV infection before developing their T-cell leukemia/lymphoma through travel into and close contacts with residents of HTLV-endemic areas.

MATERIALS AND METHODS

Serum antibodies to a disrupted whole-virus preparation were detected by a modification to the radioimmune assay (RIA) technique previously reported (17). In brief, a microtiter plate was coated with disrupted HTLV or a negative control, disrupted avian myeloblastosis virus. Thawed human serum was diluted 1:10 with phosphate-buffered saline containing 0.5% Tween 20 (PBS/Tween) and incubated on the plates. Unbound proteins were aspirated, and the plates were washed in PBS/ Tween three times. The plates were incubated again with rabbit anti-human IgG. Aspiration and washing repeated as before. Iodinated Staphlococcus Protein A (Pharmacin) was added to each well, incubated, aspirated, and washed. Individual wells were separated and counted in a gamma counter. After subtraction of control values, sera that bound significantly to disrupted HTLV were scored as positive only if their reactivity could be abolished by competition with extracts of HTLV-producing cells but not by extracts of non-HTLV-producing cells or by fetal calf serum.

Natural antibody to the major core protein p24 of HTLV was detected by a radioimmune precipitation as previously described (9). Serial twofold dilutions of thawed serum were made using 20 microliters of buffer (200 mM Tris-HCl, pH 7.5; 200 mM NaCl; 1 mM EDTA; 0.3% Triton X-100, 0.1 mM phenylmethyl sulfonyl fluoride, and 2 mg/ml bovine serum albumin). The reaction mixture was incubated for 2 hr at 37°C and overnight at 4°C with purified, homogenous, iodinated HTLV p24. Immune complexes were precipitated by adding a 20-fold excess of goat anti-human IgG, diluting with buffer to 500 microliters, and centrifuging. The supernatant was aspirated, and the pellet was counted on a gamma counter. Specificity for HTLV p24 has been demonstrated for this assay by competition experiments using disrupted retroviruses and cellular extracts (4).

In some cases a competitive binding assay with a monoclonal anti-p19 (20) was performed to demonstrate natural antibody to HTLV p19. Briefly, dilutions of human sera were mixed with an equal volume of a 1:50,000 dilution of mouse ascites fluid containing monoclonal anti-p19. Fifty-μl aliquots were incubated for 45 min at 37°C on a microtiter plate coated with disrupted HTLV. The plate was washed, and 50,000 cpm of goat anti-mouse IgG was added to detect binding of the mouse monoclonal anti-p19 to p19 in the HTLV preparation. The titer of natural human anti-p19 was expressed as the reciprocal of the dilution of serum able to compete 50% of the binding of the monoclonal p19 in the presence of a pooled normal human serum.

Samples from various patient and normal populations were submitted as frozen serum or plasma except for samples from Japan, which were sent lyophilized and were reconstituted to the original serum volume before assay. The clinical and pathologic diagnoses were as recorded by the submitting investigator, except for certain cases where slides or blocks were reviewed by E. S. Jaffe.

HTLV-DISEASE ASSOCIATIONS

To evaluate the relationship between HTLV infection and disease, sera from more than 900 cases of adult and childhood malignancies from diverse geographic areas have been tested. As shown in Table 1, only 53 of the 906 cases were positive. None of 80 nonlymphoreticular neoplasms was positive, indicating that HTLV is trophic for cells of the lymphoreticular compartment. The bulk of positive sera (44/

TABLE 1. *HTLV-specific antibodies in lymphoid and nonlymphoid malignancy[a]*

Disease type[b]	Country of origin			
	U.S. or Europe	West Indies	Japan	Total
T-lymphoid				
CTCL	2/251	0/1	NT	2/252
T-LCL/ATL	1/1	8/8[d]	23/26	32/35
T-NHL	3/27[c]	NT	6/12	9/39
T-CLL	0/40	NT	NT	0/40
T-ALL	0/16	NT	0/2	0/18
T-hairy cell leukemia	1/1	NT[e]	NT	1/1
Subtotal				44/385
Unclassified and B-lymphoid				
NHL, childhood	0/26	NT	NT	0/26
NHL, adult	NT	NT	0/14	0/14
ALL, childhood	0/77	NT	NT	0/77
ALL, adult	0/17	0/2	4/18	4/37
CLL	0/7	NT	0/7	0/14
Unclassified	0/15	NT	0/4	0/19
Hodgkin's	0/116	0/1	NT	0/117
Subtotal				4/304
Myeloid				
AML, childhood	0/18	NT	NT	0/18
AML, adult	0/32	0/2	1/9	1/43
AMoL/AMMoL	0/11	NT	1/7	1/18
CML	0/47	NT	3/11	3/58
Subtotal				5/137
Nonlymphoreticular				
Miscellaneous, childhood	0/32	NT	NT	0/32
Miscellaneous, adult	0/19	NT	NT	0/19
Melanoma	0/29	NT	NT	0/29
Subtotal				0/80
Total				53/906

[a]Sera were assayed by solid-phase whole virus RIA, or radioimmunoprecipitation of HTLV p24. Antibody-positive sera possessed HTLV-specific antibody by one or more of these methods.

[b]CTCL = cutaneous T-cell lymphoma, T-LCL = T-cell lymphosarcoma cell leukemia, ATL = adult T-cell leukemia, T-NHL = T-cell non-Hodgkin's lymphoma, T-CLL = Chronic lymphocytic leukemia of T-cells, T-ALL = acute lymphoblastic leukemia of T-cells, CLL = chronic lymphoblastic leukemia, AML = acute myelogenous leukemia, AMol = acute monocytic leukemia, AMMol = acute myelomonocytic leukemia, CML = chronic myelogenous leukemia.

[c]Two additional antibody-positive T-NHL patients treated in the United States were subsequently found to originate from elsewhere; one from Israel and one from Ecuador.

[d]Includes patient MB, whose sera were not available, but from whose cultured T-cells the second HTLV isolate was obtained (14).

[e]Number positive/number tested. NT = not tested.

385) were from patients with definite T-cell malignancy. The remaining nine were among patients from Japan with lymphoid and myeloid leukemias (see below).

Our previous reports of natural antibodies to HTLV antigens in sera from two patients with cutaneous T-cell lymphoma (CTCL) (mycosis fungoides/Sézary syndrome) (9,17) suggested an association of the virus with this form of T-cell malignancy. To pursue this association, we extended our survey for natural HTLV-specific antibodies to sera of more than 200 CTCL patients. We were surprised to find that aside from the two positive sera detected during preliminary studies, the other CTCL sera assayed were negative for HTLV antibodies. One patient, CR, was a 28-year-old Black male from Alabama, with stage IV mycosis fungoides. This case was atypical, characterized by large skin tumor masses, and was called the D'emblee variant. It was from this patient's T cells that HTLV was first isolated (14). The second patient, MJ, is a 50-year-old White male with a more typical case of the mycosis fungoides/Sézary syndrome. His history is of interest in that he traveled extensively as a merchant marine into areas where HTLV infection is prevalent.

Another CTCL patient clearly associated with HTLV is patient MB, a Black female from the West Indies with a disease resembling Sézary syndrome. In reviewing her case, however, we find that she had clinical features more typical of the newly defined syndrome called T-cell lymphosarcoma cell leukemia (T-LCL) (3) or adult T-cell leukemia (ATL). Although her serum was not available for these studies, the second HTLV isolate was obtained from her T cells (15). Recently, sera from several cases of CTCL were found to have HTLV antigen in sera that were antibody-negative, and one of these, a 72-year-old Black man, had clinical features similar to those of other HTLV-associated cases (C. Saxinger, *unpublished*).

These results establish that a small percentage of cases that would be classified as CTCL are clearly associated with HTLV. However, the absence of detectable HTLV antibody in the bulk of CTCL cases and the atypical form of disease seen in CR and MB suggest that HTLV is not usually associated with the classical form of CTCL found in the United States and Western Europe. However, validation of this conclusion awaits more systematic studies to evaluate cases for antigen and by molecular epidemiologic approaches using the cloned virus probe.

HTLV-SPECIFIC ANTIBODIES IN SERA OF JAPANESE PATIENTS WITH ADULT T-CELL LEUKEMIA

Since 1977, Japanese clinicians and pathologists have reported the occurrence of ATL, an aggressive T-cell malignancy (25). This disease has been documented to occur in a geographic cluster in southwestern Japan, particularly on the islands of Kyushu and Shikoku (23,25). The disease affects adults and frequently involves skin as well as organs. The neoplastic T cells have convoluted nuclei and ultrastructurally resemble a small-cell variant of Sézary syndrome (22). However, unlike CTCL, the cells are quite pleomorphic in morphology. Preliminary studies showed that sera of Japanese patients with ATL possessed natural antibodies to HTLV (10,21). We have now carried out a more extensive survey in which, strikingly,

23 of 26 ATL patients were positive for antibodies to HTLV (Table 1). In addition, six of 12 patients with T-cell non-Hodgkin's lymphoma (T-NHL) were also positive for HTLV-specific antibodies. The antibodies were directed against core proteins of HTLV, again suggesting that replicating virus was present in these individuals.

The nine positive cases among myeloid leukemia and unclassified lymphoreticular neoplasm are of interest in that they could represent additional examples of HTLV-associated malignancies. However, the association could be fortuitous, because some of these positive cases may come from virus-endemic areas and others may have been heavily transfused. Systematic surveys of these and other disease types should help clarify these relationships. In contrast to these data on Japanese sera, we have detected no association of HTLV with myeloid leukemias in the United States (Table 1).

HTLV-SPECIFIC ANTIBODIES IN SERA OF CARIBBEAN BLACKS WITH T-LCL

The lack of association of HTLV with typical CTCL and the strong association of the virus with the more aggressive disease of Japanese ATL have led to the hypothesis that HTLV is associated with a particular subtype of adult T-cell malignancy. Initial testing of this hypothesis has pointed to a viral involvement in T-LCL, another aggressive T-cell malignancy (3) also called adult T-cell lymphoma/leukemia (1). This malignancy is rarely diagnosed in the United States but has been found in West Indian Blacks living in the United Kingdom. The clinical, laboratory, and epidemiologic features of the Caribbean T-LCL and Japanese ATL cases are listed in Table 2.

Similarities between the two groups include the following: lymphadenopathy in almost 100% of cases; hepatosplenomegaly in 40 to 60% and leukemia in 75 to 100%; survival poor; a high incidence of hypercalcemia; and pleomorphic cytology. Cell surface marker studies confirm that all cases have a mature cell surface phenotype frequently of the "helper cell" category. However, a recent report from Japan demonstrates that some cases with "helper cell" surface markers actually inhibit *in vitro* IgG synthesis by B cells and therefore function as suppressor cells (7). The slightly younger age at onset and female predominance in the Caribbean series may reflect an ascertainment bias, because all cases emigrated to the United Kingdom from the Caribbean region.

In our preliminary studies, we have examined eight Caribbean T-LCL cases, and all eight have either natural antibodies to HTLV and/or detectable HTLV proteins or particles in cultured cells. Based on the clinical features of these Caribbean T-LCL and Japanese ATL patients, we have searched for sera of patients with similar clinical features and have found several cases from the United States and other countries who show similar symptoms and have antibodies to HTLV. Cases have now been identified in several areas of the United States, predominantly among Blacks but also one Alaskan native, one Israeli, and one Ecuadorian. Most cases exhibited lymphadenopathy and hypercalcemia. Less commonly found were hepatomegaly, splenomegaly, skin lesions, and lytic bone lesions (2,4).

TABLE 2. *Epidemiological, clinical, and laboratory features of Caribbean T-LCL and Japanese ATL patients*

Feature	T-LCL Caribbean	ATL[a] Japan
Median age (years)	46	56
Sex (M/F)	2/8	14/11
Birthplace	Caribbean Islands	Kyushu, Shikoku
Positive family history	Unknown	10%
Seasonal incidence	Unknown	Summer
Occupation	Unknown	Agriculture, fishing, forestry
Thymus	Normal	Normal
Skin involvement	30%	50%
Nodes involvement	100%	100%
Liver/spleen enlargement	40%	50–60%
Leukemia	100%	76%
Median survival	8 months	10 months
Cytology	Pleomorphic	Pleomorphic
WBC	17,000–435,000	39,000–310,000
Immunoglobulins	Normal One case poly Ig ↑	↓ IgA, ↓ IgM
Hypercalcemia	50%	24%
E rosette	100%	100%
OKT[b]	T4+, T6−, T8−, T3+, T10+/−, T11+	T4+, T8−, T3+, T10+
Functional phenotype	Unknown	Suppressor
Ia	25%	50%
TdT	Negative	Negative
HTLV antibody, antigens, and/or particles	8/8	23/26

[a]Data compiled from references 7 and 23–25.
[b]See references 3 and 7 for details of cell surface marker studies. Test for OKT 6 not performed on Japanese ATL patients.

HTLV ANTIBODIES IN CLINICALLY NORMAL PERSONS

The detection of HTLV antibodies in relatives of cases is of interest because it may reflect the infectivity of HTLV. Table 3 summarizes the data on studies of relatives in nine families. Apart from one family from Japan, in which four of eight members were antibody-positive, only one first-degree relative was found to be positive. The fact that both spouses and blood relatives were found to be positive leads us to suspect horizontal rather than vertical transmission. This conclusion is also supported by the fact that HTLV is detectable only in T, not in B cells of patient CR (5). In addition, HTLV proviral DNA is not detectable in the DNA of normal donors (18). Because relatives of these cases shared a common environment, longitudinal follow-up of exposed relatives should help to clarify the mode of HTLV transmission.

More than 1,200 persons from populations in the United States, Western Europe, Japan, and the Caribbean have been screened for antibodies to HTLV. Among the

TABLE 3. *HTLV-specific antibodies in normals[a]*

Individuals tested	United States or Europe	West Indies	Japan
Relatives of HTLV cases	2/12	3/16	8/26
Random clinical normals	3/1120[b]	12/337	12/182[c] 0/45[d]

[a]Number positive/number tested, by country of origin.
[b]The three positives were in Blacks from a sample of 130 normals from Georgia.
[c]ATL-endemic area of Japan.
[d]ATL-nonendemic area of Japan.

U.S. and West European groups, the individuals surveyed were healthy blood bank donors, healthy laboratory workers, and clinic outpatients with nonmalignant illnesses. In the majority of cases, antibodies to HTLV were not detected. The three positives were normals from the state of Georgia. Similarly, sera from the ATL-nonendemic region of Japan were antibody-negative. In contrast, 4 to 10% of clinically normal persons from the Japanese ATL-endemic region and from a normal population-based survey in the Caribbean have detectable antibodies to HTLV (Table 3). Because a characteristic form of adult T-cell leukemia/lymphoma clusters in these two areas, widespread exposure to the virus in these regions may be associated with and possibly causally related to the occurrence of this distinctive form of leukemia/lymphoma. Seroepidemiologic surveys in suspect areas should help clarify these disease relationships.

HTLV AS AN ETIOLOGIC AGENT OF HUMAN MALIGNANCY

The frustrating failures of virologists in the past to demonstrate and isolate a uniquely human type C RNA tumor virus etiologically linked with leukemia or lymphoma have tended to lead to the belief that retroviruses play no role in these or other human malignancies. HTLV is the first human virus of this class consistently identified in association with a specific type of human leukemia/lymphoma (6,14,15). The epidemiologic data summarized here demonstrate that HTLV is linked to a spectrum of T-cell, but not other, malignancies. Although the role of HTLV as an etiologic agent is far from established, it is striking that the distribution of cases is limited to a relatively narrow spectrum of mature T-cell leukemia/lymphoma cases with some shared features.

Before the discovery of HTLV and its association with Japanese ATL, clinicians and epidemiologists were intrigued by the clustering of cases in limited areas of Japan, which suggested a possible viral etiology (23,24). Several findings provide strong presumptive evidence for such an etiologic relationship: the strong association of HTLV in more than 90% of Japanese ATL cases; the isolation of virus-like particles from such cases by Japanese investigators (8,12); our demonstration that the virus of Japanese ATL is a member of the HTLV group (16); and the low but detectable occurrence of HTLV in the ATL-endemic areas and the lack of HTLV in areas where ATL is rare. A viral etiology is further supported by the finding that a disease entity with shared clinical, epidemiologic, and laboratory features also clusters in the Caribbean region, where HTLV infection is prevalent (1,3).

The initial isolation of HTLV from T cells derived from patients with CTCL was at first misleading. The data summarized here suggest that HTLV is infrequently associated with this disease and is rarely associated with hematopoietic malignancies in the United States. This is consistent with the observation that cases resembling Japanese ATL are rare in the United States and the occurrence of antibody in the normal population is low. However, the predominance of positives in Black cases from the southeastern United States in our series suggests the possibility of a virus endemic focus in this area, and systematic population-based surveys are currently under way.

In summary, we postulate that HTLV is not widespread in its distribution but rather is limited to certain regions (e.g., Japan and the Caribbean). In both areas, HTLV-associated disease is a mature adult T-cell leukemia/lymphoma that occurs in clusters and is characterized by a clinically aggressive course, poor prognosis, hypercalcemia, and visceral involvement. Moreover, in the bulk of cases examined, HTLV proteins and/or frank viral particles have been detected when the T cells were cultured with TCGF. Other areas of the world with similar geographic features may also represent endemic areas for this virus. Although further studies will be needed to establish a causal relationship, the story thus far is similar to that of the retrovirus association with leukemia/lymphoma in animals, in which the satisfaction of Koch's postulates has established an etiologic role for type C retroviruses.

ACKNOWLEDGMENTS

We thank Eric C. Vonderheid, Yoshinobu Nakao, Kazumasa Yamada, Yohei Ito, Nancy Gutensohn, Sharon Murphy, Paul A. Bunn, Jr., Daniel Catovsky, M. F. Greaves, W. F. H. Jarrett, Harald zur Hausen, M. Seligmann., J. C. Brouet, Barton F. Haynes, Brian V. Jegasothy, Jeffrey Cossman, Samuel Broder, Richard I. Fisher, David W. Golde, Audrey E. Evans, Byron Fossieck, Geraldine Schechter, Anne Lanier, Trashant K. Rohatgi, and M. H. Crawford for providing serum samples. We acknowledge the excellent technical assistance of Katherine Fahey and Maureen Jarvis. Dianna Jessee typed the manuscript.

REFERENCES

1. Blattner, W. A., Kalyanaraman, V. S., Robert-Guroff, M., Lister, T. A., Galton, D. A. G., Sarin, P., Crawford, M. H., Catovsky, D., Greaves, M., and Gallo, R. C. (1983): The human type C retrovirus, HTLV, in Blacks from the Caribbean region, and relationship to adult T-cell leukemia/lymphoma. *Int. J. Cancer.* 30:257–264.
2. Blayney, D. W., Jaffe, E. S., Fisher, R. I., Schechter, G. P., Cossman, J., Robert-Guroff, M., Kalyanaraman, V. S., Blattner, W. A., and Gallo, R. C. (1983): The human T-cell leukemia/lymphoma virus (HTLV), lymphoma, lytic bone lesions, and hypercalcemia. *Ann. Intern. Med.* 98:144–151.

3. Catovsky, D., Greaves, M. F., Rose, M., Galton, D. A. G., Goolden, A. W. G., McCluskey, D. R., White, J. M., Lampert, I., Bourikas, G., Ireland, R., Brownell, A. I., Bridges, J. M., Brownell, A. I., Blattner, W. A., and Gallo, R. C. (1982): Adult T-cell lymphoma-leukaemia in Blacks from the West Indies. *Lancet*, 1:639–642.

4. Gallo, R. C., Kalyanaraman, V. S., Sarngadharan, M. G., Sliski, A., Vonderheid, E. C., Maeda, M., Nakao, Y., Yamada, K., Ito, Y., Gutensohn, N., Murphy, S., Bunn, P. A., Jr., Catovsky, D., Greaves, M. F., Blayney, D. W., Blattner, W. A., Jarrett, W. F. H., zur Hausen, H., Seligmann, M., Grouet, J. C., Haynes, B. F., Jegasothy, B. V., Jaffe, E., Cossman, J., Broder, S., Fisher, R. I., Golde, D. W., and Robert-Guroff, M. (1983): The human type-C retrovirus: Association with a subset of adult T-cell malignancies. *Cancer Research (in press)*.

5. Gallo, R. C., Mann, D. L., Broder, S., Ruscetti, F. W., Maeda, M. K., Kalyanaraman, V. S., Robert-Guroff, M., and Reitz, M. S. (1982): Human T-cell leukemia lymphoma virus (HTLV) is in T but not B lymphocytes from a patient with cutaneous T-cell lymphoma. *Proc. Natl. Acad. Sci. USA*, 79:5680–5683.

6. Gallo, R. C., Poiesz, B. J., and Ruscetti, F. W. (1981): Regulation of human T-cell proliferation: T-cell growth factor and isolation of a new class of type-C retroviruses from human T-cells. *Haematology and Blood Transfusion, Vol. 26: Modern Trends in Human Leukemia, Vol. 4*, pp. 502–514. Springer-Verlag, New York.

7. Hattori, T., Uchiyama, T., Toibana, T., Takatsuki, K., and Uchino, H. (1981): Surface phenotype of Japanese adult T-cell leukemia cells characterized by monoclonal antibodies. *Blood*, 58:645–647.

8. Hinuma, Y., Nagata, K., Misoka, M., Nakai, M., Matsumoto, T., Kinoshita, K. I., Shirakawa, S., and Miyoshi, I. (1981): Adult T-cell leukemia: antigen in an ATL cell line and detection of antibodies to the antigen in human sera. *Proc. Natl. Acad. Sci. USA*, 78:6476–6480.

9. Kalyanaraman, V. S., Sarngadharan, M. G., Bunn, P. A., Minna, J. D., and Gallo, R. C. (1981): Antibodies in human sera reactive against an internal structural protein (p24) of human T-cell lymphoma virus. *Nature*, 294:271–273.

10. Kalyanaraman, V. S., Sarngadharan, M. G., Nakao, Y., Ito, Y., Aoki, T., and Gallo, R. C. (1982): Natural antibodies to the structural core protein (p24) of the human T-cell leukemia (lymphoma) retrovirus (HTLV) found in sera of leukemia patients in Japan. *Proc. Natl. Acad. Sci. USA*, 79:1653–1657.

11. Kalyanaraman, V. S., Sarngadharan, M. G., Poiesz, B. J., Ruscetti, F. W., and Gallo, R. C. (1981): Immunological properties of a type-C retrovirus isolated from cultured human T-lymphoma cells and comparison to other mammalian retroviruses. *J. Virol.*, 38:906–915.

12. Miyoshi, I., Kubonishi, I., Yoshimoto, S., Akagi, T., Ohtsuki, Y., Shiraishi, Y., Nagata, K., and Hinuma, Y. (1981): Type C virus particles in a cord T-cell line derived by co-cultivating normal human cord leukocytes and human leukaemic T cells. *Nature*, 294:770–771.

13. Oroszlan, S., Sarngadharan, M. G., Copeland, T. D., Kalyanaraman, V. S., Gilden, R. V., and Gallo, R. C. (1982): Primary structure analysis of the major internal protein p24 of human type C T-cell leukemia virus. *Proc. Natl. Acad. Sci. USA*, 79:1291–1294.

14. Poiesz, B. J., Ruscetti, F. W., Gazdar, A. F., Bunn, P. A., Minna, J. D., and Gallo, R. C. (1980): Detection and isolation of type-C retrovirus particles from fresh and cultured lymphocytes of a patient with cutaneous T-cell lymphoma. *Proc. Natl. Acad. Sci. USA*, 77:7415–7419.

15. Poiesz, B. J., Ruscetti, F. W., Reitz, M. S., Kalyanaraman, V. S., and Gallo, R. C. (1981): Isolation of a new type-C retrovirus (HTLV) in primary uncultured cells of a patient with Sezary T-cell leukemia. *Nature*, 294:268–271.

16. Popovic, M., Kalyanaraman, V. S., Sarngadharan, M. G., Robert-Guroff, M., Nakao, Y., Reitz, M. D., Jr., Miyoshi, I., Ito, Y., Minowada, J., and Gallo, R. C. (1983): HTLV is the virus of Japanese adult T-cell leukemia. *Nature. (in press)*.

17. Posner, L. E., Robert-Guroff, M., Kalyanaraman, V. S., Poiesz, B. J., Ruscetti, F. W., Bunn, P. A., Minna, J. D., and Gallo, R. C. (1981): Natural antibodies to the human T-cell virus in patients with cutaneous T-cell lymphomas. *J. Exp. Med.*, 154:333–346.

18. Reitz, M. S., Poiesz, B. J., Ruscetti, F. W., and Gallo, R. C. (1981): Characterization and distribution of nucleic acid sequences of a novel type-C retrovirus isolated from neoplastic human T-lymphocytes. *Proc. Natl. Acad. Sci. USA*, 78:1887–1891.

19. Rho, H. M., Poiesz, B. J., Ruscetti, F. W., and Gallo, R. C. (1981): Characterization of the reverse transcriptase from a new retrovirus (HTLV) produced by a human cutaneous T-cell lymphoma cell line. *Virology*, 112:355–360.

20. Robert-Guroff, M., Fahey, K. A., Maeda, M., Nakao, Y., Ito, Y., and Gallo, R. C. (1982): Identification of HTLV p19 specific natural human antibodies by competition with monoclonal antibody. *Virology*, 122:297–305.
21. Robert-Guroff, M., Nakao, Y., Notake, K., Ito, Y., Sliski, A., and Gallo, R. C. (1982): Natural antibodies to the human retrovirus, HTLV, in a cluster of Japanese patients with adult T-cell leukemia. *Science*, 215:975–978.
22. Shamoto, M., Murakami, S., and Zenke, T. (1981): Adult T-cell leukemia in Japan: an ultrastructural study. *Cancer*, 47:1804–1811.
23. Tajima, K., Tominaga, S., Kuroishi, T., Shimizu, H., and Suchi, T. (1979): Geographical features and epidemiological approach to endemic T-cell leukemia/lymphoma in Japan. *Jpn. J. Clin. Oncol.*, 9(Suppl.):495–504.
24. The T- and B-cell Malignancy Study Group (1981): Statistical analysis of immunologic, clinical and histopathologic data on lymphoid malignancies in Japan. *Jpn. J. Clin. Oncol.*, 11:15–38.
25. Uchiyama, T., Yodoi, J., Sagawa, K., Takatsuki, K., and Uchino, H. (1977): Adult T-cell leukemia: clinical and hematologic features of 16 cases. *Blood*, 50:481–492.

Pathogenesis of Leukemias and Lymphomas:
Environmental Influences, edited by
I. T. Magrath, G. T. O'Conor, and B. Ramot.
Raven Press, New York © 1984.

Oncogene Expression in Human Lymphoid Neoplasms

Susan M. Astrin and Ugo G. Rovigatti

The Institute for Cancer Research, Fox Chase Cancer Center,
Philadelphia, Pennsylvania 19111

In this chapter, we discuss an animal model system, the induction of bursal lymphomas in chickens by avian leukosis virus, and then relate the results of the animal model system to human lymphoid neoplasms.

THE PROMOTER INSERTION MECHANISM OF ONCOGENESIS

When the avian leukosis viruses, RAV-1 or RAV-2, are injected into day-old chicks, they cause bursal lymphomas four to 12 months after injection (15). These tumors metastasize to the liver, spleen, and/or kidney, killing the bird.

For a number of reasons, oncogenesis by the avian leukosis viruses probably differs from the mechanism involved in other oncogenic retroviruses such as Rous sarcoma virus. The properties of the acute transforming viruses such as Rous are as follows (5): All these viruses cause tumor formation two to three weeks after inoculation of susceptible animals. There is often a single target tissue for tumor induction; for example, Rous sarcoma virus causes exclusively fibrosarcomas in inoculated animals. These viruses have been shown to transform appropriate target cells in culture; for example, Rous transforms fibroblasts. Finally, the tumors produced by these viruses are polyclonal. All of these properties can be explained by the fact that each of these viral genomes contains an oncogene, that is, a gene that codes for a protein that transforms cells. In contrast to the properties of the acute transforming viruses, the avian leukosis viruses have the following properties: The latent period for tumor induction is four to 12 months. The viruses are multipotent; that is, they sometimes induce sarcomas and nephroblastomas as well as bursal lymphomas in inoculated animals. None of these viruses has been shown to transform cells in culture. The tumors produced by these viruses are clonal; that is, they result from the outgrowth of a single transformed cell (13,14). In addition, no oncogene has been identified in the genome of avian leukosis viruses; they simply contain those genes that are necessary for viral replication and reproduction.

To date, the oncogenes carried by the acute transforming viruses number over 15; that is, there are at least 15 distinct transforming genes [for reference list, see Coffin et al. (2)]. The avian retroviral oncogenes are listed in Table 1. Seven such

TABLE 1. *Avian retroviral oncogenes*

Virus	Oncogene	Neoplasm	Oncogene homolog Chicken	Oncogene homolog Human
Rous sarcoma virus (RSV)	*src*	Fibrosarcoma	+	+
Fujinami virus (FSV)	*fps*	Fibrosarcoma	+	+
Avian myeloblastosis virus (AMV)	*myb*	Myeloblastic leukemia	+	+
Avian erythroblastosis virus (AEV)	*erb*	Erythroid leukemia, fibrosarcoma	+	+
Myelocytomatosis virus (MC29)	*myc*	Myelocytic leukemia, fibrosarcoma, carcinoma, B-cell lymphoma	+	+
Avian sarcoma virus (UR-2)	*ros*	Fibrosarcoma	+	+
Avian sarcoma virus (Y73 and Esh)	*yes*	Fibrosarcoma	+	+

genes have thus far been identified: the *src* gene, carried by Rous sarcoma virus; the *fps* gene, carried by Fujinami virus; the *myb* gene, carried by avian myeloblastosis virus; the *erb* gene, carried by avian erythroblastosis virus; the *myc* gene, carried by myelocytomatosis virus; the *ros* gene, carried by avian sarcoma virus UR2; and the *yes* gene, carried by Y73 avian sarcoma virus. Table 1 shows the type of neoplasm caused by each of these viruses. Another feature of the viral oncogenes in Table 1 is that there are homologs for each of these genes in normal vertebrate cells. Thus, in addition to Rous sarcoma virus *src*, there is also chicken *src* and human *src*. The oncogene homologs appear to be very well conserved throughout evolution and are found not only in all vertebrate species but have been documented in some invertebrate species as well. It thus appears that the oncogenes carried by acute transforming viruses have derived from cellular genes by a type of recombinational process.

What is the function of the cellular homologs of the retroviral oncogenes? As mentioned above, these genes are highly conserved in evolution. They are found throughout vertebrate species and in invertebrates as well. Such conservation indicates an essential function. Current evidence indicates that these genes are expressed early in the development of selected tissues (1,6,18,19). They may therefore function as regulators of cell proliferation and/or differentiation. In addition, their function may be tissue-specific. The cellular oncogenes appear to be the progenitors of the retroviral oncogenes. The virus apparently transforms by "overloading" the cell with an otherwise normal gene product. Given the above information, it seems likely that transformation could also be achieved by activating the cellular oncogene itself.

Is it possible that the avian leukosis viruses cause tumors by activating cellular oncogenes? Figure 1 shows a diagram of the integrated form of a retroviral provirus. The viral genes are flanked by a direct repeat of approximately 350 nucleotides,

DOES AVIAN LEUKOSIS VIRUS TURN ON CELLULAR GENES?

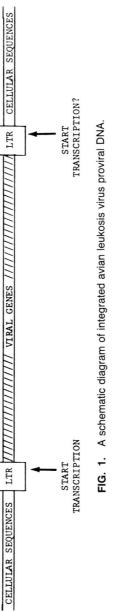

FIG. 1. A schematic diagram of integrated avian leukosis virus proviral DNA.

termed the long terminal repeat (LTR). The LTR contains the promotor for transcription of the viral genes; transcription begins within the left LTR (101 nucleotides from the right end) and proceeds through the genome into the right LTR, where it terminates. Because the identical promotor sequence is contained within the right LTR, transcripts could begin within this region, resulting in expression of the flanking cellular sequences. If these sequences contain an oncogene, expression of that gene could result in neoplastic transformation.

The following predictions may be made from this model. First, integration of the provirus next to a cellular oncogene would be expected to be a rare event, because no apparent specificity for integration has been demonstrated. Therefore, one would expect to see only one or a very small number of transformed cells within the infected bursa, and the resultant tumors would be clonal—resulting from proliferation of a single transformed cell. Second, the number of cellular oncogenes that could be activated in the bursa would be expected to be small. Therefore, tumors from different birds would have integration sites in common, that is, integration sites adjacent to the same oncogene. Third, all the tumors would contain the viral LTR, but that is the only viral sequence they would necessarily contain, because it is the only element necessary for activating the cellular gene. Finally, transcripts of the activated oncogene would be found in the tumors; these transcripts would contain 101 nucleotides of viral sequence covalently linked to oncogene sequences.

To test the model, bursal lymphomas were induced in 36 chickens, the primary tumors and metastases were excised, and DNA and RNA were prepared. The DNAs were analyzed for the sites of integration of proviruses, using restriction endonuclease cleavage and Southern blot analysis as well as molecular cloning. The RNA samples were analyzed for transcripts of oncogene sequences. The data and results from these analyses are presented elsewhere (7,13,16) but may be summarized as follows: First, in 30 of 36 tumors, an avian leukosis virus provirus was found to be integrated adjacent to the c-*myc* gene, that is, the cellular homolog of the v-*myc* gene, the transforming gene of MC29 virus. The orientation of the insert was such that transcription initiated within the viral LTR would read into the *myc* sequences. The inserts clustered in five regions located within 2 kilobases (kb) from the start of the gene. More than half of the insertions took place in a 200 base pair region just in front of the gene. In addition, the tumors contained elevated (30- to 100-fold) levels of *myc* RNA. These transcripts contained viral sequences as well as *myc* sequences, indicating that transcription was initiated within the viral LTR. We concluded from the above that transformation and tumor formation are the result of integration of an avian leukosis virus provirus adjacent to a cellular oncogene. This event results in activation of the cellular gene by providing a strong upstream transcriptional promoter (the viral LTR). We have termed this mechanism "promoter insertion," and it is the first example of tumorigenesis involving activation of the cellular homolog of a viral oncogene. The promoter insertion mechanism is shown diagrammatically in Fig. 2.

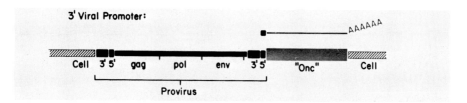

FIG. 2. A cartoon of the promotor insertion mechanism of avian leukosis virus oncogenesis. The avian leukosis virus provirus is shown schematically (black), with the long terminal repeat (LTR) enlarged. Although an intact provirus is shown, current data indicate that the proviruses usually have a deletion of 5′ sequences (16). A proposed structure for a new RNA containing both viral and cellular sequences is shown above the provirus structure. A poly-A sequence is shown at the 3′ end of the transcript. The cellular (gray) sequence adjacent to the LTR is designated as "onc" to indicate its proposed role in oncogenesis. In a majority of our lymphomas, this cellular sequence is *myc*, the endogenous counterpart of the transforming gene of the avian acute leukemia virus MC29.

MYC GENE EXPRESSION IN HUMAN LEUKEMIC CELLS

Does oncogene expression play a role in human cancer? To approach this question, we have been analyzing RNA samples from "lymphocytes" of leukemic patients for expression of the human *myc* gene. We have chosen neoplasms that are primarily of the B-cell type—acute lymphoblastic leukemia (ALL), chronic lymphocytic leukemia (CLL), and non-Hodgkin's lymphoma (diffuse, poorly differentiated NHL). We have collected peripheral blood lymphocytes and lymphoblasts from 15 patients, whose white cell counts were as follows: three ALL patients had counts ranging from 27,000 to 75,000 per cubic millimeter, eight CLL patients had counts ranging from 51,000 to 480,000, and four NHL patients had ranges of 68,000 to 108,000. DNA and RNA were extracted from the lymphoid cell samples, and the RNA was analyzed by dot blots, in which serial twofold dilutions of the sample are spotted onto nitrocellulose (20) and hybridized to radiolabeled *myc* probe. Three probes were used: chicken c-*myc*, MC29 v-*myc* (8), and a subclone of the human *myc* gene. The three probes gave very similar results. In addition to the patient samples, lymphocyte RNA from eight normal individuals (cell counts ranging from 5,000 to 8,000 per lambda) were also analyzed.

Typical results are shown in Fig. 3. Three conclusions may be drawn from the data. First, the normal samples and some of the patient samples show no detectable signal with the *myc* probe. We estimate that the level of *myc* expression in these samples is low—fewer than 10 transcripts per cell. Second, a number of the patient samples give strong signals with the probe. Based on comparison with *myc* RNA levels in ALL induced bursal lymphomas, we estimate that these samples contain more than 100 transcripts per cell, levels comparable to those seen in the bursal tumors. Third, a sample obtained from one of the *myc*-positive ALL patients while he was in remission (sample 3R) shows no detectable *myc* transcription. Thus, *myc* expression is apparently associated with the leukemic cells in that patient. The normal cells remaining after chemotherapy are negative. Results from the 24 samples are summarized in Table 2. These results are consistent with *myc* expression playing

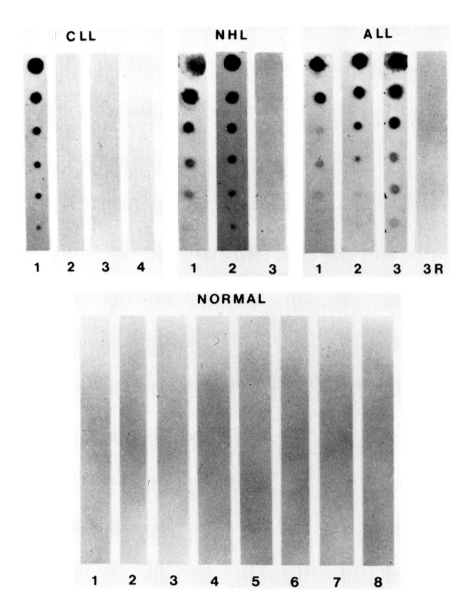

FIG. 3. Analysis of c-*myc* expression in RNA from peripheral blood leukocytes from normal donors and from patients with leukemia or lymphoma. "Dot blot" analysis was performed as described by Thomas (20). The amount of RNA in the uppermost sample was 0.5 μg (normal donors) or 1 μg (leukemics), and serial twofold dilutions were then spotted onto the paper. The probe used was the v-*myc* clone kindly provided by T. Papas (8). ALL samples 3 and 3R correspond to the same ALL patient at diagnosis and after chemotherapy and remission, respectively.

TABLE 2. *myc Gene expression in peripheral blood lymphocytes*

Samples	Number analyzed	Number of positives
Normal donors (PBL)	9	0
Chronic lymphocytic leukemia	8	3
Acute lymphoblastic leukemia	3	3
Non-Hodgkin's lymphoma	4	3
Total (tumor samples only)	15	9

a role in the development of leukemia, at least in some patients. If oncogene expression is a general phenomenon in cancer, then those patients with undetectable levels of *myc* may be positive for expression of another oncogene.

This possibility remains to be tested. In addition, the role of *myc* expression in normal lymphocyte differentiation remains to be determined. Most important, however, forging a convincing link between *myc* expression and a primary oncogenic event requires evidence of a genetic change in association with the expression. Experiments designed to detect such a genetic change at the *myc* locus are currently in progress.

Our working hypothesis can thus be stated as follows: Malignant transformation is a complex chain of events triggered by a primary oncogenic event—activation of an endogenous oncogene. We propose that oncogene expression triggers not only uncontrolled cell proliferation but other events as well, resulting in an accumulation of genetic and epigenetic changes in the tumor cells.

What types of genetic changes might result in high levels of oncogene expression? First, one must consider promoter insertion by a retrovirus. It seems likely that if human tumor viruses exist, they might function by promoter insertion. A second mechanism for oncogene activation might be inactivation of a negative effector (repressor). Because current evidence indicates that the oncogenes are expressed only at low levels in terminally differentiated tissues, a type of repression mechanism is likely to be operating. Inactivation of such a system could be accomplished by mutation in a gene coding for the negative effector itself or by genetic rearrangement resulting in relocation of the oncogene to an active transcription unit. Inactivation of a repressor would require two hits in a diploid cell. This type of mechanism could easily be accommodated by the two-hit theory that has evolved for certain cancers (12), including those for which a genetic predisposition has been described. Relocation resulting in activation is an especially interesting possibility in light of the nonrandom chromosomal translocations associated with certain cancers (17) and the recent finding that active immunoglobulin genes occupy chromosomal loci that are frequently involved as breakpoints for the translocations (10). A third possibility is mutation in the regulatory region of the oncogene, resulting in either more efficient polymerase recognition or less efficient repressor recognition. This type of mechanism may be operating in the case of enhanced *ras* gene expression seen in the human bladder carcinoma cell line (21). In this case a genetic change in the 5' flanking sequences of the oncogene may differentiate the activated *ras* gene in the carcinoma from its inactive homolog in normal cells. A fourth mechanism for enhancing oncogene expression might be gene amplification at the DNA level. For example, HL60, a human promyelocytic cell line, has been shown to have a 20-fold amplification of *myc* DNA sequences (3; U. Rovigatti and S. M. Astrin, *unpublished*) accompanied by a 20-fold elevation in expression at the RNA level (U. Rovigatti and S. M. Astrin, *unpublished*). One final mechanism for activation is demethylation. Hypomethylation has been associated with expression of a number of genes (4,9,11), and the possibility exists that some chemical carcinogens may effect DNA methylation.

In conclusion, many questions about oncogene expression and function are currently being examined experimentally. The future in this area promises to be productive and exciting.

ACKNOWLEDGMENTS

This research was supported by grants CA-27797-03, CA-06927, and RR-05539 from the National Institutes of Health and by an appropriation from the Commonwealth of Pennsylvania.

REFERENCES

1. Chen, J. H. (1980): Expression of endogenous avian myeloblastosis virus information in different chicken cells. *J. Virol.*, 36:162–170.
2. Coffin, J. M., Varmus, H. E., Bishop, J. M., Essex, M., Hardy, W. D., Jr., Martin, G. S., Rosenberg, N. E., Scolnick, E. M., Weinberg, R. A., and Vogt, P. K. (1981): Proposal for naming host cell-derived inserts in retrovirus genomes. *J. Virol.*, 40:953–957.
3. Collins, S., and Groudine, M. (1983): Amplification of endogenous *myc-related* DNA sequences in the human myeloid leukemia cell line HL-60. *Nature. (in press).*
4. Derosiers, R. C., Mulder, C., and Fleckenstein, B. (1979): Methylation of *Herpesvirus saimiri* DNA in lymphoid tumor cell lines. *Proc. Natl. Acad. Sci. USA*, 76:3839–3843.
5. Fishinger, P. J. (1979): Type C RNA transforming viruses. In: *Molecular Biology of RNA Tumor Viruses*, edited by J. P. Stephenson, pp. 163–198. Academic Press, New York.
6. Gonda, T. J., Sheiness, D. K., and Bishop, J. M. (1982): Transcripts from the cellular homologs of retroviral oncogenes: Distribution among chicken tissues. *Mol. Cell. Biol.*, 2:617–624.
7. Hayward, W. W., Neel, B. G., and Astrin, S. M. (1981): Activation of a cellular *onc* gene by promoter insertion in ALV-induced lymphoid leukosis. *Nature*, 290:475–480.
8. Lautenberger, J. A., Schulz, R. A., Garon, C. F., Tsichlis, P. N., and Papas, T. S. (1981): Molecular cloning of avian myelocytomatosis virus (MC29) transforming sequences. *Proc. Natl. Acad. Sci. USA*, 78:1518–1522.
9. Mandel, J. L., and Chambon, P. (1979): DNA methylation: organ specific variations in the methylation pattern within and around ovalbumin and other chicken genes. *Nucleic Acids Res.*, 7:2081–2103.
10. McBride, O. W., Hieter, P. A., Hollis, G. F., Swan, D., Otey, M. C., and Leder, P. (1982): Chromosomal location of human kappa and lambda immunoglobulin light chain constant region genes. *J. Exp. Med.*, 155:1480–1490.
11. McGhee, J. D., and Ginder, G. D. (1979): Specific DNA methylation sites in the vicinity of the chicken β-globin genes. *Nature*, 280:419–420.
12. Moolgavkar, S. H., and Knudson, A. G., Jr. (1981): Mutation and cancer: a model for human carcinogenesis. *JNCI*, 66:1037–1052.
13. Neel, B. G., Hayward, W. S., Robinson, H. L., Fang, J., and Astrin, S. M. (1981): Avian leukosis virus-induced tumors have common proviral integration sites and synthesize discrete new RNAs: oncogenesis by promoter insertion. *Cell*, 23:323–344.
14. Payne, G. S., Courtneidge, S. A., Crittenden, L. B., Fadly, A. M., Bishop, J. M., and Varmus,

H. E. (1981): Analysis of avian leukosis virus DNA and RNA in bursal tumors: viral gene expression is not required for maintenance of the tumor state. *Cell*, 23:311–322.

15. Purchase, H. G., and Burmester, B. R. (1978): Neoplastic diseases: leukosis/sarcoma group. In: *Diseases of Poultry*, edited by M. S. Hofstad, B. W. Calnek, C. Helmboldt, W. M. Reid, and H. W. Yoder, Jr., pp. 502–568. Iowa State University Press, Ames.

16. Rovigatti, U. G., Rogler, C. E., Neel, B. G., Hayward, W. S., and Astrin, S. M. (1983): Expression of endogenous oncogenes in tumor cells. In: *Tumor Cell Heterogeneity: Origins and Implications*. Fourth Annual Bristol-Myers Symposium on Cancer Research. Academic Press, New York.

17. Rowley, J. D. (1980): Chromosome abnormalities in human leukemia. *Annu. Rev. Genet.*, 14:17–39.

18. Scolnick, E. M., Weeks, M. O., Shih, T. Y., Ruscetti, S. K., and Dexter, T. M. (1981): Markedly elevated levels of an endogenous *sarc* protein in a hemopoietic precursor cell line. *Mol. Cell. Biol.*, 1:66–74.

19. Shibuya, M., Hanafusa, H., and Balduzzi, P. C. (1982): Cellular sequences related to three new *onc* genes of avian sarcoma virus (*fps*, *yes*, and *ros*) and their expression in normal and transformed cells. *J. Virol.*, 42:143–152.

20. Thomas, P. S. (1980): Hybridization of denatured RNA and small DNA fragments transferred to nitrocellulose. *Proc. Natl. Acad. Sci. USA*, 77:5201–5205.

21. Weinberg, R. A. (1982): Oncogenes of human tumor cells. *Trends in Biochemical Sciences*, 7:135–136.

Pathogenesis of Leukemias and Lymphomas:
Environmental Influences, Vol. 27, edited by
I. T. Magrath, G. T. O'Conor, and B. Ramot.
Raven Press, New York © 1984.

Human Hematopoietic Cell Expression of Retroviral Related Cellular *onc* Genes

E. H. Westin, F. Wong-Staal, and R. C. Gallo

Laboratory of Tumor Cell Biology, National Cancer Institute,
National Institutes of Health, Bethesda, Maryland 20205

Transforming genes contained in retroviruses are derived from normal cellular genes (c-*onc*) that are conserved among vertebrates (1). Although the function(s) of these cellular gene products has not been defined, there is evidence that virus-induced transformation is correlated with enhanced levels of expression of these genes. Because of the high degree of conservation of these genes among divergent species, clones of avian, murine, and simian retroviruses containing *onc* genes (v-*onc*) can be used as probes to study human c-*onc* gene organization at the DNA level and determine the level of RNA expression (2,6).

To study the role of several of these *onc* gene homologs in normal and neoplastic growth and differentiation of human cells, we have examined their expression in human hematopoietic cells. Both fresh blood cells and human cell lines of myeloid, lymphoid, and erythroid origin at various stages of differentiation have been examined for expression of cellular genes homologous to the transforming genes of avian myelocytomatosis virus strain MC29, avian myeloblastosis virus (AMV), Abelson murine leukemia virus (Ab-MuLV), Harvey murine sarcoma virus (Ha-MuSV), feline sarcoma virus (FeSV), and simian sarcoma virus (SSV). Table 1 summarizes the host of origin of these viruses, the types of disease caused, and the nomenclatures used in reference to the virus-related human cellular *onc* genes.

TABLE 1. *onc Genes containing retroviruses used as probes*

Virus of origin	Host	Natural tumors produced	Cellular homolog
MC29	Avian	Bursal lymphomas, sarcomas, and carcinomas	c-*myc*
AMV	Avian	Acute myeloblastic leukemia	c-*amv*
Abelson (MuLV)	Rodent	Lymphomas	c-*abl*
Harvey MuSV	Rodent	Sarcomas and erythroleukemia	c-Harvey-*ras*
FeSV	Feline	Sarcomas	c-*fes*
SSV	Primate	Sarcomas	c-*sis*

Nick translated DNA probes of *onc*-containing segments from molecularly cloned viral genomes were hybridized to poly-A-containing RNAs by RNA gel blotting techniques. The results obtained with each probe differ with respect to cell specificity and number or size of mRNA species.

LACK OF EXPRESSION OF C-*SIS* AND C-*FES* IN HUMAN HEMATOPOIETIC CELLS

Table 2 summarizes the cell lines and fresh leukemic and normal cells used and the results obtained in qualitative terms of level of expression and size of RNA species present using FeSV and SSV as probe. No detectable expression of c-*fes* and c-*sis* was found in any hematopoietic cell with the exception of c-*sis* in HUT102, a human mature malignant T-cell line known to produce human T-cell leukemia/lymphoma virus (HTLV). The transcript is identical in size (4.2 kb) to c-*sis* gene transcripts in human fibrosarcoma cell lines not infected with SSV (2). Studies are in progress to determine whether integration of the HTLV provirus correlates with activation of c-*sis*, which is usually not transcribed in hematopoietic cells.

WIDE DISTRIBUTION OF EXPRESSION OF MULTIPLE mRNA SPECIES OF THE C-*ABL* AND C-HARVEY-*RAS* GENES

The *abl* and Harvey-*ras* probes detected multiple-size species of mRNA, generally at low levels of expression based on band intensity. The *abl* probe detected four

TABLE 2. *Expression of* onc *genes in human hematopoietic cells*

Cell type	Source	v-*fes*	v-*sis* (4.2 kb)	v-*abl* (7.2, 6.4, 3.8, and 2.0 kb)	v-Harvey-ras (6.5 and 5.8 kb)	v-*myc* (2.7 kb)	v-*amv* (4.5 kb)
Myeloid	KG-1	−	−	+ +	+	+ +	+ +
	HL60	−	−	+ +	+	+ + + +	+ +
	HL60 differentiated[a]	−	−	+ +	+	±	±
	Fresh AML cells (four patients)	NT[b]	−	+ +	+	+ +	+
Erythroid	K562	−	−	+ +	+	+ +	+
Lymphoid							
T-cells	RPMI8402	−	−	+ +	+	+ +	+
	CCRF-CEM	−	−	+ +	+	+ +	+ + +
	Molt 4	−	−	+ +	+	+ +	+ + +
	HUT78	−	−	+ +	+	+ +	−
	HUT102	−	+	+ +	+	+ +	−
	ALL (one patient)	NT	−	+ +	NT	+ +	+ +
	PHA-stimulated	NT	NT	NT	NT	+ +	−
B cells	Raji	−	−	+ +	+	+ +	−
	Daudi	−	−	+ +	+	+ +	−
	NC37	−	−	+ +	+	+ +	−

[a]HL60 differentiated with either Me_2SO or retinoic acid.
[b]NT = not tested.
kb = kilobase(s).

different transcripts of 7.2, 6.4, 3.8, and 2.0 kb (Table 2). The Harvey-*ras* probe detected two faintly hybridizing transcripts of 6.5 and 5.8 kb and perhaps lower molecular weight species as well. The intensity of these bands varied within a narrow range from one sample to another.

WIDE DISTRIBUTION OF EXPRESSION OF A SINGLE RNA SPECIES OF C-*MYC*

The *myc* probe detected only a single transcript of 2.7 kb in all hematopoietic cells examined, including normal peripheral blood lymphocytes and phytochem-agglutin-stimulated peripheral blood lymphocytes (Table 2). With one exception, the signal intensity of this band varies less than twofold to fourfold across the spectrum of cell types examined. The exception was HL60, a human promyelocytic leukemic cell line that showed expression of *myc*-related sequences at approximately a 10-fold greater level than other cell types. Because HL60 can be induced to differentiate with a variety of agents including Me_2SO and retinoic acid, the level of *onc* gene expression was studied under these conditions. Expression of c-*myc* was markedly reduced on induction of differentiation. However, expression of c-Harvey-*ras* and c-*abl* did not change.

LIMITED DISTRIBUTION OF EXPRESSION OF A SINGLE RNA SPECIES OF C-*AMV*

The *amv* probe detected a single transcript of 4.5 kb in all immature myeloid, T-lymphoid, and erythroid cell types examined with a fivefold to 10-fold higher level of expression seen in the immature T-cell lines Molt 4 and CCRF-CEM (Table 2). Detectable levels of expression were not found in mature T cells HUT102 and HUT78, normal peripheral blood lymphocytes either resting or PHA-stimulated or B-cell lines, including Raji and Daudi derived from patients with Burkitt's lymphoma. In addition, when HL60 was induced to differentiate, the level of expression of c-*amv* decreased.

SUMMARY

Several studies have implicated derepression of cellular *onc* genes in retrovirus-induced tumorigenesis. In B-cell lymphomas of chickens induced by two distinct viruses—avian leukosis virus and avian syncytia virus—the exogenous proviruses are integrated in the vicinity of c-*myc* and, as a result, expression of c-*myc* is greatly enhanced (3–5). As yet, however, there is no evidence for activation with high-level expression of *onc* genes in nonviral-induced tumors in animal systems. Our studies do not implicate high-level expression of the *onc* genes evaluated in the causation of human hematopoietic neoplasms. Possible exceptions are c-*myc* in promyelocytic leukemia and c-*amv* in immature T-cell lymphoma/leukemia. However, more examples of these diseases need to be examined. Our findings are also compatible with the hypothesis that certain *onc* genes, such as c-*amv* and c-*myc*, may be activated only during particular stages of normal hematopoietic cell differentiation, and others, such as c-*abl* and c-Harvey-*ras*, are constitutively expressed. Whether or not any of these genes also plays a role in transformation of human hematopoietic cells remains to be determined.

REFERENCES

1. Bishop, J. M. (1978): Retroviruses. *Annu. Rev. Biochem.*, 47:35–88.
2. Eva, A., Robbins, K. C., Andersen, P. R., Srinivasan, A., Tronick, S. R., Reddy, E. P., Ellmore, N., Galen, A. T., Lautenberger, J. A., Papas, T. S., Westin, E. H., Wong-Staal, F., Gallo, R. C., and Aaronson, S. A. (1982): Cellular genes analogous to retroviral *onc* genes are transcribed in human tumor cells. *Nature*, 295:116–119.
3. Fung, Y. K., Fadly, A. M., Crittenden, L. B., and Kung, H. I. (1981): On the mechanism of retrovirus-induced avian lymphoid leukosis: deletion and integration of the proviruses. *Proc. Natl. Acad. Sci. USA*, 78:3418–3422.
4. Hayward, W., Neel, B. G., and Astrin, S. M. (1981): Activation of a cellular *onc* gene by promoter insertion in ALV-induced lymphoid leukosis. *Nature*, 290:475–480.
5. Neel, B. G., Hayward, W. S., Robinson, H. L., Fang, J., and Astrin, S. M. (1981): Avian leukosis virus-induced tumors have common proviral integration sites and synthesize discrete new RNAs: oncogenesis by promoter insertion. *Cell*, 23:323–334.
6. Westin, E. H., Wong-Staal, F., Gelmann, E. P., Dalla-Favera, R., Papas, T. S., Lautenberger, J. A., Eva, A., Reddy, E. P., Tronick, S. R., Aaronson, S. A., and Gallo, R. C. (1982): Expression of cellular homologues of retroviral *onc* genes in human hematopoietic cells. *Proc. Natl. Acad. Sci. USA*, 79:2490–2494.

Pathogenesis of Leukemias and Lymphomas:
Environmental Influences, edited by
I. T. Magrath, G. T. O'Conor, and B. Ramot.
Raven Press, New York © 1984.

Expression of c-*myc* Sequences in Human Lymphomas

*Nancy Zeller, **Jeffrey Cossman, **Elaine S. Jaffe,
and *Philip Tsichlis

*Laboratory of Tumor Virus Genetics and **Laboratory of Pathology, National Cancer
Institute, National Institutes of Health, Bethesda, Maryland 20205*

Both the avian and the mammalian retroviruses can be divided into two distinct groups; the transforming and the nontransforming viruses. This classification is based on the genetic structure and the biological properties of individual virus strains (2,15,16). The transforming viruses carry, in addition to or in place of certain replicative genes, nonstructural genetic information (transforming or *onc* gene) that seems to be important in the initiation and maintenance of the transformed state (2,8,21). Seventeen virus-associated transforming genes (v-*onc* genes) have been identified so far (4). It has been conclusively shown that these genes have normal cellular homologs (c-*onc* genes) and that the transforming viruses arose by transduction of c-*onc* genes by the nontransforming retroviruses (2,4,7,9,11,13,25,27,33). The function of the c-*onc* genes is unknown. However, several observations indicate that they play an important functional role in normal cells—they are highly conserved through evolution, appearing in species as diverse as drosophila and humans (4,7,9,11–13,25,27,31–33), and evidence exists indicating that their expression depends on the state of differentiation of a particular cell type (3,26,38).

The transforming viruses induce polyclonal tumors that arise after a short incubation period. In contrast, the nontransforming viruses induce monoclonal tumors after a long latency period (23,24). These tumors produce only nontransforming viruses at least in the majority of cases, so it is unlikely that the tumors arise because of newly generated transforming viruses by transduction of cellular *onc* genes (24). Based on this information and a genetic analysis of the nontransforming viruses, a model was proposed suggesting that nontransforming viruses induce disease by introducing the viral promotor next to a c-*onc* gene allowing its high-level constitutive expression (35–37). This model, which is now known as the promotor insertion model of oncogenesis, has been shown to be correct in the case of bursal lymphomas induced in chickens by avian leukosis viruses. The c-*onc* gene activated in these tumors is called c-*myc*, and it was originally identified as the transforming gene of the highly oncogenic virus MC29 (9,17,22).

We reasoned that if activation of c-*myc* is specific for B-cell lymphomas, B-cell tumors induced by a variety of oncogenic agents may show a similar activation. In the experiments presented here, we have examined the expression of c-*myc* sequences in human lymphomas and human nonneoplastic tissues. The results indicate a modest elevation of the levels of c-*myc*-specific RNA in human B-cell lymphomas. The significance of these results is discussed.

MATERIALS AND METHODS

Identification and Classification of Lymphoid Tumors

Tissues involved by malignant lymphomas were classified according the scheme of Rappaport by standard histopathologic criteria (1). Representative portions were teased apart in RPMI 1640 (GIBCO Lab., Grand Island, NY), minced finely, and pressed through a stainless-steel wire mesh sieve. Cell suspensions were characterized by standard immunologic techniques as previously described (5,18). B-cell tumors were defined as those in which the neoplastic cells bore surface immunoglobulins (sIg) with a single light chain class. In T-cell tumors, the neoplastic cells lack sIg and are able to form E rosettes. A representative portion of each tumor was immediately snap-frozen in a mixture of isopentane and Dry Ice and stored in the vapor phase over liquid nitrogen until further use for RNA isolation.

B-cell tumors studied included the following histopathologic subtypes: nodular follicular lymphomas, diffuse large-cell ("histiocytic") lymphomas, Burkitt's lymphoma, hairy cell leukemia, and chronic lymphocytic leukemia. T-cell tumors studied included lymphoblastic lymphoma and peripheral T-cell lymphoma. Miscellaneous lymphoreticular tumors studied included Hodgkin's disease, thymoma, and null-cell acute leukemia; nonneoplastic controls included spleens, thymus, liver, muscle, and tonsils with reactive follicular hyperplasia.

Preparation of RNA

RNA was extracted from tissues by a modification of the technique of Edmonds and Caramela (10). Briefly, the tissue was homogenized directly in a 1:1 mixture of water-saturated phenol and buffer consisting of 0.1 M Tris-HCl, pH 9; 1 mM EDTA, and 0.5% SDS. After three phenol extractions and one chloroform/isoamyl alcohol extraction, the RNA was ethanol-precipitated overnight. The RNA pellet was precipitated again in 3 M sodium acetate, pH 5, at 4°C. The final pellet was resuspended in sterile, distilled water. Polyadenylated RNA was selected using oligo(dT)-cellulose chromatography.

Analysis of the RNA Samples

The RNA samples and cloned DNA were applied on nitrocellulose filters using the technique described by Thomas (34). The samples were dissolved in 20 µl of 10 mM sodium phosphate, pH 7, and twofold serial dilutions of the samples were spotted on dry nitrocellulose filters (Schleicher and Schuell BA 85) previously soaked in 20 × SSC. The filters were hybridized in 50% formamide and 5 × SSC overnight at 42°C. After four initial washes in $2 \times$ SSC plus 0.1% SDS at room temperature, the filters were washed twice in $0.1 \times$ SSC and 0.1% SDS at 45°C.

Probes

The *myc* probe we used was a 1.7 kb Pst 1 fragment containing 80% of the v-*myc* sequence. This fragment was subcloned into PBR 322 from the MC38 clone of the MC29 virus generously provided by J. M. Bishop (29); v-HA-*ras* and v-Ki-*ras* were donated by R. Ellis (11); v-*abl* was supplied by D. Baltimore (14); v-*fes* was provided by C. Sherr (30); v-*src* was supplied by J. M. Bishop (6). The probes were ^{32}P-labeled by nick translation to a specific activity of 1 to 2×10^8 cpm/μg of DNA.

RESULTS

c-*myc* Expression in Normal and Tumor Tissues

The RNA extracted from the tumor and normal tissues was spotted on nitrocellulose filters and hybridized as described above. The largest amount of mRNA from each RNA sample spotted on the filters was 2 μg, followed by serial twofold dilutions out to 15 ng. Serial dilutions of the cloned v-*myc* DNA were also applied on each filter as an internal hybridization standard. Thus, the amount of each sample mRNA that hybridized with the *myc* probe could be calculated by comparing the highest dilution of the sample RNA with the highest dilution of the *myc* DNA of known picogram amounts that hybridized to the same degree. So if, for example, 78 pg of cloned v-*myc* DNA gives the same hybridization intensity as 500 ng of an mRNA sample, then approximately 78 pg of the total 500 ng of mRNA hybridizes to the *myc* probe. Stated slightly differently, there is 0.156 ng *myc*-specific RNA per microgram of total mRNA.

In each experiment, the following controls were used. RNA extracted from the Q5 MC29 transformed nonproducer quail cell line was used as the positive control. This cell line was found to have 1.2 ng of *myc*-specific RNA per microgram mRNA. Poly-A (−) ribosomal RNA from normal, uninfected cells was used as the negative control. The amount of *myc*-specific RNA in each sample was compared to the amount observed in a variety of nonneoplastic human tissues we examined, including five spleens, two thymuses, three tonsils with reactive follicular hyperplasia, phytochemagglutinin (PHA)-stimulated and nonstimulated peripheral blood lymphocytes, skeletal muscle, and liver.

The amount of *myc*-specific RNA per microgram of mRNA in each sample examined is shown in Fig. 1. Nodular and diffuse B-cell lymphomas as well as B-cell chronic lymphocytic leukemia showed similar levels of c-*myc* expression. These levels were in general two to five times as high as those observed in nonneoplastic tissues. The differences were statistically significant, using the student's *t*-test at $p < 0.05$. Higher levels of c-*myc* expression were specific for B-cell lymphomas. The level of c-*myc* expression in non-B-cell tumors was comparable to the level

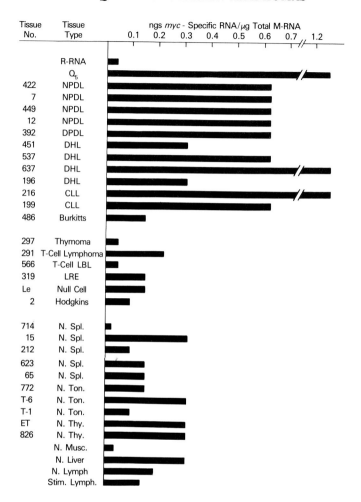

FIG. 1. Expression of MC29 *myc*-related sequences in human nonneoplastic and tumor tissues. The positive control is Q₅, an MC29 transformed nonproducer cell line, and the negative control is ribosomal RNA (R-RNA). The tissue mRNA samples tested are divided into three groups. The top group is the B-cell tumors, which include nodular lymphomas (NPDL), diffuse nodular lymphomas (DPDL), chronic lymphocytic leukemias (CLL), diffuse histiocytic lymphomas (DHL), and a Burkitt's lymphoma. The middle group includes different types of lymphoreticular neoplasms such as thymoma, peripheral T-cell lymphomas, T-cell lymphoblastic lymphoma (T-cell LBL), null-cell acute leukemia, and Hodgkin's disease. One case of lymphoreticuloendotheliosis (LRE) is also included in this group. The bottom group contains the normal tissue samples (N.), including spleens (spl.), tonsils (ton.), thymus (thy.), skeletal muscle (musc.), liver, and PHA-stimulated (stim. lymph.) and nonstimulated peripheral lymphocytes (N. lymph.).

observed in the control normal tissues. In addition, PHA stimulation of lymphocytes did not seem to affect the level of c-*myc* expression. Both PHA-stimulated and nonstimulated lymphocytes showed similar levels of *myc*-specific RNA.

Specificity of Elevated *myc* Expression in B-cell Lymphomas

The same nonneoplastic tissues and tumor samples examined for c-*myc* expression were also tested for hybridization with a variety of other v-*onc* probes, including the v-*fes*, v-*abl*, v-Ha-*ras*, v-Ki-*ras*, and v-*src* described above. To exclude hybridization to PBR-322 sequences, we also examined several samples with a PBR-322 probe. The results are shown in Table 1. The v-*fes*, v-*abl*, and v-Ki-*ras* probes did not hybridize to the human mRNA samples. The v-Ha-*ras* detected very low levels of RNA in the non-B-cell tumors and the nonneoplastic controls. The v-*src* probe detected v-*src*-specific RNA in all tissues examined, but no correlation could be made between the type of tissue and the level of expression. Finally, the PBR-322 control gave no hybridization to any of the samples tested.

DISCUSSION

Normal tissues from a variety of species as diverse as drosophila and man contain genetic information that is homologous to the transforming genes originally identified in transforming retroviruses (4,7,9,11–13,25,27,31–33). The expression of these genes in normal tissues varies depending on a variety of factors: (a) the nature of the gene itself; certain genes like c-*mos* are not known to be expressed (21), whereas others, like c-*myc*, are expressed in a relatively high copy number (28); (b) the tissue examined; the c-*src* gene, for example, is expressed at relatively high levels in brain tissue (J. Brugge, *personal communication*); and (c) the state of differentiation of the cells examined (3,26,38).

Constitutive high-level expression of transforming genes is associated with transformation. This is observed in the case of cells infected by transforming retroviruses as well as in cells transfected with DNA of cellular *onc* genes activated by retrovirus control elements *in vitro* (21). The constitutive high-level expression of *onc* genes appears to be necessary for the initiation as well as the maintenance of the transformed phenotype (2,8,21).

The significance of these phenomena in oncogenesis was fully realized when it was discovered that the cellular homolog of the transforming gene of the highly oncogenic virus MC29 (c-*myc*) was constitutively expressed at high levels in chicken bursal lymphomas induced by avian leukosis viruses. The expression of c-*myc* was caused by the introduction of the viral promotor in the vicinity of this gene (17,19,22). The expression of c-*myc* is specific for bursal lymphomas; it is not seen in other tumors induced by avian leukosis virus (23; H. Robinson, *personal communication*), while bursal lymphomas induced by reticuloendotheliosis virus also express c-*myc* sequences (20).

We have presented evidence that expression of c-*myc* sequences is elevated in the majority of human B-cell lymphoid malignancies, including nodular follicular lymphomas, diffuse large-cell or "histiocytic" lymphomas, and B-cell chronic lymphocytic leukemias. However, increased expression was not present in all types of B-cell tumors. One Burkitt's lymphoma and one leukemic reticuloendotheliosis

TABLE 1. Expression of retroviral onc sequences in human nonneoplastic and tumor tissues[a]

Tissue	MC29 myc	FeSV fes	Abelson abl	Harvey Ha-ras	Kirsten Ki-ras	Rous src	PBR control
Nodular lymphomas	0.62 (5)	neg (3)	neg (3)	neg (4)	neg (3)	0.35 (2)	neg (2)
Diffuse histiocytic lymphomas	0.62 (5)	neg (2)	neg (3)	neg (2)	neg (3)	0.31 (2)	neg (2)
Non-B-cell tumors	0.12 (7)	neg (2)	neg (3)	0.01 (2)	neg (2)	0.62 (2)	neg (2)
Nonneoplastic control tissues	0.18 (13)	neg (2)	neg (3)	0.01 (2)	neg (2)	0.47 (2)	ND
Retroviral transformed nonproducer cells	1.25	ND	ND	0.32	0.16	ND	ND
pg Cloned DNA detected[b]	78	39	78	39	78	78	78

[a]ng onc-specific RNA per μg of total mRNA. Numbers in parentheses are number of tissue samples. ND = not done.
[b]The amount of cloned onc DNA detected with the appropriate hybridization probe after overnight film exposure.

showed normal levels of c-*myc*-specific mRNA. The level of c-*myc* expression in the B-cell lymphomas was significantly higher than in the group of non-B-cell tumors, which showed levels comparable to those found in the nonneoplastic controls. The level of expression does not appear to correlate directly with the rate of cellular proliferation. For example, a single case of Burkitt's lymphoma, a rapidly proliferating B-cell tumor of childhood, was not associated with increased expression. Tonsils with florid follicular hyperplasia showed levels of c-*myc* expression comparable to those found in other controls. Finally, PHA-stimulated lymphocytes did not demonstrate increased levels of c-*myc* expression compared to unstimulated lymphocytes. The specificity of c-*myc* expression was strengthened by the observation that other transforming genes, including Ha-*ras*, Ki-*ras*, *abl*, *fes*, and *src*, were expressed at levels comparable to those in the nonneoplastic controls.

These results are based on samples extracted from surgically removed human tissue and not cell lines. We have purposely avoided the use of cell lines derived from human tumors because of the possibility that secondary events during cultivation of the cells may have altered the primary picture.

The elevation of c-*myc* expression that we observed in the human B-cell lymphomas was modest. However, the level of c-*myc* expression necessary for the induction and maintenance of transformation is not known. Therefore, it is possible that only a modest increase in its expression would suffice for transformation to occur in lymphoid cells. Before we can understand the significance of these results and the role the c-*myc* gene product may play in human malignancy, it will be necessary to determine the normal function and regulation of this gene.

ACKNOWLEDGMENT

We would like to thank Dr. George Khoury for the samples he provided and the helpful suggestions he made during the course of this study.

REFERENCES

1. Berard, C. W., and Dorfman, R. F. (1974): Histopathology of malignant lymphomas. *Clin. Haematol.*, 3:39–76.
2. Bishop, J. M. (1978): Retroviruses. *Annu. Rev. Biochem.*, 47:35–38.
3. Chen, J. H. (1980): Expression of endogenous avian myeloblastosis virus information in different chicken cells. *J. Virol.*, 36:162–170.
4. Coffin, J. M., Varmus, H. E., Bishop, J. M., Essex, M., Hardy, W. D., Martin, G. S., Rosenberg, N. E., Scolnick, E. M., Weinberg, R. A., and Vogt, P. K. (1981): Proposal for naming host cell-derived inserts in retroviruses genomes. *J. Virol.*, 40:953–957.
5. Cossman, J., and Jaffe, E. S. (1981): Distribution of complement receptor subtypes in non-Hodgkin's lymphomas of B-cell origin. *Blood*, 58:20–26.
6. Czernilowsky, A. P., Levinson, A. D., Varmus, H. E., Bishop, J. M., Tischer, E., and Goodman, H. M. (1980): Nucleotide sequence of an avian sarcoma virus oncogene (src) and proposed amino acid sequence for gene product. *Nature*, 287:198–203.
7. Dalla Favera, R., Gelman, E. P., Gallo, R. C., and Wong-Staal, F. (1981): A human onc gene homologous to the transforming gene (v-sis) of simian sarcoma virus. *Nature*, 292:31–35.
8. Deng, C.-T., Stehelin, D., Bishop, J. M., and Varmus, H. E. (1977): Characteristics of virus-specific RNA in avian sarcoma virus transformed BHK-21 cells and revertants. *Virology*, 76:313–330.

9. Duesberg, P. H. (1979): Transforming genes of retroviruses. *Cold Spring Harbor Symp. Quant. Biol.*, 44:13–30.

10. Edmonds, M., and Caramela, M. G. (1969): The isolation and characterization of adenosine monophosphate-rich polynucleotides synthesized by Ehrlich ascites cells. *J. Biol. Chem.*, 244:1314–1324.

11. Ellis, R. W., Defeo, D., Shis, T. Y., Gonda, M. A., Young, H. A., Tsuchida, N., Lowy, D. R., and Scolnick, E. M. (1981): The p21 *src* genes of Harvey and Kirsten sarcoma viruses originate from divergent members of a family of normal vertebrate genes. *Nature*, 292:506–511.

12. Frankel, A. E., and Fischinger, P. J. (1976): Nucleotide sequences in mouse DNA and RNA specific for Moloney sarcoma virus. *Proc. Natl. Acad. Sci. USA*, 78:3705–3709.

13. Goff, S. P., Gilboa, E., Witte, O. N., and Baltimore, D. (1980): Structure of Abelson murine leukemia virus genome and the homologous cellular gene: Studies with cloned viral DNA. *Cell*, 22:777–785.

14. Goff, S. P., Witte, O. N., Gilboa, E., Rosenberg, N., and Baltimore, D. (1981): Genome structure of Abelson murine leukemia virus variants: Proviruses in fibroblasts and lymphoid cells. *J. Virol.*, 38:460–468.

15. Graf, T., and Beug, H. (1978): Avian leukemia viruses: Interactions with their target cells. *Biochim. Biophys. Acta*, 516:269–299.

16. Hanafusa, H. (1977): Cell transformation by RNA tumor viruses. In: *Comprehensive Virology*, edited by H. Fraenkel-Conrat and R. Wanger, pp. 408–483. Plenum Press, New York.

17. Hayward, W. S., Neel, B. G., and Astrin, S. M. (1981): Activation of a cellular *onc* gene by promoter insertion in avian leukosis virus-induced lymphoid leukemias. *Nature*, 290:475–480.

18. Jaffe, E. S., Braylan, R. K., Frank, M. M., Green, I., and Berard, C. W. (1976): Heterogeneity of immunologic markers and surface morphology in childhood lymphoblastic lymphoma. *Blood*, 48:213–222.

19. Neel, B. G., Hayward, W. S., Robinson, H. L., Fang, J. M., and Astrin, S. M. (1981): ALV-induced tumors have common proviral integration sites and synthesize discrete new RNAs: Oncogenesis by proviral insertion. *Cell*, 23:323–334.

20. Noori-Daloii, M. R., Swift, R. A., Kung, H.-J., Crittenden, L., and Witter, R. L. (1981): Specific integration of REV proviruses in avian bursal lymphomas. *Nature*, 294:574–576.

21. Oskarsson, M., McClements, W. L., Blair, D. L., Vande Woude, G. F., and Maizel, J. V. (1980): Properties of a normal mouse cell DNA sequence (sarc) homologous to the src sequence of Moloney sarcoma virus. *Science*, 207:1222–1224.

22. Payne, G. S., Bishop, J. M., and Varmus, H. E. (1982): Multiple arrangements of viral DNA and an activated host oncogene in bursal lymphomas. *Nature*, 295:209–214.

23. Robinson, H. L., Blais, B. M., Tsichlis, P. N., and Coffin, J. M. (1982): At least two regions of the viral genome determine the oncogenic potential of avian leukosis viruses. *Proc. Natl. Acad. Sci. USA*, 79:1225–1229.

24. Robinson, H. L., Pearson, M. N., DeSimone, D. W., Tsichlis, P. N., and Coffin, J. M. (1979): Subgroup-E avian leukosis virus associated disease in chickens. *Cold Spring Harbor Symp. Quant. Biol.*, 44:1133–1142.

25. Roussel, M., Saule, S., Lagrou, C., Rommens, C., Beug, H., Graf, T., and Stehelin, D. (1979): Three new types of viral oncogenes of cellular origin specific for hemapoietic cell transformation. *Nature*, 281:452–455.

26. Scolnick, E. M., Weeks, M. O., Shih, T. Y., Ruscetti, S. K., and Dexter, T. M. (1981): Markedly elevated levels of an endogenous sarc protein in a hemopoietic precursor cell line. *Mol. Cell. Biol.*, 1:66–74.

27. Sheiness, D., and Bishop, J. M. (1979): Uninfected vertebrate cells contain nucleotide sequences related to the putative transforming gene of avian myeloblastosis virus. *J. Virol.*, 31:514–521.

28. Sheiness, D., Hughes, S. H., Varmus, H. E., Stubblefield, E., and Bishop, J. M. (1980): The vertebrate homolog of the putative transforming gene of AMV: Characteristics of the DNA locus and its RNA transcript. *J. Virol.*, 105:415–424.

29. Sheiness, D., Vennstrom, B., and Bishop, J. M. (1981): Virus-specific RNAs in cells infected by avian myeloblastosis virus and avian erythroblastosis virus: Modes of oncogene expression. *Cell*, 23:291–300.

30. Sherr, C. J., Fedele, L. A., Donner, L., and Turek, L. P. (1979): Restriction endonuclease mapping of unintegrated proviral DNA of Snyder-Theilen feline sarcoma virus: Localization of sarcoma-specific sequences. *J. Virol.*, 32:860–875.

31. Shilo, B.-Z., and Weinberg, R. A. (1981): DNA sequences homologous to vertebrate oncogenes are conserved in *Drosophila melanogaster*. *Proc. Natl. Acad. Sci. USA*, 78:6789–6792.

32. Spector, D. H., Varmus, H. E., and Bishop, J. M. (1978): Nucleotide sequences related to the transforming gene of avian sarcoma virus are present in uninfected vertebrates. *Proc. Natl. Acad. Sci. USA*, 75:4102–4106.

33. Stehelin, D., Varmus, H. E., Bishop, J. M., and Vogt, P. K. (1976): DNA related to the transforming genes of avian sarcoma viruses is present in normal avian DNA. *Nature*, 260:170–173.

34. Thomas, P. S. (1980): Hybridization of denatured RNA and small DNA fragments transferred to nitrocellulose. *Proc. Natl. Acad. Sci. USA*, 77:5201–5205.

35. Tsichlis, P. N., and Coffin, J. M. (1979): Recombination between the defective component of an acute leukemia virus and Rous associated virus O, an endogenous virus of chickens. *Proc. Natl. Acad. Sci. USA*, 76:3001–3005.

36. Tsichlis, P. N., and Coffin, J. M. (1980): Recombinants between endogenous and exogenous avian tumor viruses: Role of the C region and other portions of the genome in the control of replication and transformation. *J. Virol.*, 33:238–249.

37. Tsichlis, P. N., and Coffin, J. M. (1980): Role of the C region in relative growth rates of endogenous and exogenous avian oncoviruses. *Cold Spring Harbor Symp. Quant. Biol.*, 44:1123–1132.

38. Westin, E. H., Gallo, R. C., Arya, S. K., Eva, A., Souza, L. M., Baluda, M. A., Aaronson, S. A., and Wong-Staal, F. (1982): Differential expression of the avian myeloblastosis virus gene in human hematopoietic cells. *Proc. Natl. Acad. Sci. USA*, 79:2194-2198.

*Pathogenesis of Leukemias and Lymphomas:
Environmental Influences*, edited by
I. T. Magrath, G. T. O'Conor, and B. Ramot.
Raven Press, New York © 1984.

Recent Advances and New Approaches in the Search for a Viral Etiology of Human Lymphoid Neoplasia: Summary and Comments

A. S. Levine

National Institute of Child Health and Human Development, National Institutes of Health, Bethesda, Maryland 20205

This section of this volume begins with introductory chapters by H. S. Kaplan (Chapter 32) and M. Essex (Chapter 33), who emphasize the increasing relevance of animal models in the study of human lymphoid malignancies, in view of the fact that in nature most such malignancies are induced by retroviruses. Moreover, a retrovirus has recently—and for the first time—been consistently associated with a human lymphoid malignancy. Naturally occurring models for retrovirus-induced leukemia and/or lymphoma include the chicken, mouse, cat, cow, and gibbon ape.

MOLECULAR ANATOMY AND BIOLOGY OF RETROVIRUSES

Retroviruses bind to specific cell receptors, which probably explains the exquisite target cell specificity associated with these agents. After binding, the virus penetrates the cell, is uncoated, and—employing the reverse transcriptase encoded by the viral genome—a complementary DNA (cDNA) copy of the RNA viral genome is synthesized. This cDNA is then integrated as a provirus genome in linear continuity with cellular DNA. Reading from 5' to 3', a prototypical retrovirus genome comprises a long terminal repeat (LTR); *gag, pol,* and *env* coding regions; and another LTR. The *gag, pol,* and *env* regions direct the synthesis of viral core proteins (with group-specific antigens), the polymerase, and the envelope proteins, respectively. The LTRs contain transcription controls for the adjoining DNA.

Retroviruses may be of two types, endogenous or exogenous. The endogenous retroviruses are inherited vertically as proviruses in the germ line. These viruses do not normally replicate, and their provirus genomes are not transcribed or translated to any significant extent. Consequently, endogenous viruses are not ordinarily released by the cell. Moreover, they do not cause any known disease. However, endogenous proviral genomes can apparently move easily within the host cell genome and recombine with other endogenous proviral sequences or with cellular

DNA sequences. In this regard, the endogenous proviruses act as if they were transposons, and they are able to "transduce" cell DNA segments. The new virus-virus, or virus-cell DNA recombinants replicate readily; they are released by the cell and are able to infect other cells exogenously. Moreover, these exogenous recombinants are able to induce leukemia and/or lymphoma in appropriate target cells. The exogenous, recombinant retroviruses thus have two new properties—a new cell tropism, and the ability to induce lymphoid malignancies.

The exogenous retroviruses are of two subtypes, nondefective and defective. Nondefective exogenous retroviruses are exemplified by the avian sarcoma virus, the genome of which reads LTR-*gag-pol-env-sarc*-LTR. This genome has, in addition to the prototypical sequences, an *onc* gene *(sarc)* that it incorporated historically from an avian cell genome. Defective exogenous retroviruses are exemplified by the avian erythroblastosis virus, the genome of which reads LTR-*gag-onc-env*-LTR. Since this genome is missing the *pol* coding region, it is able to replicate only in the presence of a helper virus. Moreover, portions of the *gag* and *env* regions are also missing, such that the antigenic determinants usually associated with these regions cannot be detected serologically.

Certain murine leukemia viruses, such as the radiation leukemia virus and the virus that induces "spontaneous" AKR leukemia, are virus-virus DNA recombinants. Their genomes read LTR-*gag-pol-env*(rec)-LTR. The recombinational event of interest has thus occurred in the *env* region, with a contribution from each of two endogenous retroviruses. It is this *env* recombination that creates new envelope proteins and endows the murine virus with a new cell tropism as well as the ability to induce lymphoid malignancies, e.g., in the thymus. The ability to induce the disease may simply be a consequence of viral genetic material gaining access to a cell from which it was formerly excluded. Interestingly, these murine leukemia viruses are associated with a long latency before the occurrence of disease, undoubtedly because each parent of the recombinant must accumulate in sufficient quantities to mathematically favor a recombinational event.

onc GENES AND THE MECHANISM OF ONCOGENESIS

It is now apparent that *onc* genes are conserved in normal cells throughout evolution, from drosophila through humans. Where their products have been examined, *onc* genes frequently encode a protein kinase that phosphorylates tyrosine and is found in contiguity with the nuclear and surface plasma membranes. Given this function and location, it is reasonable to propose that the function of the *onc* gene is to control normal DNA replication, cellular proliferation, differentiation, and/or relationships with neighboring cells. Retrovirus infection may bring about the insertion into the cell genome of extra *onc* gene copies (which had been incorporated historically by the virus). In this circumstance, transcription from the extra *onc* gene would be highly promoted by its adjoining LTR. Alternatively, only the viral LTR might be inserted immediately upstream from a resident cellular *onc* gene. The normal *onc* gene would then be promoted constitutively, also resulting in uncontrolled cellular proliferation and possibly affecting differentiation as well (as predicted by the above hypothesis). Finally, the viral *onc* gene may be mutated with respect to the normal cell *onc* gene, and the mutant sequences may be necessary and sufficient for oncogenesis.

"VIRUS-NEGATIVE" TUMORS

These mechanisms suggest an explanation for "virus-negative" lymphoid malignancies that have been, in fact, induced by retroviruses. A defective virus may gain entry into a cell with a helper virus, but then lose the helper. The defective virus would have transformed the cell but is not able to replicate. Moreover, the provirus cannot readily be detected, because it only elaborates extra copies of normal cellular *onc* gene products and has altered *env/gag* proteins that cannot be detected serologically. Alternatively, only the LTR of the retrovirus may have been integrated in the host cellular genome and can only be detected with a specific and highly sensitive molecular probe.

A naturally occurring example of a "virus-negative" lymphoid malignancy induced by a retrovirus is feline leukemia. As the virus replicates in cats acutely infected with feline leukemia virus, it yields new cell surface antigens that are recognized by the host; cells bearing such antigens are then lysed by antibody. About 2% of such infected cats develop a chronic viremia, and some of these animals eventually die with virus-positive lymphoid malignancy. However, about 0.2% of acutely infected cats develop a virus-negative leukemia or lymphoma. One explanation for this circumstance is that a small number of cells contain a defective feline leukemia virus that does not replicate and does not yield new cell surface antigens. As a consequence, cells containing this defective virus are not lysed but are transformed. Again, the important lesson for the study of human lymphoid malignancy is that only with the use of highly sensitive and specific cDNA probes would the true explanation for "virus-negative" lymphoid malignancy in the cat become apparent.

ADULT T-CELL LYMPHOID MALIGNANCY AND THE HUMAN T-CELL LEUKEMIA VIRUS

Following the discussion of retrovirus biology, M. S. Reitz et al. (Chapter 34), W. A. Blattner et al. (Chapter 35), and T. Suchi and K. Tajima (Chapter 39) review their data on a human T-cell leukemia virus (HTLV). This virus was originally isolated by Dr. Robert Gallo's laboratory from a patient with a cutaneous, mature T-cell lymphoma. The patient's blasts had been grown *in vitro* in the presence of T-cell growth factor (TCGF). After chronic culture, virus particles were visualized by electron microscopy, a 70S RNA was found in the cell supernate, and reverse transcriptase activity was also present. Taken together, these findings indicate that a retrovirus had been present in this patient's malignant cells. From serologic and other tests, it now appears that an identical or virtually identical virus has infected patients from southwestern Japan and the Caribbean basin with adult T-cell leukemia/lymphoma; moreover, the virus has an endemic distribution in these two areas but appears to cause infection sporadically elsewhere in the world. The syndrome that has been associated with infection by this virus primarily involves patients between 40 and 50 years old, who may have leukemia as well as lymphoma (the blasts being small and "Sézary-like" in appearance), and who have a prevalence of adenopathy, hepatosplenomegaly, and skin infiltration. Severe hypercalemia is also prevalent. This mature T-lymphoid syndrome seems to be distinguishable from classical mycosis fungoides/Sézary disease, but it is evident that as further observations accumulate, the clinical spectrum may be broader than the syndrome so far defined. By molecular hybridization and protein analysis, HTLV appears to be a unique retrovirus, although it is distantly related to the bovine leukemia virus, and both viruses may have had a common ancestor historically. HTLV proviral DNA has not been found in B lymphocytes from patients with this T-cell malignancy, nor even in other T lymphocytes from the same patient. It is evident, therefore, that the virus is present in only one subset of the T-lymphocyte population (an OKT $4+$/OKT $8-$ phenotype). Therefore, this retrovirus is not endogenous but rather must be an acquired, horizontally transmitted virus analogous to the known horizontally transmissible leukemia-inducing retroviruses of animals.

Virtually all patients with this adult T-cell lymphoid malignancy within the endemic area of Japan and all patients in the endemic area of the Caribbean basin have antibody directed against HTLV. However, 5 to 10% of the normal population within these endemic areas is also serologically positive, and this figure can range as high as 50% in older people within certain endemic regions. Moreover, a small fraction of bone marrow cells from clinically normal people in these areas may contain HTLV. Members of the primary families of adult T-cell lymphoid malignancy patients have a somewhat higher incidence of seropositivity than the random population within the endemic areas, suggesting a low level of contagion. Preliminary observations suggest that the peak antibody titers are not different in seropositive normals and seropositive patients.

In other preliminary observations, it appears that there is a summer incidence peak in the clinical onset of the lymphoid malignancy. Moreover, the endemic areas of virus distribution are rural, and the prevalent occupations are fishing, farming, and forestry. These facts suggest the possibility of an insect vector and an animal reservoir for the virus, although the incidence of seropositivity allows the alternative explanation that humans themselves are the reservoir.

The adult T-cell lymphoma/leukemia syndrome described here is rare; only one in 2,000 to 3,000 seropositive individuals has the disease. No known seropositive individual has yet developed the disease, and no known seronegative individual has yet become positive. Finally, there may well be an individual genetic susceptibility to this disease beyond whatever ethno/racial genotypes may be implicated, because 10% of patients with the adult T-cell lymphoid malignancy have a family history of a similar illness.

The strongest observations favoring an etiologic rather than a passenger role for HTLV in this newly described mature T-cell malignancy include (a) the restricted distribution of HTLV, (b) clusters of the disease within the endemic areas of virus distribution, (c) the fact that proviral DNA appears to be integrated monoclonally only in the patient's tumor cells, with the integration site being the same in all cells of any one patient's tumor but different among tumors from different patients (suggesting that the virus causes the disease, rather than that the disease permits the virus to be a passenger in malignant cells), (d) the fact that HTLV infection has been consistently identified in virtually all patients with the syndrome, and (e) the fact that HTLV transforms cord T lymphocytes *in vitro*, and the transformed cells yield tumors in immunosuppressed hamsters. These data, taken together, provide strong circumstantial evidence that the virus is the cause of the disease, but definitive proof would be at hand if a vaccine (possibly developed against viral or *onc* gene proteins) were to result in the elimination of the disease. Whether this type of proof will become available, however, probably depends on questions of vaccine feasibility, costs, and efficacy. In any event, it is clear that mere infection does not induce this disease and that a particular genotype and/or an accumulation of additional risk factors is required. If HTLV is the cause of the disease, it is interesting to speculate that the viral LTR may be promoting transcription from the TCGF gene constitutively, with that gene conceptualized as an *onc* gene.

onc GENE EXPRESSION IN HUMAN CELLS

In the final part of this section of this volume, S. M. Astrin and U. G. Rovigatti (Chapter 36) describe experiments using the avian leukosis virus to induce bursal lymphoid malignancies in chickens. Hypothetically, either the whole viral genome (containing an *onc* gene) may be implicated in tumor induction, or just a viral LTR, integrated upstream of a normal chick cell *onc* gene and promoting its transcription. In chickens, the *onc* gene has been identified as "c-*myc*"; this gene appears to have been incorporated by the MC29 strain of avian leukosis virus, and within the viral genome, it is identified as "v-*myc*." Astrin and Rovigatti's results indicate that the 3′ viral LTR is necessary and sufficient to produce the bursal malignancy when it is integrated immediately upstream of c-*myc*. In that circumstance, the transcription of c-*myc* mRNA is enhanced as much as 100-fold [Varmus et al. *(unpublished)* have shown that bidirectional promotion can also occur, such that the LTR may be inserted downstream of the *onc* gene and still enhance its expression].

With the knowledge that c-*myc* is virtually identical in structure to a human *onc* gene, Astrin and Rovigatti employed v-*myc* and c-*myc* probes to study transcription in normal human lymphoid cells and in malignant lymphoid cells from patients with chronic lymphocytic leukemia (CLL), acute lymphoblastic leukemia (ALL), and non-Hodgkin's lymphoma. Nine of 15 such patients demonstrated a 10- to 30-fold enhancement of *myc*-like mRNA transcription compared with normal donors or an ALL patient in complete remission.

Zeller et al. (Chapter 38) confirm these results in patients with nodular lymphoma, diffuse histiocytic lymphoma, or CLL, but not in patients with T-cell lymphoid malignancies, nor in normal lymphocytes stimulated *in vitro* with PHA. Thus, promotion of the *onc* gene in humans may relate to the induction of lymphoid malignancy, and these data are suggestive but do not provide proof. Moreover, the most important objective of Astrin and Rovigatti's experiments is simply to deter- mine whether human *onc* genes are being highly promoted, and if so, to study their structure in an attempt to establish why, in fact, their transcription has now become constitutive.

E. H. Westin et al. (Chapter 37) report that they also have employed retrovirus probes for *onc* gene transcription in malignant cells from patients with lymphoid tumors and in cells from normal human cultured hematopoietic cell lines. With certain of the diverse probes employed, only immature T lymphocytes and myeloid cells demonstrated enhanced transcription. Moreover, Westin et al. examined HL-60, a human acute promyelocytic leukemia line, and found that as it differentiates *in vitro* (under the influence of chemical inducers), *onc* gene transcription diminishes, suggesting that this expression may relate merely to the stage of differentiation rather than to leukemogenesis per se. This distinction will be hard to establish, given the difficulty of obtaining populations of undifferentiated, nonmalignant hematopoietic cells, but the problems raised here may be resolved as further insight is gained into the molecular function of *onc* genes in human cells.

Pathogenesis of Leukemias and Lymphomas:
Environmental Influences, edited by
I. T. Magrath, G. T. O'Conor, and B. Ramot.
Raven Press, New York © 1984.

Appendix:
Selected Epidemiological Data Pertinent to Topics Discussed in this Volume

Ian Magrath

National Cancer Institute, National Institutes of Health, Bethesda, Maryland 20205

ACUTE LEUKEMIAS

The proportion of patients with acute myeloblastic as opposed to acute lymphoblastic leukemia differs markedly with age in the United States (Fig. 1). Because of differences in the representation of different age groups in the population, the shapes of the curves depicting *actual numbers of cases* differ considerably from those depicting *incidence* by age group (Figs. 2 and 3). Of interest is the high incidence of acute lymphoblastic leukemia (ALL) in the United States in individuals over the age of 80 years—a small and rapidly diminishing age group in most

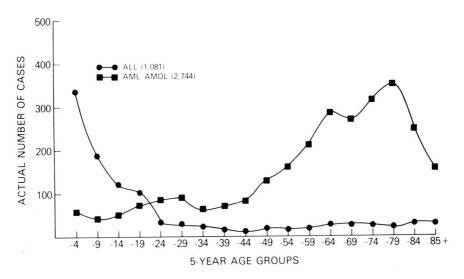

FIG. 1. Actual numbers of patients with either acute lymphoblastic leukemia (ALL) or acute myeloblastic (AML)/acute monocytic (AMOL) leukemia in five-year age groups (designated by the highest age in the group), all races in the United States. Data from the SEER Program, NCI, 1973–1977.

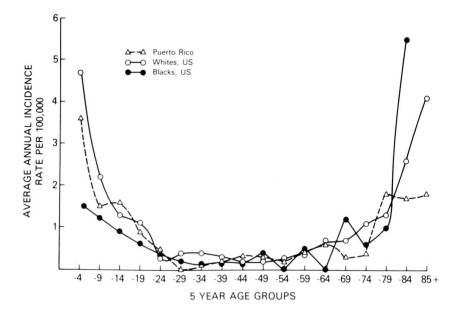

FIG. 2. Incidence of acute lymphoblastic leukemia in Blacks, Whites, and Puerto Ricans by age group. Both sexes are included. Data from the SEER Program, NCI, 1973–1977.

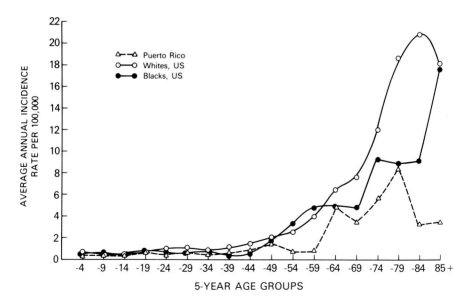

FIG. 3. Incidence of acute myelocytic (granulocytic) leukemia in Blacks, Whites, and Puerto Ricans by age group. Both sexes are included. Data from the SEER Program, NCI, 1973–1977.

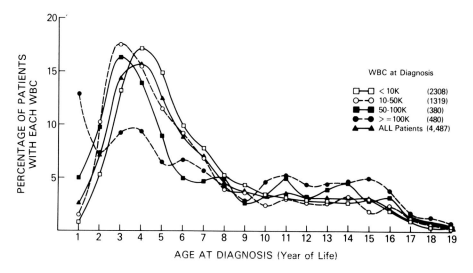

FIG. 4. Percentage distribution of ALL patients (4,487) with various total white cell counts by age 1972–1982. Data kindly provided by H. Sather, Children's Cancer Study Group statistical office.

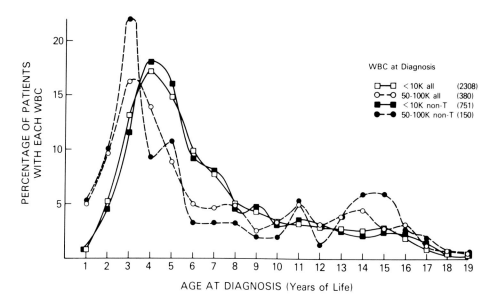

FIG. 5. Percentage distribution of ALL patients (4,487) with various total white cell counts by age, according to leukemia phenotype, i.e., T-cell or non-T-cell, determined on the basis of E-rosette formation in a subgroup of 901 patients tested between 1978–1982. Data kindly provided by H. Sather, Children's Cancer Study Group statistical office.

developing countries—and the gradually increasing incidence of acute myeloblastic leukemia (AML) in the United States in individuals more than 50 years old. This increase in the incidence of AML is not nearly as prominent in Puerto Rico and appears to be essentially absent in many of the countries represented in this volume. The early age peak in ALL, which has been shown to be caused by common ALL, is well shown in these figures.

The possibility that underdiagnosis of ALL in developing countries accounts for the apparent paucity of this disease and the lack of an early age peak in such populations, although very difficult to exclude completely, seems unlikely, because such an explanation would presuppose selective underdiagnosis of patients with common ALL. This might be tenable if patients with common ALL tended to have lower total white blood cell counts than other leukemic phenotypes, for it is reasonable to assume that the patients most likely to be missed are those with normal or low white counts. Yet this in itself, although consistent with the predominance of high-risk patients in developing countries, is clearly an inadequate explanation for the lack of an early age peak, because

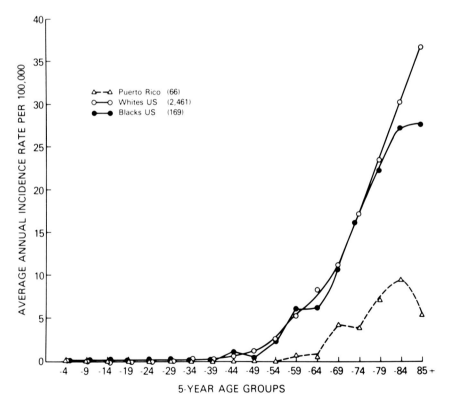

FIG. 6. Incidence of chronic lymphocytic leukemia in Blacks, Whites, and Puerto Ricans by age group. Both sexes are included. Data from the SEER Program, NCI, 1973–1977.

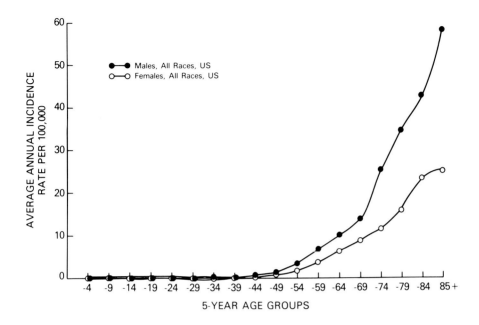

FIG. 7. Incidence of chronic lymphocytic leukemia in U.S. males and females, all races, by age group. Data from the SEER Program, NCI, 1973–1977.

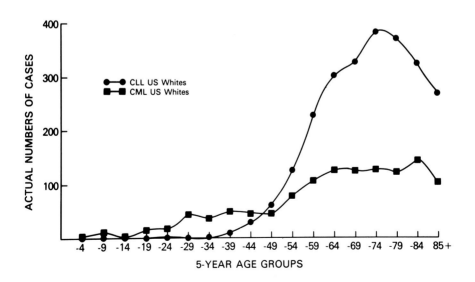

FIG. 8. Actual numbers of cases of chronic lymphocytic (CLL) and chronic myelocytic leukemia (CML) in U.S. Whites by age group. Both sexes are included. Data from the SEER Program, NCI, 1973–1977.

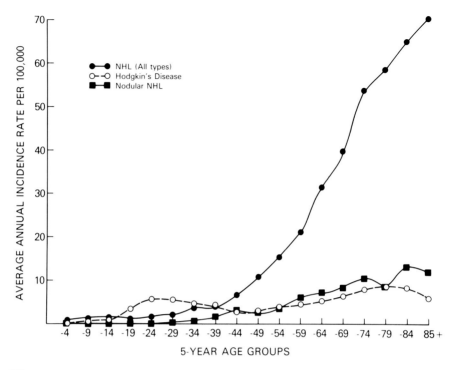

FIG. 9. Incidence of non-Hodgkin's lymphoma (NHL) (all types), Hodgkin's disease, and nodular NHL in White U.S. males by age group. Data from the SEER Program, NCI, 1977–1979.

in data from the Children's Cancer Study Group, an early age peak is present at all white counts up to 100,000/mm³ (Figs. 4 and 5).

CHRONIC LEUKEMIAS

The paucity of chronic lymphocytic leukemia (CLL) in countries outside the United States and Europe has been clearly demonstrated in this volume and elsewhere. Incidence rates by age group for the United States are shown in Fig. 6 for Blacks, Whites, and Puerto Ricans, and in Fig. 7 for males and females. The incidence rates for Blacks and Whites are identical, but females and Puerto Ricans have a low incidence of CLL. The CLL of middle-aged women described in Nigeria and northern India stands in marked contrast to this age-related incidence pattern. Actual numbers of cases of CLL and chronic myelocytic leukemia in U.S. Whites by age group are shown in Fig. 8.

MALIGNANT LYMPHOMAS

Incidence rates for Hodgkin's disease, all non-Hodgkin's lymphomas, and nodular lymphomas in white males and females in the United States are shown in Figs. 9 and 10. Differences in incidence at different ages of these diseases are

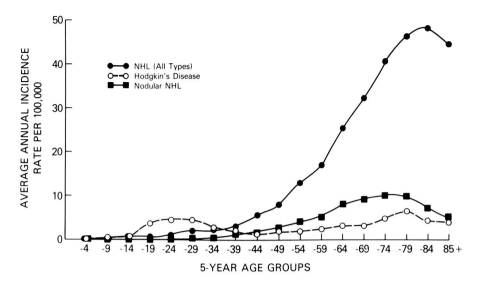

FIG. 10. Incidence of non-Hodgkin's lymphoma (NHL) (all types), Hodgkin's disease, and nodular NHL in White U.S. females by age group. Data from the SEER Program, NCI, 1977–1979.

TABLE 1. *Non-Hodgkin's lymphoma: Distribution of diffuse and nodular categories by race and sex[a]*

Race Sex	Total	Diffuse		Nodular	
Whites					
Males	2,724	2,144	(79%)	580	(21%)
Females	2,693	2,042	(76%)	651	(24%)
Blacks					
Males	146	129	(88%)	17	(12%)
Females	119	97	(82%)	22	(18%)

[a]United States, 1977–1979 (SEER Program).

apparent. Nodular lymphomas are uncommon outside Europe and the United States, and it is of interest that the incidence of nodular lymphomas in U.S. Blacks is higher than in developing countries but not as high as in U.S. Whites (Tables 1 and 2). At first sight this argues against a genetic predisposition of Caucasian races to nodular lymphoma, but U.S. Blacks are not genetically identical to, for example, African Blacks, and the relative importance of interbreeding in U.S. Blacks and Whites versus environmental factors in giving rise to the current incidence of nodular lymphomas in Blacks will be difficult if not impossible to compute. To resolve this issue of "nature versus nurture," it will be important to observe over time the incidence of nodular lymphomas in different populations throughout the world, particularly those undergoing marked socioeconomic changes.

TABLE 2. *Age adjusted incidence rates per
100,000 (1970 population) of diffuse and
nodular subtypes by race and sex[a]*

Race Sex	Diffuse	Nodular	Ratio[b]
Whites			
Males	8.93	2.36	3.37
Females	6.49	2.19	
Blacks			
Males	6.62	0.83	6.34
Females	4.04	0.82	

[a]United States, 1977–1979 (SEER Program).
[b]Ratio of diffuse to nodular.

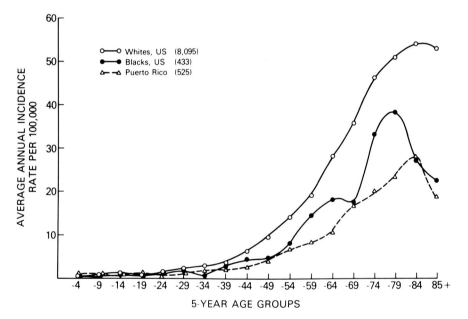

FIG. 11. Incidence of non-Hodgkin's lymphoma (all types) in Blacks, Whites, and Puerto Ricans. Both sexes are included. Data from the SEER Program, NCI, 1973–1977.

The incidence of all non-Hodgkin's lymphomas by age group in Whites, Blacks, and Puerto Ricans is shown in Fig. 11. The decreasing order of incidence in these three racial groups is demonstrated. In Blacks, this is predominantly because of a paucity of nodular lymphomas, for the incidence of diffuse lymphomas is 1.46 times higher in Whites, whereas the incidence of nodular lymphomas is 2.74 times higher in Whites than in Blacks.

Subject Index

Subject Index